BOLD fMRI

Scott H. Faro, MD

Professor and Vice-Chairman of Radiology, Director of Functional Brain Imaging Center, Director of Radiology Research and Academics, and Clinical MRI, Temple University School of Medicine, Philadelphia, Pennsylvania

Feroze B. Mohamed, PhD

Associate Professor of Radiology, Associate Director of Functional Brain Imaging Center, Temple University School of Medicine, Philadelphia, Pennsylvania

Editors

BOLD fMRI

A Guide to Functional Imaging for Neuroscientists

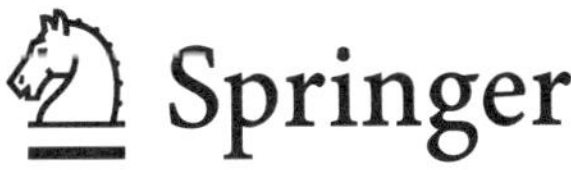 Springer

Scott H. Faro, MD
Professor and Vice-Chairman
    of Radiology
Director of Functional Brain
    Imaging Center
Director of Radiology Research
    and Academics, and Clinical MRI
Temple University School of Medicine
Philadelphia, PA 19140
USA

Feroze B. Mohamed, PhD
Associate Professor of Radiology
Associate Director of Functional
    Brain Imaging Center
Temple University School of Medicine
Philadelphia, PA 19140
USA

ISBN 978-1-4419-1328-9   e-ISBN 978-1-4419-1329-6
DOI 10.1007/978-1-4419-1329-6
Springer New York Dordrecht Heidelberg London

Library of Congress Control Number: 2010929273

Preface

Functional magnetic resonance imaging (fMRI) represents one of the most advanced and enlightening functional imaging techniques that has ever been developed. One major area of research interest in fMRI is within the field of Cognitive Neuroscience, which focuses on understanding all aspects of the mental processes involved in awareness, reasoning, and acquisition of knowledge and behavior. This book includes selected chapters from *Functional MRI: Basic Principles and Clinical Applications* (S. Faro and F. Mohamed, Eds. New York: Springer Science+Business Media, LCC 2006) that the editors feel are of particular interest to neuroscientists, as the focus is primarily on describing the basic principles of Blood Oxygen Level Dependent (BOLD) imaging and the developing clinical applications of fMRI in the neurosciences.

The first section of the book is an introduction to the physics principles of BOLD imaging as well as a review of fMRI scanning methodologies, data analysis, experimental design, and clinical challenges. The second section reviews some current and future clinical applications of fMRI, including the clinical fields of Language, Memory, fMRI WADA, and Brain Mapping. The third and final section is a pictorial neuroanatomical atlas of the basic motor, sensory, and cognitive activation sites within the brain. This section will give neuroscientists a familiarity with some of the more clinically relevant brain activation sites that are discussed in other chapters.

There has been a discovery of a tremendous body of knowledge in the relatively young field of fMRI. Functional imaging has quickly grown to be a vital tool for clinical and cognitive neuroscience research. It is the hope of the editors that this book will give a thorough introduction to this exciting field and will serve as a concise reference to all cognitive neuroscientists for the emerging clinical applications of fMRI.

Contents

Preface v

Contibutors ix

Part I   BOLD Functional MRI

1   Principles of Functional MRI 3
    Seong-Gi Kim and Peter A. Bandettini

2   fMRI Scanning Methodologies 23
    Alexander B. Pinus and Feroze B. Mohamed

3   Experimental Design and Data Analysis for fMRI 55
    Geoffrey K. Aguirre

4   Challenges in fMRI and Its Limitations 71
    R. Todd Constable

5   Clinical Challenges of fMRI 93
    Nader Pouratian and Susan Y. Bookheimer

Part II   fMRI Clinical Applications

6   Brain Mapping for Neurosurgery and Cognitive Neuroscience 119
    Joy Hirsch

7   fMRI of Memory in Aging and Dementia 161
    Andrew J. Saykin and Heather A. Wishart

8   fMRI of Language Systems: Methods and Applications 183
    Jeffrey R. Binder

9   fMRI Wada Test: Prospects for Presurgical Mapping
    of Language and Memory 215
    *Brenna C. McDonald, Andrew J. Saykin, J. Michael Williams,
    and Bassam A. Assaf*

10 Cognitive Neuroscience Applications 249
    Mark D'Esposito

Part III   Neuroanatomical Atlas

11   Neuroanatomical Atlas.. 277
     Feroze B. Mohamed and Scott H. Faro

Index.. 287

Contributors

Geoffrey K. Aguirre, MD, PhD
Department of Neurology Center for Cognitive Neuroscience, University of Pennsylvania, Philadelphia, PA, USA

Bassam A. Assaf, MD
Department of Neurology, University of Illinois College of Medicine at Peoria, Peoria, IL, USA

Peter A. Bandettini, PhD
Section on Functional Imaging Methods, Laboratory of Brain and Cognition, National Institute of Mental Health, Bethesda, MD, USA

Jeffrey R. Binder, MD
Department of Neurology; and Language Imaging Laboratory, Medical College of Wisconsin, Milwaukee, WI, USA

Susan Y. Bookheimer, PhD
Department of Psychiatry and Biobehavioral Sciences, Brain Research Institute, UCLA School of Medicine, Los Angeles, CA, USA

R. Todd Constable, PhD
Department of Diagnostic Radiology, Neurosurgery, and Biomedical Engineering; and the Magnetic Resonance Research Center, Yale University School of Medicine, New Haven, CT, USA

Mark D'Esposito, MD
Henry H. Wheeler, Jr. Brain Imaging Center, Helen Wills Neuroscience Institute and Department of Psychology, University of California, Berkeley, CA, USA

Scott H. Faro, MD
Department of Radiology, Functional Brain Imaging Center and Clinical MRI, Temple University School of Medicine, Philadelphia, PA, USA

Joy Hirsch, PhD
Departments of Radiology, Neuroscience, and Psychology; and Program for Imaging & Cognitive Sciences, Columbia University, New York, NY, USA

Seong-Gi Kim, PhD
Departments of Neurobiology and Radiology, University of Pittsburgh, Pittsburgh, PA, USA

Brenna C. McDonald, PsyD, MBA
Department of Radiology; and Center for Neuroimaging, Indiana University School of Medicine, Indianapolis, IN, USA

Feroze B. Mohamed, PhD
Department of Radiology, Functional Brain Imaging Center, Temple University School of Medicine, Philadelphia, PA, USA

Alexander B. Pinus, PhD
Department of Diagnostic Radiology, Magnetic Resonance Research Center, Yale University School of Medicine, New Haven, CT, USA

Nader Pouratian, MD, PhD
Department of Neurological Surgery; and Functional Movement Disorder Program, UCLA School of Medicine, Los Angeles, CA, USA

Andrew J. Saykin, PsyD
Department of Radiology; and Center for Neuroimaging, Indiana University School of Medicine, Indianapolis, IN, USA

J. Michael Williams, PhD
Department of Psychology, Drexel University, Philadelphia, PA, USA

Heather A. Wishart, PhD
Brain Imaging Laboratory, Department of Psychiatry, Dartmouth Medical School , Lebanon, NH, USA

Part I

BOLD Functional MRI

1

Principles of Functional MRI

Seong-Gi Kim and Peter A. Bandettini

Introduction

The idea that regional cerebral blood flow (CBF) could reflect neuronal activity began with experiments of Roy and Sherrington in 1890.[1] This concept is the basis for all hemodynamic-based brain imaging techniques being used today. The focal increase in CBF can be considered to relate directly to neuronal activity because the glucose metabolism and CBF changes are coupled closely.[2] Thus, the measurement of CBF change induced by stimulation has been used for mapping brain functions. Because cerebral metabolic rate of glucose (CMR_{glu}) and CBF changes are coupled, it is assumed that cerebral metabolic rate of oxygen ($CMRO_2$) and CBF changes also are coupled. However, based on positron emission tomographic measurements of CBF and $CMRO_2$ in humans during somatosensory and visual stimulation, Fox and colleagues reported that an increase in CBF surpassed an increase in $CMRO_2$.[3,4] Consequently, a mismatch between CBF and $CMRO_2$ changes results in an *increase* in the capillary and venous oxygenation level, opening a new physiological parameter (in addition to CBF change) for brain mapping. In 1990, based on rat brain studies during global stimulation at 7 Tesla (T), Ogawa and colleagues at AT&T Bell Laboratories reported that functional brain mapping is possible by using the venous blood oxygenation level-dependent (BOLD) magnetic resonance imaging (MRI) contrast.[5–7] The BOLD contrast relies on changes in deoxyhemoglobin (dHb), which acts as an endogenous paramagnetic contrast agent.[5,8] Therefore, changes in the local dHb concentration in the brain lead to alterations in the signal intensity of magnetic resonance images.[5–7,9]

Application of the BOLD contrast to human functional brain mapping followed shortly thereafter.[10–12] Since then, functional magnetic resonance imaging (fMRI) has been the tool of choice for visualizing neural activity in the human brain. The fMRI has been used extensively for investigating various brain functions, including vision, motor, language, and cognition.

This chapter previously appeared in *Functional MRI: Basic Principles and Clinical Applications*, edited by S. Faro and F. Mohamed. New York: Springer Science + Business Media, LCC 2006.

From: *BOLD fMRI: A Guide to Functional Imaging for Neuroscientists*
Edited by: S.H. Faro and F.B. Mohamed, DOI 10.1007/978-1-4419-1329-6_1
© Springer Science+Business Media, LLC 2010

The BOLD imaging technique is used widely because of its high sensitivity and easy implementation. Because the BOLD signal is dependent on various anatomical, physiological, and imaging parameters,[13] its interpretation with respect to physiological parameters is qualitative or semi-quantitative. Thus, it is difficult to compare the BOLD signal changes in different brain regions, from the different imaging laboratories, and/or from different magnetic fields. Alternatively, change in CBF can be measured using MRI. Because these fMRI signals are related to a single physiological parameter, its quantitative interpretation is more straightforward.

Functional MRI is a very powerful method to map brain functions with relatively high spatial and temporal resolution. In order to utilize fMRI techniques efficiently and interpret fMRI data accurately, it is important to examine underlying physiology and physics. In this introductory chapter, we will discuss the source of the BOLD signal and improvement of BOLD fMRI techniques.

Physiological Changes

Because fMRI measures the vascular hemodynamic response induced by increased neural activity, it is important to understand a chain of events from task to fMRI (see Figure 1.1). Task and/or stimulation induce synaptic and electric activities at localized regions, which will trigger an increase in CBF, cerebral blood volume (CBV), $CMRO_2$, and CMR_{glu}. Although the exact relationship between neural activity and vascular physiology change is not known, it is well-accepted that the change in CMR_{glu} is a good indicator of neural activity. Since the CMR_{glu} change is correlated linearly with the CBF change, a change in CBF is a good alternative secondary indicator of neural activity.

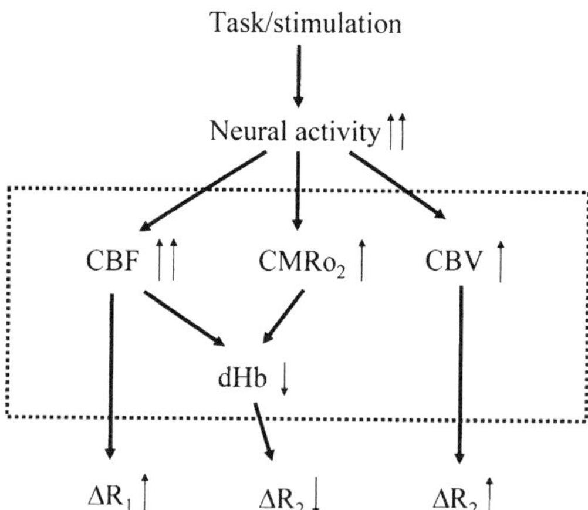

Figure 1.1. A schematic of fMRI signal changes induced by stimulation. Task/stimulation increases neural activity and increases metabolic (cerebral metabolic rate of oxygen) and vascular responses (cerebral blood flow and volume). Increase in CBF enhances venous oxygenation level, whereas increase in $CMRO_2$ decreases venous oxygenation level. Because an increase in CBF exceeds an increase in $CMRO_2$, venous oxygenation level increases. These vascular parameter changes will modulate biophysical parameters. Increases in CBF and CBV increase R_1 $(= 1/T_1)$ and R_2 $(= 1/T_2)$, respectively, whereas decrease in dHb contents reduces R_2. Changes in biophysical parameters affect MRI signal changes.

Cerebral blood flow and CBV changes are correlated because change in CBF is a multiple of CBV and velocity changes. The relationship between CBF and CBV obtained in monkeys during CO_2 modulation can be described as

$$\Delta CBV/CBV = (\Delta CBF/CBF + 1)^{0.38} - 1, \tag{1.1}$$

where $\Delta CBV/CBV$ and $\Delta CBF/CBF$ are relative total CBV and CBF changes.[14] The similar relationship was observed in rat brain during hypercapnia (see Figure 1.2A).[15] Recently, Ito and colleagues measured relative CBF and CBV

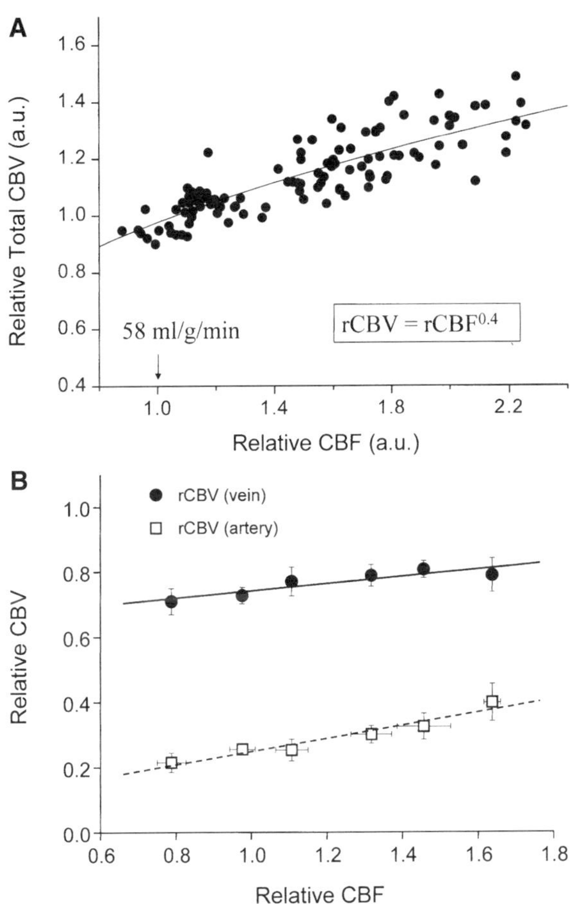

Figure 1.2. Relationship between CBF and CBV in rat brain.[15] Cerebral blood flow and CBV were measured using arterial spin labeling and ^{19}F NMR after injection of blood-substitute perflurocarbons during hypercapnia. Cerebral blood volume values were normalized with the CBV value at normocapnia (CBF = 58mL/100g/min). (A) Relationship between CBF and total CBV. The change in total rCBV was correlated linearly with the change in rCBF in a CBF range of 50–130mL/100g/min ($rCBV(total)/rCBF$ = 0.31). (B) Relationship between CBF and arterial/venous CBV. Arterial and venous CBV can be separated by using diffusion-weighted ^{19}F NMR.[69] The contribution of venous CBV changes to total CBV change is ~36%. Reprinted from Lee S-P, Duong T, Yang G, Iadecola C, Kim S-G. Relative changes of cerebral arterial and venous blood volumes during increased cerebral blood flow: Implications for BOLD fMRI. *Magn Reson Med.* 2001;45:791–800. Copyright © 2001. Reprinted with permission of Wiley-Liss, Inc., a subsidiary of John Wiley & Sons, Inc.

changes in human visual cortex during visual stimulation and found that the above relationship is reasonably applicable to human stimulation studies.[16] Thus, change in total blood volume can be a good index of the CBF change. Change in total blood volume can be measured by using contrast agents because contrast agents distribute in all vascular system. Because venous blood volume constitutes of 75% of the total blood volume,[15] it is conceivable that the venous blood volume change is dominant. However, based on separate measurements of arterial and venous blood volume changes during hypercapnia by a novel ^{19}F NMR technique and video-microscopy, a relative change in venous blood volume is approximately half of the relative total CBV change (see Figure 1.2B).[15]

In the context of BOLD contrast, only venous blood can contribute to activation-induced susceptibility changes because venous blood contains deoxyhemoglobin. The venous oxygenation level is dependent on a mismatch between oxygen supply by CBF and oxygen utilization in tissue. Assuming an arterial oxygen saturation of 1.0, the relative change of venous oxygenation level (Y) can be determined from the relative changes of both CBF and $CMRO_2$ in the following manner[17]:

$$\frac{\Delta Y}{1-Y} = \frac{(\Delta CMR_{O_2} / CMR_{O_2} + 1)}{(\Delta CBF / CBF + 1)} \tag{1.2}$$

From Equation (1.2), a relative change in $CMRO_2$ can be obtained from information of relative CBF and Y changes. It also is important to recognize that relationship between oxygenation change and blood flow change is linear at low CBF changes,[18,19] but nonlinear at very high CBF changes.[20,21]

Functional Imaging Contrasts

Magnetic resonance imaging signal in a given voxel can be described as a vector sum of signals from different compartments weighted by functions of T_1^* and T_2^*. Thus, MRI signal intensity is

$$S = \sum_i So_i fn(T_{1i}^*) fn(T_{2i}^*), \tag{1.3}$$

where S_{0i} is the spin density of compartment i in a given voxel, and T_{1i}^* and T_{2i}^* are apparent longitudinal and transverse relaxation times of compartment i, respectively. Thus, the signal change can be induced by a change in spin density, T_1^* and/or T_2^*. Changes in T_1^* can be induced by CBF changes, and changes in T_2^* can be induced by modulation in paramagnetic contents.

T_1 Weighted fMRI

An inflow effect into the region of interest will shorten apparent T_1. Using this property, time-of-flight angiographic images can be obtained. When the inflow time is relatively long, such as one second, the inflow effect exists not only in arterial vessels, but also in capillaries and the surrounding tissue. Thus, CBF can be measured noninvasively using arterial water as a perfusion tracer.[22-27] The general principle behind the arterial spin labeling (ASL) techniques is to differentiate the net magnetization of endogenous arterial water

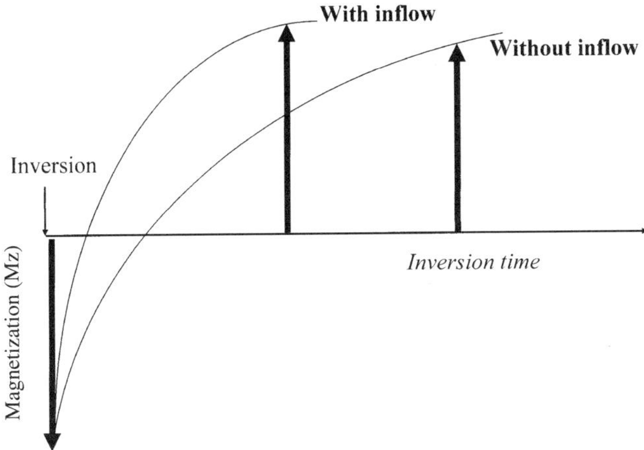

Figure 1.3. Hypothetical longitudinal magnetization with and without inflow effect after application of an inversion pulse (IR). Inflow effects relax spins faster.

flowing proximally to the region of interest from the net magnetization of tissue. Labeled spins by radio frequency (RF) pulse(s) move into capillaries in the imaging slice and exchange with tissue water spins. These techniques include continuous arterial spin tagging,[22] flow-sensitive alternating inversion recovery (FAIR),[23–25] and various other techniques.[26–28] In all of these techniques, two images are acquired, one with arterial spin labeling and the other without labeling. Among many available techniques, FAIR is most widely utilized because of its simple implementation. Two inversion recovery (IR) images are acquired in FAIR; one with a non-slice–selective inversion pulse and the other with a slice-selective inversion pulse. The longitudinal magnetization following a non-selective inversion pulse and a slice-selective inversion pulse recover by R_1 $(= 1/T_1)$ and $R_1^*(= 1/T_1^*)$, respectively, where R_1^* is equal to $R_1 + CBF/\lambda$ where λ is the tissue–blood partition coefficient ([g water/g tissue]/[g water/mL blood]). Figure 1.3 shows hypothetical relaxation recovery curves after the inversion pulse, with and without the inflow effect. Cerebral blood flow can be estimated by determinations of T_1 and T_1^*. In functional activation studies, two IR images are alternately and repeatedly acquired during both control and task periods. Then the differences between each pair of slice-selective and non-selective IR images are calculated during control periods (ΔS_{cont}) and stimulation periods (ΔS_{st}). Relative CBF changes during task periods can be described as $CBF_{st}/CBF_{cont} = \Delta S_{st}/\Delta S_{cont}$, where CBF_{st} and CBF_{cont} are CBF values during task and control periods, respectively. Functional brain mapping has been obtained successfully during motor, vision, and cognitive tasks (see Figure 1.4 for finger movements). Relative CBF changes measured by FAIR agree extremely with those measured by $H_2^{15}O$ positron emission tomography (PET) in the same region and subject during the identical stimulation task.[29] Thus, the perfusion-weighted MRI technique is an excellent approach to detect relative CBF changes induced by neural activity or other external perturbations. Furthermore because small arterioles and capillaries are very close to neuronally active tissue, it is expected that a tissue-specific CBF

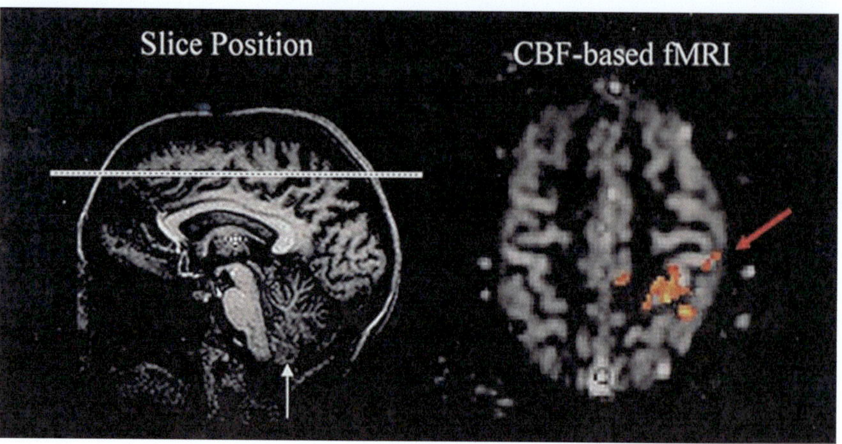

Figure 1.4. Cerebral blood flow-weighted functional image during left finger movements.[70] To obtain the perfusion contrast, flow direction (indicated by an up-arrow) has to be considered. Thus, 5-mm–thick transverse planes were selected for CBF-based fMRI studies. The background image was perfusion-weighted; higher signal areas have higher inflow rates. Functional activity areas are located at gray matter in the contralateral primary motor cortex, indicated by a red arrow. Interestingly, no large signal changes were observed at the edge of the brain, which often was seen in conventional BOLD functional maps. Adapted from Kim S-G, Tsekos NV, Ashe J. Multi-slice perfusion-based functional MRI using the FAIR technique: Comparison of CBF and BOLD effects. *NMR in Biomed*. 1997;10:191–196.

signal improves a spatial specificity of functional images. Figure 1.5 demonstrates the signal specificity of the perfusion-weighted fMRI technique in an anesthetized cat during single-orientation stimuli. Based on previous 2-DG glucose studies,[30] CMR_{glu} showed patchy, irregular columnar structures with an average inter-column distance of 1.1 to 1.4 millimeters. Cerebral blood flow-based fMRI maps showed similar activation patterns and intercluster distance, suggesting that the CBF response is specific to areas with metabolic increase.[31] It should be noted that the sagittal sinus running between two hemispheres does not show signal changes in CBF-based studies, contrary to conventional BOLD measurements, which has showed the largest signal change in the draining sagittal sinus.[32,33]

Although perfusion-based approaches can be utilized for fMRI studies, there are many shortcomings. First, large vascular contribution exists because labeled blood fill up arterial vasculature before it travels into capillaries (see also Figure 1.6).[34] This arterial vascular contribution can be reduced by using spin-echo data collection (see Figure 1.6) or eliminated using bipolar gradients, but this reduces SNR of perfusion-weighted images. Because the dilation of *large* arterial vessels is small,[15] no activation at large vessel areas was found.[35] Thus, for mapping purpose, it may not be necessary to remove large vessel contributions (see Figure 1.5). Second, the proper perfusion contrast is achieved only when enough time is allowed for the labeled arterial spins to travel into the region of interest and exchange with tissue spins. This makes it difficult to detect changes in CBF with a temporal resolution greater than T_1 of arterial blood, resulting in ineffective signal averaging. Third, in multi-slice application, transit times to different slices are different, which may cause errors in quantification of relative CBF changes.[28,36] Relative CBF

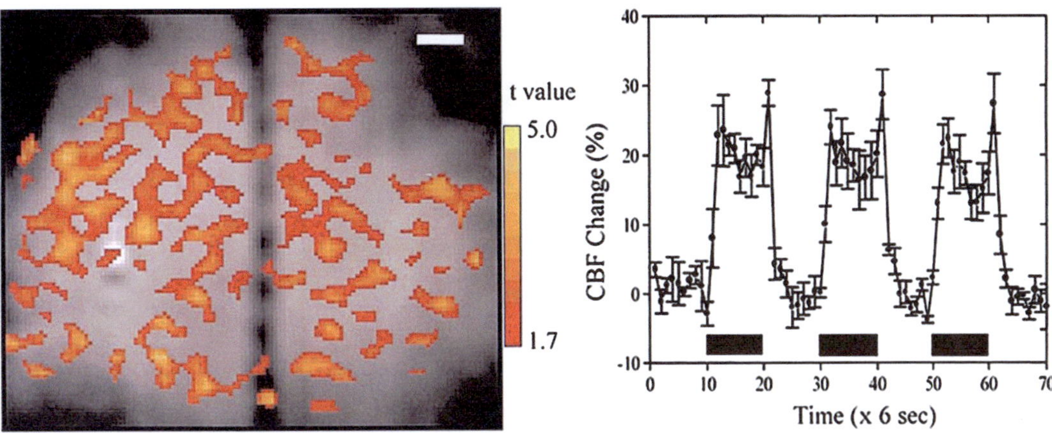

Figure 1.5. Application of the CBF-based (FAIR) fMRI technique to isoflurane-anesthetized cat's orientation column mapping.[31] Moving gratings with black and white rectangular single-orientation bars were used for visual stimulation. Unlike the conventional BOLD technique, CBF-weighted fMRI is specific to tissue, not draining vessels. More importantly, active clusters are irregular and column-like based on the size of clusters and the interval between clusters. In addition, single-condition functional regions activated by two orthogonal orientation stimuli are complementary. Scale bar = 1mm; color vertical bar = t value. Time course of activation area is shown. Boxes underneath the time course indicate one-minute–long stimulation periods. Typical CBF change induced by visual stimulation ranges between 15 and 50%. Reprinted with permission from Duong TQ, Kim DS, Ugurbil K, Kim SG. Localized cerebral blood flow response at submillimeter columnar resolution. *Proc Natl Acad Sci USA* 98:10904–10909. Copyright © 2001, National Academy of Sciences, U.S.A.

changes measured by multi-slice FAIR agree extremely with those measured by $H_2{}^{15}O$ PET, suggesting that the change in transit time is not a significant confound.[29]

T_2^* and T_2 Based fMRI

It is well known that, with typical fMRI acquisition parameters, the BOLD response is particularly sensitive in and around large draining veins because the BOLD effect is sensitive to baseline venous blood volume and vessel size.[17,37] To understand the spatial resolution of BOLD-based fMRI, it is important to examine the anatomical source of the BOLD signal. The BOLD contrast induced by dHb arises from both intravascular (IV) and extravascular (EV) components. Because the exchange of water between these two compartments (typical lifetime of the water in capillaries greater than 500 milliseconds) is relatively slower compared with the imaging time (echo time less than 100 milliseconds), MRI signals from these are treated as separate pools.

Intravascular Component

During fMRI measurements, water rapidly exchanges between red blood cells (RBC) with paramagnetic dHb and plasma (average water residence time in RBC's equals approximately five milliseconds) and move along space with different fields by diffusion (e.g., diffusion distance [i.e., (6 × diffusion

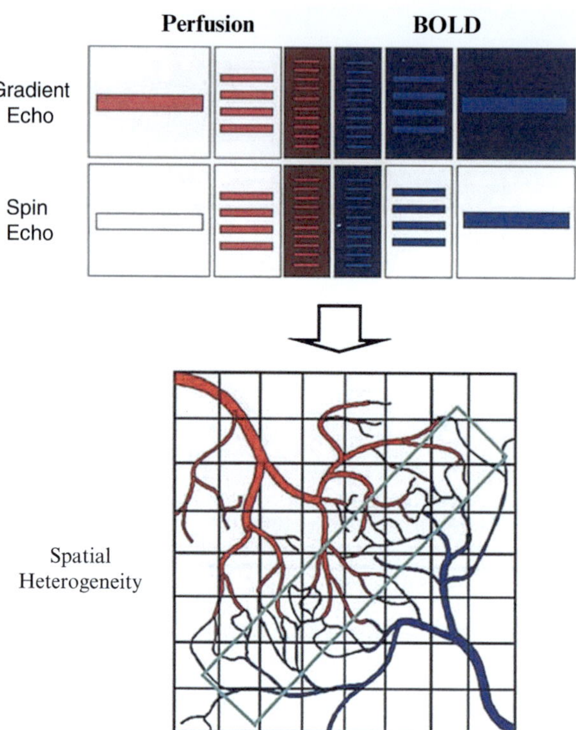

Figure 1.6. Intravascular and extravascular signal contributions to perfusion and BOLD signals.[71] In perfusion-weighted images, the IV component of all arterial vessels (red color) and EV component (pink) of capillaries will constitute. When spin-echo data collection is used, spins in large vessels will not be refocused, removing very large artery contribution. Further removal can be achieved by using bipolar flow-crushing gradients. In BOLD images, IV (blue color) and EV (black) components of all size venous vessels will contribute when gradient-echo data collection is used. When spin-echo data collection is utilized, EV effect of large vessels can be minimized. Spatial heterogeneity of vascular distributions exists; in some pixels, large vessels are dominant, whereas some pixels contain mostly capillaries. When neural activity occurs at tissue level, demarked by a green rectangle, only capillary-level signal change will locate the actual neural activity area. Containing large vessels will misleadingly deviate activation to non-specific vessel area. Adapted with permission from Bandettini PA. The temporal resolution of Functional MRI. In: Moonen CTW, Bandettini PA, eds. Functional MRI. New York: Springer 1999:204–220.

constant $\times$ diffusion time)$^{1/2}$] during ~50 milliseconds measurement time = ~17 micrometers (μm) with diffusion constant of ~1μm^2 per millisecond). Thus, dynamic (time irreversible) averaging occurs over the many different fields induced by dHb. All water molecules inside the vessel will experience the similar dynamic averaging, resulting in reduction of T_2 of blood water in the venous pool. A transverse relaxation rate of blood water is affected by exchange of water and diffusion. In both cases, blood T_2 can be written as

$$1/T_2 = A_o + K(1-Y)^2 , \tag{1.4}$$

where A_o is a field-independent constant term and K would scale quadratically with the magnetic field and depend also on the echo time used in a spin-echo measurement.[38] T_2 of blood water at 1.5T is ~127ms for $Y = 0.6$[38], whereas T_2 is ~12–15ms at 7T[39,40] and 5ms at 9.4T.[41] These experimental values are consistent with predictions based on Equation (1.4). T_2 values of gray matter water at 1.5T, 7T, and 9.4T are 90ms,[42] 55ms,[40] and 40ms,[41] respectively. When spin-echo time is set to T_2 of gray matter, it is evident that the blood contribution to MRI signal decreases dramatically when the magnetic field increases.

In addition to the T_2 change induced by deoxyhemoglobin, frequency shift is observed. When a blood vessel is considered as an infinite cylinder, frequency shift $\Delta\omega$ induced by dHb within and around the vessel is depicted at Figure 1.7. It should be noted that frequency and magnetic field are interchangeable because $\omega = \gamma B$, where γ is the gyromagnetic ratio and B is the magnetic field. Inside the blood vessel, the frequency shift is expressed by

$$\Delta\omega_{in} = 2\pi\Delta\chi_o(1-Y)\omega_o(\cos^2\theta - 1/3), \tag{1.5}$$

where $\Delta\chi_o$ is the maximum susceptibility difference between fully oxygenated and fully deoxygenated blood, Y is the fraction of oxygenation in venous blood, ω_o is the applied magnetic field of magnet in frequency units $\omega_o = \gamma B_0$), and θ is the angle between the applied magnetic field (B_0) and vessel orientation. $\Delta\chi_o$ is dependent on a hematocrit level. Assuming a hematocrit level of 0.38 and the susceptibility difference between 100% oxyhemoglobin and 100% dHb of 0.27ppm,[8] $\Delta\chi_o$ in whole blood is 0.1ppm. In a given voxel, many vessels with different orientations exist. Rather than inducing a net phase shift, the random orientations cause a phase dispersion, therefore causing a reduction in T_2^*. However, a very large vessel will have its own phase depending on oxygenation level and orientation. Using this property, Haacke and his colleagues determined a venous oxygenation level[43] from a vessel that they determined to be perpendicular to B_0.

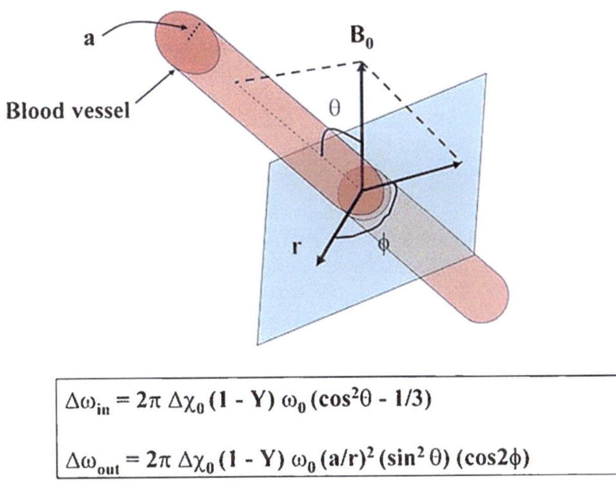

$$\Delta\omega_{in} = 2\pi\,\Delta\chi_0(1-Y)\,\omega_0(\cos^2\theta - 1/3)$$

$$\Delta\omega_{out} = 2\pi\,\Delta\chi_0(1-Y)\,\omega_0(a/r)^2(\sin^2\theta)(\cos 2\phi)$$

Figure 1.7. Diagram of a blood vessel and the parameters that determine the susceptibility effect induced by dHb irons in red blood cells at a distance r from the center of a vessel. The vessel with a radius of a is oriented at angle θ from the main magnetic field B_0. ϕ is the angle between r and plane defined by B_0 and the vessel axis. Reprinted from *Methods*, Vol. 30, Kim SG, Ugurbil K, High-resolution functional MRI in the animal brain, 28–41. Copyright © 2003, with permission from Elsevier.

Extravascular Component

At any location outside the blood vessel, the frequency shift can be described by

$$\Delta\omega_{out} = 2\pi\Delta\chi_O(1-Y)\omega_o(a/r)^2(\sin^2\theta)(\cos 2\phi) \qquad (1.6)$$

where a is the radius of blood vessel, r is the distance from the point of interest to the center of the blood vessel, and ϕ is the angle between r and plane defined by B_0 and the vessel axis. The dephasing effect is dependent on the orientation of vessel. Vessels running parallel to the magnetic field do not have the EV effect, whereas those orthogonal to B_0 will have the maximal effect (see Figure 1.8). At the lumen of vessels ($r = a$), $\Delta\omega_{out}$ is identical and independent of vessel sizes. At $r = 5a$, the susceptibility effect is four percent of the maximally available $\Delta\omega_{out}$. The same frequency shift will be observed at 15µm around a 3-µm radius capillary and 150µm around a 30-µm radius venule (see Figure 1.9). This shows that the dephasing effect around a larger vessel is more spatially extensive because of a smaller susceptibility gradient. The EV contribution from large vessels to conventional BOLD signal is significant, regardless of magnetic field strength.[41] During echo time for fMRI studies (e.g., ~50ms), water molecules diffuse ~17µm, which covers a space with the entire range of susceptibility effects around the 3-µm radius capillary, but with a small range of static susceptibility effects around the 30-µm radius venule. Thus, tissue water around *capillaries* will be dynamically averaged over the many different fields (i.e., no net phase change like the IV component). However, because tissue water around *large vessels* will be averaged locally during an echo time, the static dephasing effect is dominant (see small circles with dephasing information in Figure 1.9). The dephasing effect around large vessels can be refocused by the 180-degree RF pulse. Therefore, the EV contribution of large vessels can be reduced by using the spin-echo technique (see Figure 1.8).

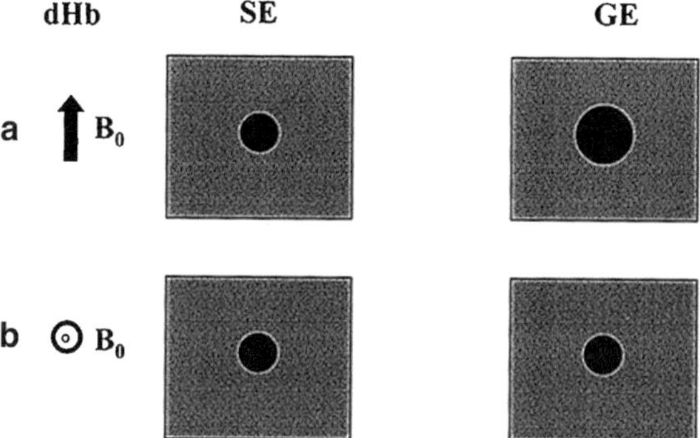

Figure 1.8. Spin-echo and gradient-echo image of a capillary filled with blood with deoxyhemoglobin.[7] Two different orientations were used. When vessel orientation is parallel to B_0 (b), no signal change outside the capillary was observed. However, when vessel is orthogonal to B_0 (a), gradient-echo signal change outside the capillary was detected. Adapted from Ogawa S, Lee T-M. Magnetic resonance imaging of blood vessels at high fields: in vivo and in vitro measurements and image simulation. *Magn Reson Med.* 1990;16:9–18.

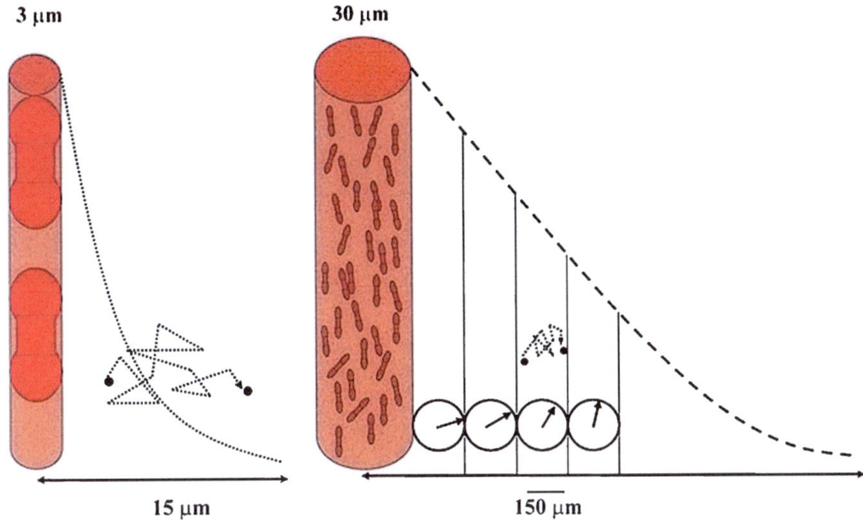

Figure 1.9. Extravascular dephasing effects from a 3-μm radius capillary and a 30-μm radius venule. Magnitude of dephasing effect (dashed decay lines from vessels) is shown as a function of distance. Hypothetical displacement of a water molecule is shown. Refocusing RF pulse in the spin-echo sequence cannot refocus dephasing effects around a small vessel because of dynamic averaging, whereas it can refocus static dephasing (shown in averaged phases in circles). Reprinted from *Methods*, Vol. 30, Kim SG, Ugurbil K, High-resolution functional MRI in the animal brain, 28–41. Copyright © 2003, with permission from Elsevier.

In a given voxel, MRI signal intensity with dephasing effects (i.e., frequency shifts) induced by numerous vessels will be summed, resulting in a decrease in T_2^* and a decrease in MRI signal. Signal in the voxel can be described, according to equation

$$S(TE) = \sum_i So_i e^{-TE/T_{2i}} e^{-i\omega_i TE} , \tag{1.7}$$

where the summation is performed over the parameter i, which designates small volume elements within the voxel (e.g., hypothetically a volume with a small circle with phase shift), the time-averaged magnetic field experienced within these small volume elements. $\omega_i TE$ indicates the phase shift of location i at echo time TE. This signal loss occurs from *static averaging*. If the variation ω_i within the voxel is relatively large, the signal will be decayed approximately with a single exponential time constant T_2^*. Based on Monte Carlo simulation, the dephasing effect within a voxel can be simplified into R_2' (in order to separate measured $R_2^* = $ intrinsic $R_2 + R_2'$ induced by contrast agent) change as

$$R_2' = \alpha \cdot CBV \{\Delta\chi_O \omega_O (1-Y)\}^\gamma \tag{1.8}$$

where α and γ are constants.[17,44,45] The power term γ is 1.0 for static averaging domain and 2.0 for time-irreversible averaging domain.[17,44,45] All venous vessels will have a power term of 1.0 to 2.0; γ is 1.0 to 2.0 for the gradient-echo sequence, and 1.5 to 2.0 for spin-echo sequence.[17,44,45] If diffusion-related travel distance of water molecules during echo time is sufficient to effectively average frequency shifts (also related to magnetic field), γ will be 2.0.

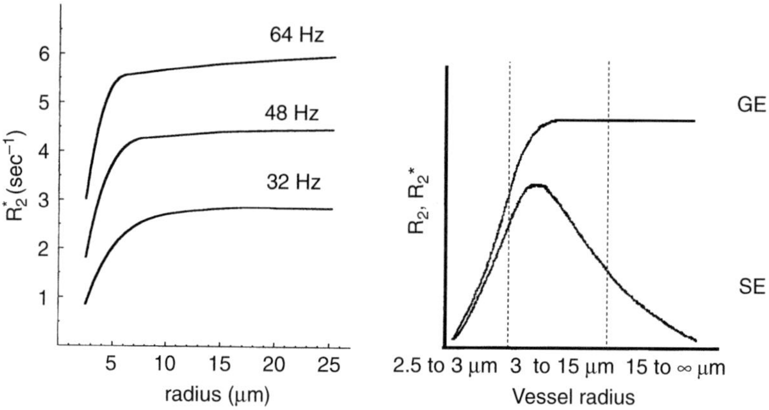

Figure 1.10. R_2^* and R_2 changes as a function of vessel radius.[17,46] Monte Carlo simulation was performed to calculate R_2^* change induced by three frequency shifts.[17] Reprinted with permission from Ogawa S, Menon RS, Tank DW, Kim SG, Merkle H, Ellermann JM and Ugurbil. Functional brain mapping by blood oxygenation level-dependent contrast magnetic resonance imaging. A comparison of signal characteristics with a biophysical model. *Biophys. J*, 64:803–812;1993.

Thus, a longer echo time (i.e., longer diffusion distance) and a higher magnetic field (i.e., large susceptibility gradient) will reduce a vessel size for dynamic averaging. Figure 1.10 shows the R_2' dependency on vessel size and frequency shift, which was obtained from Monte Carlo simulation with CBV of two percent and echo time of 40 milliseconds. R_2' increases linearly with venous CBV.[17] Frequency shift at $Y = 0$ is 40 hertz at 1.5T and 107 hertz at 4T. Let us examine vessels with 3μm and 30μm radii. When a frequency shift increases from 32 to 64 hertz (due to an increase in magnetic field and/or a decrease in oxygenation level), R_2^* values of 3μm and 30μm radius vessels change from 1.2 to 3.5 sec^{-1} and from 2.8 to 6.0 sec^{-1}, respectively. A power term γ will be 1.5 for a 3-μm vessel and 1.1 for a 30-μm vessel, showing that a smaller size vessel is more sensitive to the frequency shift (such as induced by magnetic field). Spin-echo and gradient-echo BOLD signal changes in a function of vessel size can be seen in Figure 1.10.[46] At capillaries, a change in R_2 is similar to that of R_2^*. However, when vessel size increases above five- to eight-micrometer radius (which is related to diffusion time and susceptibility gradient), R_2 change is reduced, but R_2^* change remains high. Thus, spin-echo BOLD signals predominantly originate from small-size vessels, including capillaries, whereas gradient-echo BOLD signals are contributed from large draining veins.

Spin Echo versus Gradient Echo BOLD

As has been discussed previously, gradient-echo BOLD signals consist of EV and IV components of venous vessels, regardless of the vessel size (see Figure 1.6). Spin echo refocuses the dephasing effect around large vessels, and thus the spin-echo BOLD image contains the EV effect of vessels with time-irreversible diffusion effect (i.e., small-size vessel) and the IV component of all sizes of vessels. It is important to differentiate parenchyma signals (see a green rectangular box) from large vessel signals because the venous vasculature, including large draining veins, can be distant from the site of elevated neuronal activity (see also Figure 1.6).[32,47–50] Dilution by blood draining from inactive areas should ultimately diminish this non-specific draining-vein effect and thus limit its extent; however, before this occurs, substantial less-specific activation can be generated.[51] Therefore, it is important to minimize draining-vein signals from both intravascular and extravascular contributions for high-resolution studies.

The intravascular component can be reduced by setting an echo time of greater than 3 T_2^* or $3T_2$ of blood. Thus, at ultrahigh fields, the IV component can be reduced significantly because venous blood T_2^* and T_2 decreases faster than tissue T_2^* / T_2 when magnetic field increases. The intravascular contribution to the BOLD responses can be examined using bipolar gradients.[52] These gradients induce velocity-dependent phase shifts in the presence of flow and consequently suppress signals from blood because of inhomogeneous velocities within a vessel and the presence of blood vessels of different orientations within a voxel. Based on bipolar gradient studies, the BOLD fMRI signals at 1.5T originate predominantly from the IV component (70–90%),[44,53,54] whereas those at 7T and 9.4T come predominantly from the EV component (see Figure 1.11).[41,55] When bipolar gradients increased to greater than $400s/mm^2$, relative percent BOLD signal change maintained constant, even though signal intensity decreased. With relatively high sensitivity of spin-echo BOLD at high fields, high-resolution functional maps can be obtained from human brain at 7T (see Figure 1.11).

After removing the IV component in the BOLD signal, the EV component remains. In gradient-echo BOLD fMRI, the EV effect around large vessels is linearly dependent on magnetic field, whereas the EV effect around small vessels is supra-linearly dependent on the magnetic field. Even at 9.4T, the EV effect around large vessels is significant. In spin-echo BOLD fMRI, the EV effect around small vessels is supra-linearly dependent on the magnetic field, whereas that around large vessels is reduced. Thus, the spin-echo technique is more specific to parenchyma than gradient-echo BOLD fMRI. However, because the dephasing effect around vessels is refocused, the sensitivity of spin-echo BOLD signal is reduced significantly. For example, $\Delta R_2 / \Delta R_2^*$ is 0.3–0.4 at 1.5T,[56,57] and also at 9.4T.[21] Even if respective optimized echo times are used for gradient-echo and spin-echo BOLD fMRI, the gradient-echo BOLD technique provides the higher signal change, even at 9.4T. For most applications, the gradient-echo BOLD technique is the choice of tools because of high sensitivity, even if its spatial specificity compromises.

Contrast-to-Noise Ratio

Important consideration of fMRI is contrast-to-noise ratio (neural activity-induced signal change relative to signal fluctuation). Increase of neural activity-induced MRI signal and decrease of noise are important aspects for high-resolution fMRI. Neural activity-induced signal is dependent on both image contrast and imaging techniques used for fMRI. In the T_2^*-based measurements, the signal change induced by neural activity (ΔS) can be described by

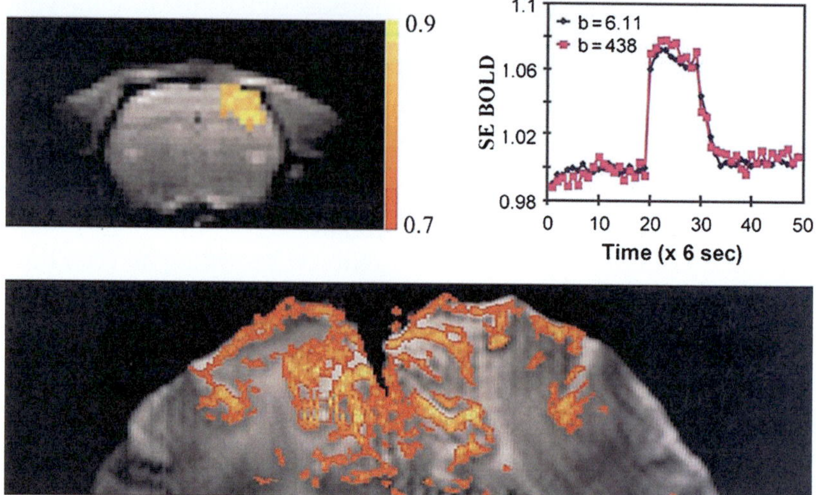

Figure 1.11. Spin-echo BOLD-based fMRI at 9.4T and 7T.[41,72] (top) An α-chloralse anesthetized rat was used for somatosensory forelimb stimulation. Color indicates a cross-correlation value. Localized activation is observed at the forelimb S1. Functional MRI time courses of spin-echo BOLD signal in the primary somatosensory region. To investigate the IV component, flow-crushing gradients (in a unit of b value) were used. The higher b value will result in the more reduction of the moving blood signal. If the IV component is significant, a much lower BOLD signal change is expected when a larger b value is used. However, any reduction of relative BOLD signals was not observed, suggesting that spin-echo BOLD signal does not contain a significant IV component. Somatosensory stimulation was performed during image number 20 to 29. (bottom) High-resolution spin-echo BOLD image was obtained from a human during visual stimulation at 7T. At high fields, sensitivity of SE BOLD signal is sufficient for high-resolution mapping of human brain. Spatial resolution is $1 \times 1 \times 2mm^3$. Reprinted from Duong TQ, Yacoub E, Adriany G, et al. High-resolution, spin-echo BOLD and CBF fMRI at 4 and 7T. *Mag Reson Med.* 2002;48:589–593. Copyright © 2002. Reprinted with permission of Wiley-Liss, Inc., a subsidiary of John Wiley & Sons, Inc.

$$\Delta S = \rho \cdot S_{cont} \cdot (e^{-TE \cdot \Delta R_2^*} - 1), \tag{1.9}$$

where ρ is the fraction of a voxel that is active, S_{cont} is the signal intensity during the control period, TE is the echo time, and ΔR_2^* is the change in the apparent transverse relaxation rate in the active partial volume. Signal change is maximal when a gradient echo time is set to T_2^* of tissue at resting conditions. When spin-echo imaging techniques are used, ΔR_2^* is replaced by ΔR_2. ΔR_2^* is equivalent to $\Delta R_2 + \Delta R_2'$, where $\Delta R_2'$ is the relaxation rate induced by local inhomogenous magnetic fields. ΔS for spin-echo BOLD fMRI will be maximal by setting TE of T_2 of tissue. In CBF-based techniques, $TE\Delta R_2^*$ is substituted by $TI\Delta R_1^*$, where TI is the spin labeling time (i.e., the inversion time for pulsed labeling methods), and ΔR_1^* is the change in the apparent longitudinal relaxation rate. ΔS is maximized by setting TI of T_1 of tissue. In any technique, contribution of large vessels increases ΔS. Depending on constraints of spatial specificity for each measurement, the technique with the highest ΔS should be chosen. Because contribution of small intracortical veins is likely localized within 1.5 millimeters to the site of activation,[58] contribution of small veins can improve SNR for supramillimeter spatial resolution. In typical fMRI studies with supramillimeter spatial resolution, the removal of only large surface arteries and veins may be necessary.

Sources of noise include random white noise, physiological fluctuations, bulk head motion, and system instability if it exists. Random noise is independent between voxels, whereas other noise sources may be coherent among voxels, resulting in spatial and temporal correlation. In fMRI, coherent noises are the major source of signal fluctuation. Bulk head motion can be eliminated by head holders. Physiological motion, which is due mainly to respiration and cardiac pulsation, can be minimized by gating data acquisition and/or reduced by post processing.[59,60]

Spatial and Temporal Resolution of fMRI

Spatial Resolution

Spatial resolution of high-resolution fMRI is dependent on signal-to-noise ratio (SNR) and intrinsic hemodynamic response. The intrinsic limit of spatial specificity of hemodynamic-based fMRI can be dependent on how finely CBF is regulated. It has been suggested, based on optical imaging studies, that CBF regulation is widespread beyond neuronally active areas.[61] However, recent studies have suggested that intrinsic CBF changes are specific to submillimeter functional domains.[31] The highest CBF change was observed in the middle of the rat somatosensory cortex, cortical layer IV, not at the surface of the cortex during somatosensory stimulation.[21,62] This observation is consistent with invasive 2-DG and ^{14}C-iodoantipyrine autoradiographic studies in the barrel cortex.[63] To further examine the specificity of CBF response, the perfusion-based FAIR technique has been utilized.[23]From this study, it was found that CBF is regulated to submillimeter layer-specific and laminar-specific functional domains.[21,31] Among the available hemodynamic fMRI approaches, the CBF-based signal is the most specific to neuronal active sites because most signals originate from tissues and capillaries. Tissue-specific BOLD signal without large vessel contribution will have a similar spatial specificity to the CBF-weighted signal.[21]

Temporal Resolution

Because hemodynamic responses are sluggish, it is difficult to obtain very high temporal resolution, even if images can be obtained rapidly. Typically, hemodynamic signal changes are observed at one to two seconds after the onset of neural stimulation and reaches maximum at four to eight seconds (see Figure 1.12). The exact time of neural activity from hemodynamic responses cannot be obtained easily because hemodynamic response varies depending on vascular structures (see Figure 1.12). The important issue is to determine sequential neural activities of different cortical regions or pixels. If the hemodynamic response times in all regions and in all subjects were the same, neuronal activities could be inferred directly from fMRI time courses. However, this may not be true in all regions and in all subjects (see Figure 1.12); thus, differences in fMRI time courses may be simply related to intrinsic hemodynamic response time differences, hampering temporal studies. Thus, temporal resolution of fMRI is limited. Alternative approaches to

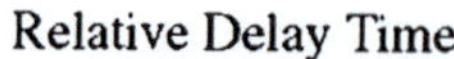

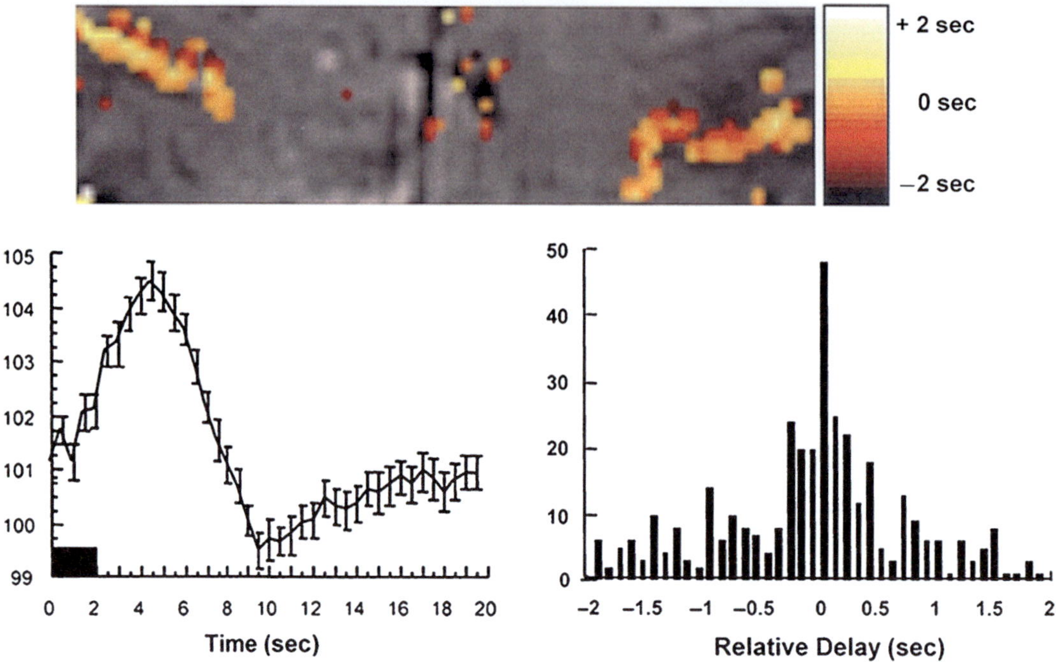

Figure 1.12. Heterogeneity of hemodynamic responses.[71] Delay time of T_2^*-weighted fMRI signal changes was obtained in the motor cortical areas. Two-second bilateral finger movements were performed at 3T. Although average delay time is approximately one second, there is a large variation in delay time shown in color map, as well as histogram. In histogram and the delay map, relative hemodynamic delay time (not actual delay time) was calculated, which means average of all delay times of zero seconds. Adapted with permission from Bandettini PA. The temporal resolution of Functional MRI. In: Moonen CTW, Bandettini PA, eds. Functional MRI. New York: Springer 1999:204–220.

overcome these problems have been proposed. To separate intrinsic hemodynamic differences from neural activity differences, a time-resolved event-related fMRI technique can be utilized.[64–67] The idea is to examine how fMRI parameters vary with behavioral correlates and thus requires multiple behavioral outcome measures. Subsequently, temporal characteristics of fMRI responses can be correlated with behavioral data such as response time. Differences in the underlying temporal behavior of neuronal activity can be distinguished from hemodynamic response time variations between subjects and brain areas (see a review article[68]). This approach allows the experimenter to obtain higher temporal resolution. Dynamic fMRI studies can be feasible using standard gradient-echo BOLD fMRI. The issues related to spatial and temporal characteristic is further discussed in detail in chapter 4 of this book.

Conclusions

Advancement of imaging technologies allows detections of various vascular physiological parameters induced by neural activity. Fortunately, tissue-based hemodynamic response is relatively specific to neuronal active sites.

Thus, spatial resolution of fMRI can be achieved up to on an order of a column. Because hemodynamic response is slow, its temporal resolution cannot be reached easily at a level of neural activity time scale. By using an approach with multiple experiments with different stimulus intervals or durations, temporal resolution can be improved up to on the order of 100 milliseconds.

References

1. Roy CS, Sherrington CS. On the regulation of blood supply of the brain. *J Physiol.* 1890;1:85–108.
2. Raichle ME. Circulatory and metabolic correlates of brain function in normal humans. In: Handbook of Physiology—The Nervous System. Vol. V. Bethesda, MD: American Physiological Society; 1987:643–674.
3. Fox PT, Raichle ME. Focal physiological uncoupling of cerebral blood flow and oxidative metabolism during somatosensory stimulation in human subjects. *Proc Natl Acad Sci USA.* 1986;83:1140–1144.
4. Fox PT, Raichle ME, Mintun MA, Dence C. Nonoxidative glucose consumption during focal physiologic neural activity. *Science.* 1988;241:462–464.
5. Ogawa S, Lee T-M, Nayak AS, Glynn P. Oxygenation-sensitive contrast in magnetic resonance image of rodent brain at high magnetic fields. *Magn Reson Med.* 1990;14:68–78.
6. Ogawa S, Lee T-M, Kay AR, Tank DW. Brain magnetic resonance imaging with contrast dependent on blood oxygenation. *Proc Natl Acad Sci USA.* 1990;87:9868–9872.
7. Ogawa S, Lee TM. Magnetic resonance imaging of blood vessels at high fields: in vivo and in vitro measurements and image simulation. *Magn Reson Med.* 1990;16:9–18.
8. Pauling L, Coryell CD. The magnetic properties and structure of hemoglobin, oxyhemoglobin and carbonmonoxyhemoglobin. Proc Natl Acad Sci USA. 1936;22:210–216.
9. Thulborn KR, Waterton JC, Mattews PM, Radda GK. Oxygenation dependence of the transverse relaxation time of water protons in whole blood at high field. *Biochem Biophys Acta.* 1982;714:265–270.
10. Ogawa S, Tank DW, Menon R, et al. Intrinsic signal changes accompanying sensory stimulation: Functional brain mapping with magnetic resonance imaging. *Proc Natl Acad Sci USA.* 1992;89:5951–5955.
11. Kwong KK, Belliveau JW, Chesler DA, et al. Dynamic magnetic resonance imaging of human brain activity during primary sensory stimulation. *Proc Natl Acad Sci USA.* 1992;89:5675–5679.
12. Bandettini PA, Wong EC, Hinks RS, Rikofsky RS, Hyde JS. Time course EPI of human brain function during task activation. *Magn Reson Med.* 1992;25:390–397.
13. Ogawa S, Menon RS, Kim S-G, Ugurbil K. On the characteristics of functional magnetic resonance imaging of the brain. *Annu Rev Biophys Biomol Struct.* 1998;27:447–474.
14. Grubb RL, Raichle ME, Eichling JO, Ter-Pogossian MM. The effects of changes in PaCO2 on cerebral blood volume, blood flow, and vascular mean transit time. *Stroke.* 1974;5:630–639.
15. Lee S-P, Duong T, Yang G, Iadecola C, Kim S-G. Relative changes of cerebral arterial and venous blood volumes during increased cerebral blood flow: Implications for BOLD fMRI. *Magn Reson Med.* 2001;45:791–800.
16. Ito H, Takahashi K, Hatazawa J, Kim S-G, Kanno I. Changes in human regional cerebral blood flow and cerebral blood volume during visual stimulation measured by positron emission tomography. *J Cereb Blood Flow Metab.* 2001;21:608–612.

17. Ogawa S, Menon RS, Tank DW, et al. Functional brain mapping by blood oxygenation level-dependent contrast magnetic resonance imaging. *Biophys J.* 1993;64:800–812.

18. Hoge RD, Atkinson J, Gill B, Crelier GR, Marrett S, G.B.P. Linear coupling between cerebral blood flow and oxygen consumption in activated human cortex. Proc *Natl Acad Sci.* 1999;96:9403–9408.

19. Kim S-G, Rostrup E, Larsson HBW, Ogawa S, Paulson OB. Simultaneous measurements of CBF and $CMRO_2$ changes by fMRI: Significant increase of oxygen consumption rate during visual stimulation. *Magn Reson Med.* 1999;41:1152–1161.

20. Silva A, Lee S-P, Yang C, Iadecola C, Kim S-G. Simultaneous BOLD and perfusion functional MRI during forepaw stimulation in rats. *J Cereb Blood Flow Metab.* 1999;19:871–879.

21. Lee S-P, Silva AC, Kim S-G. Comparison of diffusion-weighted high-resolution CBF and spin-echo BOLD fMRI at 9.4T. *Magn Reson Med.* 2002;47:736–741.

22. Detre JA, Leigh JS, Williams DS, Koretsky AP. Perfusion imaging. *Magn Reson Med.* 1992;23:37–45.

23. Kim S-G. Quantification of relative cerebral blood flow change by flow-sensitive alternating inversion recovery (FAIR) technique: application to functional mapping. *Magn Reson Med.* 1995;34:293–301.

24. Kwong KK, Chesler DA, Weisskoff RM, et al. MR perfusion studies with T1-weighted echo planar imaging. *Magn Reson Med.* 1995;34:878–887.

25. Schwarzbauer C, Morrissey S, Haase A. Quantitative magnetic resonance imaging of perfusion using magnetic labeling of water proton spins within the detection slice. *Magn Reson Med.* 1996;35:540–546.

26. Edelman RR, Siewert B, Darby DG, et al. Qualitative mapping of cerebral blood flow and functional localization with echo-planar MR imaging and signal targeting with alternating radio frequency. *Radiology.* 1994;192:513–520.

27. Helpern J, Branch C, Yongbi M, Huong N. Perfusion imaging by uninverted flow-sensitive alternating inversion recovery (UNFAIR). *Magn Reson Imaging.* 1997;15:135–139.

28. Wong E, Buxton R, Frank L. Quantitative imaging of perfusion using a single subtraction (QUIPSS and QUIPSS II). *Magn Reson Med.* 1998;39:702–708.

29. Zaini MR, Strother SC, Andersen JR, et al. Comparison of matched BOLD and FAIR 4.0T-fMRI with [^{15}O]water PET brain volumes. *Medical Physics.* 1999;26:1559–1567.

30. Lowel S, Freeman B, Singer W. Topographic organization of the orientation column system in large flat-mounts of the cat visual cortex: a 2-deoxyglucose study. *Exp Brain Res.* 1988;71:33–46.

31. Duong TQ, Kim D-S, Ugurbil K, Kim S-G. Localized cerebral blood flow response at submillimeter columnar resolution. *Proc Natl Acad Sci USA.* 2001;98:10904–10909.

32. Duong TQ, Kim D-S, Ugurbil K, Kim S-G. Spatio-temporal Dynamics of the BOLD fMRI Signals: Toward mapping submillimeter columnar structures using the early negative response. *Magn Reson Med.* 2000;44:231–242.

33. Kim D-S, Duong TQ, Kim S-G. High-resolution mapping of iso-orientation columns by fMRI. *Nature Neurosci.* 2000;3:164–169.

34. Ye FQ, Mattay VS, Jezzard P, Frank JA, Weinberger DR, McLaughlin AC. Correction for vascular artifacts in cerebral blood flow values by using arterial spin tagging techniques. *Magn Reson Med.* 1997;37:226–235.

35. Kim S-G, Tsekos NV. Perfusion imaging by a flow-sensitive alternating inversion recovery (FAIR) technique: Application to functional mapping. *Magn Reson Med.* 1997;37:425–435.

36. Buxton R, Frank L, Wong E, Siewert B, Warach S, Edelman R. A general kinetic model for quantitative perfusion imaging with arterial spin labeling. *Magn Reson Med.* 1998;40:383–396.

37. Weisskoff RM, Zuo CS, Boxerman JL, Rosen BR. Microscopic susceptibility variation and transverse relaxation: Theory and experiment. *Magn Reson Med.* 1994;31:601–610.

38. Wright GA, Hu BS, Macovski A. Estimating oxygen saturation of blood in vivo with MR imaging at 1.5T. *J Magn Reson Imag.* 1991;1:275–283.

39. Ogawa S, Lee TM, Barrere B. Sensitivity of magnetic resonance image signals of a rat brain to changes in the cerebral venous blood oxygenation. *Magn Reson Med.* 1993;29:205–210.

40. Yacoub E, Shmuel A, Pfeuffer J, et al. Imaging brain function in humans at 7 Tesla. *Magn Reson Med.* 2001;45:588–594.

41. Lee S-P, Silva AC, Ugurbil K, Kim S-G. Diffusion-weighted spin-echo fMRI at 9.4T: microvasculuar/tissue contribution to BOLD signal change. *Magn Reson Med.* 1999;42:919–928.

42. Breger RK, Rimm AA, Fischer ME, Papke RA, Haughten VM. T_1 and T_2 measurements on a 1.5 Tesla commercial imager. *Radiology.* 1989;171:273–276.

43. Haacke E, Lai S, Yablonskiy D, Lin W. In vivo validation of the BOLD mechanism: A review of signal changes in gradient echo functional MRI in the presence of flow. Int J Imaging Syst Technol. 1995;6:153–163.

44. Boxerman JL, Bandettini PA, Kwong KK, et al. The intravascular contribution to fMRI signal change: Monte Carlo modeling and diffusion-weighted studies in vivo. *Magn Reson Med.* 1995;34:4–10.

45. Kennan RP, Zhong J, Gore JC. Intravascular susceptibility contrast mechanisms in tissues. *Magn Reson Med.* 1994;31:9–21.

46. Bandettini PA, Wong EC. Effects of biophysical and physiologic parameters on brain activation-induced R2* and R2 changes: Simulations using a determistic diffusion model. *Int J Imaging Syst Technol.* 1995;6:133–152.

47. Lai S, Hopkins AL, Haacke EM, et al. Identification of vascular structures as a major source of signal contrast in high resolution 2D and 3D functional activation imaging of the motor cortex at 1.5T: preliminary results. *Magn Reson Med.* 1993;30:387–392.

48. Menon RS, Ogawa S, Tank DW, Ugurbil K. 4 Tesla gradient recalled echo characteristics of photic stimulation-induced signal changes in the human primary visual cortex. Magn Reson Med. 1993;30:380–386.

49. Kim S-G, Hendrich K, Hu X, Merkle H, Ugurbil K. Potential pitfalls of functional MRI using conventional gradient-recalled echo techniques. *NMR in Biomed.* 1994;7:69–74.

50. Frahm J, Merboldt K-D, Hanicke W, Kleinschmidt A, Boecker H. Brain or vein-oxygenation or flow? On signal physiology in functional MRI of human brain activation. *NMR in Biomed.* 1994;7:45–53.

51. Kim S-G, Ugurbil K. Functional magnetic resonance imaging of the human brain. *J Neurosci Methods.* 1997;74:229–243.

52. Stejskal EO, Tanner JE. Spin diffusion measurements: Spin echoes in the presence of a time-dependent field gradient. *J Chem Physics.* 1965;42:288–292.

53. Song AW, Wong EC, Tan SG, Hyde JS. Diffusion-weighted fMRI at 1.5T. *Magn Reson Med.* 1996;35:155–158.

54. Zhong J, Kennan RP, Fulbright RK, Gore JC. Quantification of intravascular and extravascular contributions to BOLD. *Magn Reson Med.* 1998;40:526–536.

55. Duong TQ, Yacoub E, Adriany G, Hu X, Ugurbil K, Kim S-G. Microvascular BOLD contribution at 4 and 7 Tesla in the human brain: Diffusion-weighted, gradient-echo and spin-echo fMRI. *Mag Reson Med.* In press.

56. Bandettini PA, Wong EC, Jesmanowicz A, Hinks RS, Hyde JS. Spin-echo and gradient-echo EPI of human brain activation using BOLD contrast: a comparative study at 1.5T. *NMR in Biomed.* 1994;7:12–20.

57. Lowe M, Lurito J, Mattews V, Phillips M, Hutchins G. Quantitative comparison of functional contrast from BOLD weighted spin echo and gradient-echo echo-planar imaging at 1.5 Tesla and H215O PET in the whole brain. *J Cereb Blood Flow Metab.* 2000;20:1331–1340.

58. Duvernoy H, Delon S, Vannson J. Cortical blood vessels of the human brain. *Brain Res.* 1981;7:519–579.
59. Hu X, Kim S-G. Reduction of signal fluctuations in functional MRI using navigator echos. *Magn Reson Med.* 1994;31:495–503.
60. Hu X, Le TH, Parrish T, Erhard P. Retrospective estimation and compensation of physiological fluctuation in functional MRI. *Magn Reson Med.* 1995;34:210–221.
61. Malonek D, Grinvald A. Interactions between electrical activity and cortical microcirculation revealed by imaging spectroscopy: Implication for functional brain mapping. *Science.* 1996;272:551–554.
62. Duong TQ, Silva AC, Lee S-P, Kim S-G. Functional MRI of calcium-dependent synaptic activity: Cross correlation with CBF and BOLD measurements. *Magn Reson Med.* 2000;43:383–392.
63. Woolsey TA, Rovainen CM, Cox SB, et al. Neuronal units linked to microvascular modules in cerebral cortex: Response elements for imaging the brain. *Cereb Cortex.* 1996;6:647–660.
64. Kim S-G, Richter W, Ugurbil K. Limitations of temporal resolution in fMRI. Magn Reson Med. 1997;37:631–636.
65. Richter W, Andersen PM, Georgopoulos AP, Kim S-G. Sequential activity in human motor areas during a delayed cued movement task studied by time-resolved fMRI. *Neuroreport.* 1997;8:1257–1261.
66. Richter W, Ugurbil K, Georgopoulos AP, Kim S-G. Time-resolved fMRI of mental rotation. *Neuroreport.* 1997;8:3697–3702.
67. Richter W, Somorijai R, Summers R, et al. Motor area activity during mental rotation studied by time-resolved single-trial fMRI. *J Cogn Neurosci.* 2000;12:310–320.
68. Menon R, Kim S-G. Spatial and temporal limits in cognitive neuroimaging with fMRI. *Trends Cogn Sci.* 1999;3:207–215.
69. Duong TQ, Kim S-G. In vivo MR measurements of regional arterial and venous blood volume fractions in intact rat brain. *Magn Reson Med.* 2000;43:393–402.
70. Kim S-G, Tsekos NV, Ashe J. Multi-slice perfusion-based functional MRI using the FAIR technique: Comparison of CBF and BOLD effects. *NMR in Biomed.* 1997;10:191–196.
71. Bandettini PA. The temporal resolution of Functional MRI. In: Moonen CTW, Bandettini PA, eds. Functional MRI. New York: Springer; 1999:205–220.
72. Duong TQ, Yacoub E, Adriany G, et al. High-resolution, spin-echo BOLD and CBF fMRI at 4 and 7T. *Mag Reson Med.* 2002;48:589–93.

2

fMRI Scanning Methodologies

Alexander B. Pinus and Feroze B. Mohamed

General Overview

A pervasive and constant challenge in the field of neuroscience is to advance in the understanding of working mechanisms of the human brain and what enacts such complex functions as perception, emotions, and behavior. In areas of clinical psychology, neurophysiology, and neurosciences, it is an ultimate interest to describe neuronal functions quantitatively, as well as qualitatively, under what is considered normal conditions and various disorders, and later use that knowledge for diagnostic purposes.

To investigate these complex concepts, there are a number of techniques developed to detect and characterize neuronal activity of the human brain. In recent years, technical advances in the area of magnetic resonance (MR) research and development tremendously enhanced capabilities of magnetic resonance imaging (MRI) equipment in regard to detection and characterization of minute physiological features, and unprecedentedly widened the number of applications of this modality. Such MRI and nuclear magnetic resonance (NMR) systems with superconducting magnets operating at field strengths of 8 Tesla for human[1] and up to 21 Tesla for animal studies[2, 3] have lately become available, allowing extremely fine spatial resolution and considerably improved signal-to-noise ratios (SNRs). The low-noise detection electronics coupled with ultra-fast signal collection algorithms paved the way for new sensitive imaging techniques towards imaging of highly detailed static morphological features, as well as dynamic markers of physiological events and brain functions. The latter may manifest themselves through an intertwined regional changes of such physiological parameters as blood oxygenation and cerebral metabolism, blood flow and volume, and diffusion and perfusion, all of which take place coincidentally.

In the area of the in vivo MRI, various achievements have led to the development of methods of functional MRI (fMRI). Functional MRI is a class of techniques that exploits susceptibility of the magnetic resonance

---

This chapter previously appeared in *Functional MRI: Basic Principles and Clinical Applications*, edited by S. Faro and F. Mohamed. New York: Springer Science+Business Media, LCC 2006.

From: *BOLD fMRI: A Guide to Functional Imaging for Neuroscientists*
Edited by: S.H. Faro and F.B. Mohamed, DOI 10.1007/978-1-4419-1329-6_2
© Springer Science+Business Media, LLC 2010

signal to certain physiological properties associated with neuronal activity in general and intrinsic qualities of blood in particular. The most explored and developed fMRI method—Blood Oxygenation Level Dependency (BOLD)—detects tiny changes in magnetic properties of blood caused by metabolic and vascular responses to an elicited neuronal activity.

The brain activity and, in particular, pre-synaptic firings are associated with increased energy demands and are satisfied mainly by way of an oxidative glucose consumption.[4-7] After an onset of a particular brain activity, a nearby feeding arteriole dilates, thus causing the blood flow in downstream capillaries to increase.[8,9] Although during no-stimulus (baseline) conditions, all capillaries are already perfused, brain activity increases the blood flow through the capillaries in an immediate vicinity of active neurons. Because an influx of the blood flow is larger than an increase in oxygen consumption, overall oxygen concentration in blood increases, especially on the venular side of a capillary and further down in venous vessels.[10,11]

Due to such an increase, the blood becomes more oxygenated, which implies that the oxygen dissolved in blood gets bound to partially or fully deoxygenated heme molecules, thus turning deoxyhemoglobin to oxyhemoglobin. In a configuration with bound oxygen, ferrous iron on the heme changes its conformation and becomes more diamagnetic (less paramagnetic) as more oxygen molecules are attached to the heme. Hence, the oxyhemoglobin is more diamagnetic than the deoxyhemoglobin, and, therefore, when placed in the magnetic field of an MR scanner, imparts a different, lesser magnetic susceptibility in regard to the surroundings. The numerical and statistical evaluations of image intensity differences caused by blood magnetic susceptibility during periods of stimulated or spuriously evoked neuronal activity and periods of absence thereof may show neuroanatomical markers of such an activity.

The described phenomenon is the basis of the blood oxygenation level-dependent (BOLD) contrast employed in the fMRI. A quality and an observational value of an MRI study designed to monitor a particular brain function or a number of brain functions involved in a specific physiological or behavioral event depend on assortment of parameters and factors prescribed in a form of MRI pulse sequences.

The imaging pulse sequence is a set of instructions given by a developer to the MR scanner's data acquisition system on how to collect the MR signal and sensitize it to a particular property of the target, which could be of a morphological, functional, or chemical origin. To this end, selectivity of an acquisition protocol usually is accomplished by temporal adjustments of appropriate manipulations with magnitude and phase of the sample's bulk magnetization during the data collection process.

Of particular importance in an MR experiment is to achieve a high SNR and the tissue, or function, or chemical contrast. Higher SNR is achieved by the way of adjusting pulse sequence parameters so that maximum amount of available MR signal returned by a target is captured. Higher contrast is achieved by the way of sensitizing the MR signal to a specific target and, in some cases, suppressing that of the target's surroundings. For instance, in order to perform a routine clinical morphological analysis, MR signal intensities of adjacent tissues have to differ by an amount appreciative to an unaided eye. Similarly, to gain functional information, for instance in a typical BOLD experiment, the nature, structure, and timing of the pulse sequence's manipulations are optimized collect most data when the MR signal related to a studied set of functions is the strongest.

It has been shown that dynamics of the MR signal, especially its decay (relaxation) rates, is dependent on the blood oxygen content.[12,13] In particular, increased magnetic susceptibility caused by the deoxygenation affects T_2^* and T_2 relaxation processes. Such a dependence may be taken advantage of in fMRI experiments, with pulse sequences purposefully tuned to produce T_2^* or T_2 contrast. Such sequences are designed to be sensitive to tiny variations of magnetic fields (microscopic field gradients) induced by changing blood oxygen content. Depending on application objectives, the target's relaxation and MR-related properties, gradient-echo signal formation mechanisms can be used to achieve T_2^* contrast, whereas the spin-echo signal formation algorithms are employed to produce the T_2-weighted contrast.

Spin-Echo and Gradient-Echo Imaging Methods

Conventional single-echo, spin-echo, and gradient-echo signal formation algorithms have been routinely used clinical applications for years, mainly because of their versatility to produce a number of contrasts for various targets. Spin-echo imaging pulse sequences are used in an assortment of anatomical studies to produce T_1, T_2, and proton density (PD) weighted images; gradient-echo imaging pulse sequences are more likely to be employed in formation of T_2 and T_2^* image contrasts, although they are used to render the T_1 image contrast, especially in higher-field strength systems. In addition, being sensitive to motion, gradient-echo imaging is used in MR angiography (MRA), volumetric evaluation studies, and those with contrast agents.

Both imaging mechanisms are sensitive to BOLD-associated microscopic field gradients imparted by the neuronal activity. The spin-echo MR signal is susceptible to local gradients due to inflow effects and irreversible diffusion dephasing that introduce T_2 weighting. These factors also affect the gradient-echo MR BOLD-coupled signal. Furthermore, the MR signal detected in experiments with gradient-echo pulse sequences reflects conventional reversible T_2^* losses due to the intravoxel field distribution.

Spin-Echo Formation Mechanism

To generate a spin echo, at least two radio frequency (RF) pulses are required—the first is used to deflect the initial longitudinal magnetization into the transverse plane, and the second is needed to recreate the lost spin phase coherence. Consider the evolution of the transverse magnetization and the spin phase in the rotating reference[a] frame, as illustrated in the top portion of the Figure 2.1, and the process of creating the spin echo shown in the laboratory frame[b] in the middle part of the same figure.

---

[a]A precessing frame or reference. Spin isochromats precessing at the Larmor frequency appear stationary.
[b]A stationary frame of reference. All spin isochromats are seen precessing.

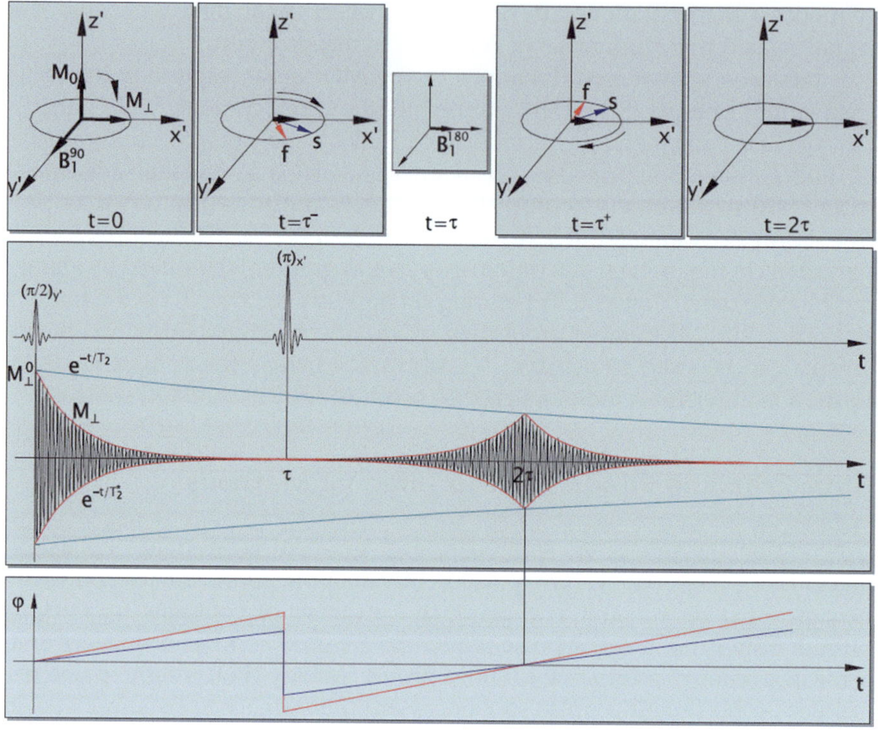

Figure 2.1. SE Echo: Evolution, MR Signal, Spin Phase Dynamics.

At the moment of time $t = 0$, a $\frac{\pi}{2}$–radian RF pulse is applied to the sample along the y' axis, forcing the bulk magnetization into the transverse plane. As the free precession ensues, two isochromats with precessional frequencies $\omega_f > \omega_s > \omega_0$ start to progressively lose coherence and deflect from their original direction along the x' axis. This process lasts until the free precession is somehow disrupted, for instance by another RF pulse applied at the time instance τ. Immediately before time τ elapses, the isochromats are separated by the phase angle $(\omega_f - \omega_s)\tau^-$; the magnetization has diminished due to the T_2^* relaxation process.

At the moment of time τ, an x'-axis–oriented π-radian pulse is applied that flips both spin isochromats over to the other half of the transverse plane. Consequently, immediately following such an operation, the vector that was ahead is now lagging behind the slower one by the same phase angle that it was leading just prior the π-radian RF pulse. Because the spin isochromats continue to precess in the same direction, clockwise in the graphics, and at the same rates (assuming the spin isochromats see the same field inhomogeneity throughout the echo formation), the faster isochromat starts to gain on the slower one, decreasing the deflection phase angle $-(\omega_f - \omega_s)t$. Because the spins get closer to each other, their coherence improves, so that the overall magnetization starts to build up. After exact same period of time τ it took to deflect them by the aforementioned phase angle, the two isochromats become aligned again at the moment of time known as the echo time, which, in this particular scenario type of the RF echo, happens at $T_E = 2\tau$.

As shown in the Figure 2.1, the refocusing RF pulse is applied after the phases of individual spins have been "scrambled" and most of the transverse magnetization has vanished. However, the refocusing pulse can be applied even before the transverse magnetization fully fades away. In either case, after the refocusing RF pulse, the magnetization grows gradually and reaches its maximum amplitude. However, the MR signal magnitude at the echo is smaller than the original amplitude immediately following the first RF pulse. This is because of the phase coherence loss encountered from random field fluctuations that cannot be recovered by the refocusing RF pulse.

Spin-Echo Imaging Pulse Sequence

The pulse sequence that implements the spin-echo measurement is shown in the Figure 2.2. In spin-echo sequences, a $\frac{\pi}{2}$–radian RF pulse typically is applied to excite samples' spin isochromats.

There are generally two excitation regimes, selective and non-selective, with the selectivity referring to a spatial preference of the excitation. The non-selective regime is invoked when no special arrangements are made to associate precessional frequencies of spin isochromats with their positions. Indeed, if all spin isochromats precess at the same frequency, namely the frequency given by the well-known Larmor Equation

$$\omega_0 = \gamma B_0 \tag{2.1}$$

imparted by the static magnetic field B_0, it is impossible to tell isochromats apart, and therefore find their position. It also remains infeasible to establish positions of the spin isochromats if precessional rates are affected by local inhomogeneities in a random fashion, or when the inhomogeneity profile is unknown. The RF pulse that affects spins non-selectively is called hard pulse.

In order to spatially differentiate and act on a selected population of spin isochromats, precessional frequencies have to be made a function of position. It typically is achieved by an augmentation of the static magnetic field B_0 with a set of supplemental magnetic fields, gradient fields, with known,

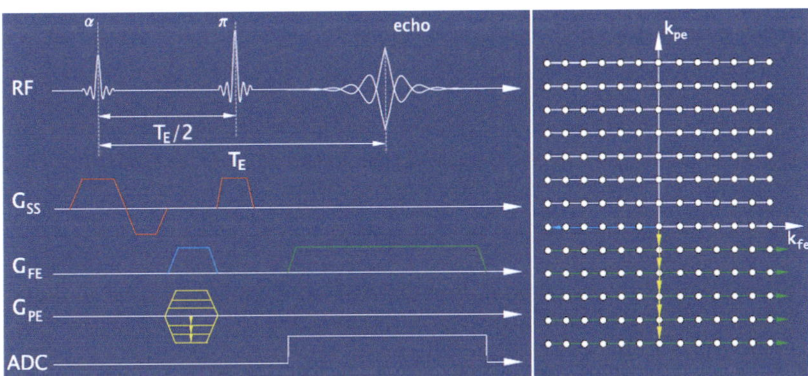

Figure 2.2. Spin Echo Timing Diagram.

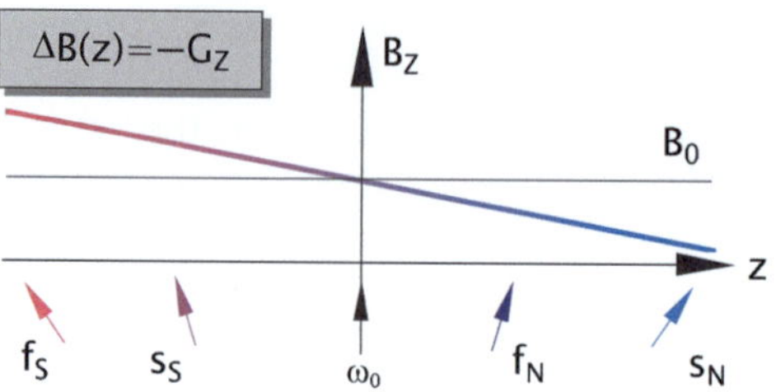

Figure 2.3. The Gradient Field.

and usually linear, spatial profiles. Such magnetic fields are a special kind of inhomogeneity that make spin precessional frequency position-dependent in a known fashion.

Indeed, the precessional frequency of the spin isochromat can be evaluated using a slightly modified version of the Equation (2.1), taking into consideration the gradient amplitude. For instance, if the gradient G_z is the field with an amplitude changing along z direction, the precessional frequency of spin isochromats follows the gradient profile, as shown in the Figure 2.3:

$$\omega(z) = \gamma(B_0 + B_{G_z}) = \gamma(B_0 + B_z z) = \gamma\left(B_0 + \frac{\partial B_G}{\partial z} z\right), \tag{2.2}$$

where the amplitude of the applied gradient G_z is given as the spatial partial derivative of the gradient field B_G. Similar expressions are valid for the gradients with amplitudes varying along two other axes:

$$\omega(x) = \gamma(B_0 + B_{G_x}) = \gamma(B_0 + G_x x) = \gamma\left(B_0 + \frac{\partial B_G}{\partial x} x\right), \tag{2.3}$$

$$\omega(y) = \gamma(B_0 + B_{G_y}) = \gamma(B_0 + G_y y) = \gamma\left(B_0 + \frac{\partial B_G}{\partial y} y\right). \tag{2.4}$$

The physical magnetic fields B_{Gx}, B_{Gy} and B_{Gz} are created by gradient coils, which are current-carrying conductors housed in the MRI system. Because the amplitudes of these fields vary in orthogonal directions, the gradient fields are said to be orthogonal.

When the linear gradient magnetic field

$$B_G = G_x x + G_y y + G_z z \tag{2.5}$$

is added to the static magnetic field B_0, precessional frequencies of spin isochromats become varied in all three directions. For a simple case of

$$B_G = G_z z = G_{ss} z,$$

the association between the precessional frequency and position of a spin isochromat, as well as the translation of the RF pulse's bandwidth into the slice thickness, is shown in the Figure 2.4. The position of the slice's center z' and its thickness Δz can be chosen by varying the central frequency f' and either the gradient's strength G_z (the slope of the line in the graphics) or the

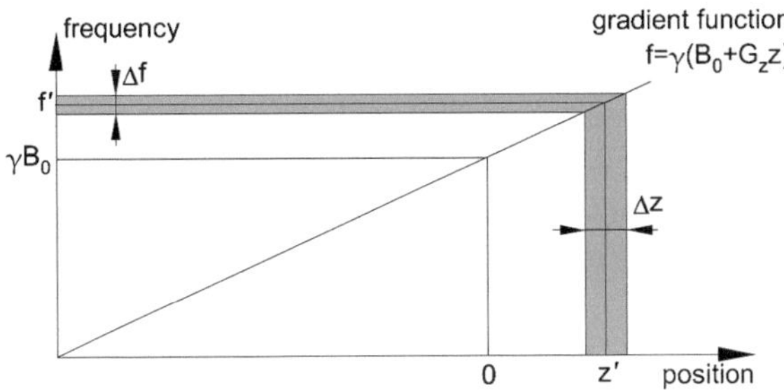

Figure 2.4. Position-Frequency Translation.

bandwidth Δf of the RF pulse, respectively. Ultimately, the effect of the gradients on spin isochromats is the separation of their precessional frequencies.

If the RF pulse with a finite bandwidth, and thus a spectrum of frequencies, is applied to a population of spin isochromats frequency-separated by acting gradients fields, only those that are exposed to the pulse and precess at frequencies found within the RF pulse's bandwidth get excited. Such an excitation regime is called selective excitation, and the excitation RF pulse is called a soft pulse.

The arrangement of physical gradients, itself a vector, applied concurrently with RF pulses establishes a direction of the logical gradient called the slice selection gradient, G_{ss}. The precessional frequency of spin isochromats follows the shape of the gradient's profile, linearly varying along the gradient's direction.

Because the slice selection gradient makes precessional frequency position-dependent only in the direction of itself, the precessional frequency in two other orthogonal directions is not affected.[c] Therefore, the localization of spin isochromats within the slice remains unfeasible. To that end, the same principle of the position dependency can be applied to localize in-plane spin isochromats.[d]

As the slice selection gradient G_{ss} modulates the precessional frequency of spin isochromats, two similar gradients, frequency encoding (G_{fe}) and phase encoding (G_{pe}) gradients, are applied to condition spin precessional frequencies in two directions orthogonal to that established by the slice selection gradient. The combination of these gradients defines the spin precessional frequency in the three-dimensional (3D) space. Because each of the gradients defines its own thickness, the trio thus establishes imaging unit volumes—voxels.

The MR signal sample produced by spin isochromats in a particular voxel can be encoded in terms of frequencies varied by the gradient fields. Every such acquired sample of the MR signal comes from spin isochromats precessing at frequencies established by the arrangement of the applied gradients. The entire series of received MR signal samples for all prescribed gradient arrangement, and thus for all necessary precessional frequencies, can be placed conveniently in a matrix. The size of such a matrix and the

---

[c]An approximation for low gradients, because Maxwell equations demand concomitant fields in orthogonal directions.
[d]That is spin isochromats that lie within the defined slice.

order in which it gets filled with MR signal samples usually is determined by spatial frequency indices.

Indeed, the precessional frequency of spin isochromats in every voxel within the prescribed slice is defined by an arrangement of in-plane G_{fe} and G_{pe} gradients. Taking into consideration that the gradient field may be a function of time, the indices corresponding to the gradients usually are expressed as integrals of gradient amplitudes over their duration times:

$$k_{ss} = \gamma \int G_{ss} dt, \tag{2.6}$$

$$k_{fe} = \gamma \int G_{fe} dt, \tag{2.7}$$

$$k_{pe} = \gamma \int G_{pe} dt, \tag{2.8}$$

The received MR signal samples are therefore arranged in a form of a matrix, $M(k_{ss}, k_{fe}, k_{pe})$. The location of each spin isochromat is frequency-encoded in such a matrix in terms of spatial frequency k indices, and thus the received MR signal is represented in the spatial frequency space called the k-space. The depiction of the MR signal samples that make up the matrix $M(k_{ss}, k_{fe}, k_{pe})$, also known as k-space diagram, is shown on the right of the Figure 2.2, where the MR signal samples are represented by solid circles.

A conversion from the frequency-encoded representation of the MR signal, known as the raw MR signal, to its spatially encoded format is performed by a 3D Fourier transformation:

$$m(r) = \frac{1}{2\pi} \int_{k_{ss}} \int_{k_{fe}} \int_{k_{pe}} M(k_{ss}, k_{fe}, k_{pe}) e^{j(k \cdot r)} dr, \tag{2.9}$$

where r is the basis of the 3D spatial coordinate system. Such a process is known as image reconstruction. This equation implies that the principle prerequisite to the image reconstruction process is the availability of the raw signal matrix, $M(k_{ss}, k_{fe}, k_{pe})$.

After a particular MR signal sample is acquired and recorded into the current element of the raw signal matrix, one or more k-indices is incremented and the next MR signal sample is acquired and stored in the successive element of matrix. As the k-indices are advanced by changing the amplitudes and timing of the gradients, the current element of the matrix propagates through the k-space. This process continues until the entire k-space matrix is filled[e] with the MR signal samples. The process of MR signal acquisition and construction of the raw signal matrix often is called the k-space coverage.

The k-space can be covered in a variety of ways. The most typical coverage path utilized in the majority of conventional pulse sequences is the sequential line-by-line traversal. Its name originates from the appearance of the k-space coverage pattern in which the order of placement of the MR signal samples in the k-space diagram gives an appearance of the line, as shown by the green arrow on the right of the Figure 2.2.

---

[e]Some pulse sequences fill only a half of the k-space, which is then used to compute the other half using a property of the Hermitian complex conjugateness.

In order to implement this type of the coverage, one of the in-plane gradients is turned on for a period of time and with the amplitude needed to get the value of the corresponding k_{pe} index advanced to the location of the necessary k-space line. Such a move is shown by yellow gradient lobes on the pulse sequence graphics and corresponding arrows in the k-space diagram. At the same time, another in-plane gradient, the frequency encoding, is applied to move the index k_{fe} along just-selected k-space line to the location of the matrix element that corresponds to a first-to-be-acquired MR signal sample. This advancement is shown by the light blue color. In order to conserve imaging time, these two gradients, respectively called y- and x-offset gradient pulses, are applied simultaneously and immediately after the slice-selective excitation. The amplitude and duration of these gradients are chosen so that they conclude forwarding corresponding indices to an assigned position in the raw signal matrix before the refocusing π-radian RF pulse is issued, which comes at the moment $t = \tau = \dfrac{T_E}{2}$ after the initial $\dfrac{\pi}{2}$ –radian excitation RF pulse.

As described in the previous section, the π-radian RF pulse is applied to rephase spins, which were so far dephasing in the transverse plane after the initial excitation pulse. Worth noting again, the effect of such a pulse is the changed character of the precession: faster moving spins now chase slower ones, closing the gap between them. Such a motion causes spins to refocus, hence the refocusing pulse, and regain their in-plane coherence with each other, forming the MR signal echo. The MR signal echo fully develops at $t = 2\tau = T_E$, as indicated in the Figure 2.1. The MR signal acquisition period usually starts immediately after the refocusing pulse, so that the echo would occur in the middle of it. Such an arrangement assures the most efficient imaging conditions with given imaging parameters.

During the signal acquisition period, the detection circuitry and the analog-to-digital converter[f] are turned on to receive and digitize the RF signal from the precessing spin isochromats. Simultaneously, the frequency encoding gradient is turned on in order to encode the precessional frequencies with position. As long as this gradient is applied, the resonance frequency of the spin isochromats is adjusted depending on the gradient's amplitude and moment of time during which a particular sample is acquired. The signal is sampled with the prescribed sampling rate and recorded into the element of the raw MR signal matrix according to the k-space indices.

Because the signal sampling takes finite time, the effect of the longitudinal and transverse relaxations on the MR signal has to be taken in to account. That is to say, if the transverse component of the MR signal deteriorates before all samples necessary to reconstruct an image adequately are acquired, the coverage of the k-space is performed in several iterations, segments.[g]

In a typical and the most simple k-space coverage, such every segment corresponds to a single line. The MR signal acquisition is completed along such a line in a single repetition period, T_R. In this case, only one of the k-space indices, for instance k_{fe}, is incremented, whereas the other in-plane index, k_{pe}, is kept constant. When all necessary MR signal samples along the line are acquired, the process moves onto the next iteration, beginning with the next

---

[f]Hence the ADC label in the Figure 2.2, and Figure 2.5.
[g]In ultra-fast imaging sequences, like echo planar imaging (EPI), the entire k-space coverage may be accomplished in a single T_R period.

excitation RF pulse. This time, the amplitude of the phase-encoding gradient is incremented between the excitation and refocusing RF pulses so that the corresponding index k_{pe} is advanced to the next k-space line. Further on, the detection circuitry is turned on in the presence of the frequency-encoding gradient, and the MR signal is sampled along that k-space line.

In the description of the spin-echo formation mechanism and the corresponding pulse sequence, it was presumed that the center of the acquisition window coincides with the center of the k-space line. The center of the k-space line corresponds to an MR signal sample that has only been encoded partially with spatial information, as one of indices, namely k_{fe}, is zero.[h] The center of the acquisition window is taken as a point of time when the phase dispersion created by the offset gradient is compensated fully by the rephasing lobe of the read-out gradient. Only in this case does it become possible to fully eliminate the phase dispersion accrued due to fixed local field inhomogeneities.

Indeed, if the first half of the read-out gradient lasts exactly as long as the x-offset gradient and has the same amplitude, the phase of spin isochromats imparted by the gradients is zero in the center of the acquisition window. On the other hand, the phase dispersion developed due to fixed local field inhomogeneities between the excitation and refocusing pulses is nullified by the rephasing following the pulse to form what was described as the spin-echo. Therefore, when the echo time coincides with the center of the k-space line, with all other sources of the phase aberrations compensated, the overall phase disturbance is imposed only by irreversible random fluctuations due to the T_2 relaxation, which are solely responsible for overall image ontrast.

However, it is not required for the echo time to match the moment when the k-space line's center MR signal sample is acquired along the acquisition window. The spin-echo can be arranged to occur slightly before or after that particular sample by respectively moving the refocusing pulse toward or away the excitation pulse. The spin-echo is then also moved with it, as it invariably trails the refocusing pulse by exactly the same time as the latter follows the excitation pulse. Therefore, for the spin-echo to occur by a time c earlier relative to the center of the k-space line, the refocusing pulse has to be transmitted by a time $\frac{\tau}{2}$ earlier than that in the typical symmetrical arrangement. Such an offset spin-echo is referred to as the asymmetric spin-echo (ASE).

No longer in an ASE pulse sequence is the phase dispersion developed out of local inhomogeneities balanced at the moment of passing the k-space line's center, thus leaving the MR signal slightly dephased at that time. Because it is the very MR signal sample located in the center of the k-space line that contributes the most to the overall image contrast, the magnetic susceptibility effects will be reflected in the final image. Therefore, besides a general T_2 contrast, an additional T_2^* weighting is introduced into the MR signal, thus making the ASE pulse sequence more sensitive to the BOLD effect.

It is possible, regardless of the echo position along the acquisition window, to cover several lines in a single iteration. The corresponding pulse sequence diagram is shown in the Figure 2.5.[i] Although there are multiple variations

---

[h]The center of the k-space lacks any spatial information, as both indices, k_{fe} and k_{pe}, are zero.

[i]The T_R has to be adequately short and sampling rate high to allow sufficient amount of the decaying MR signal be detected during the entire acquisition period.

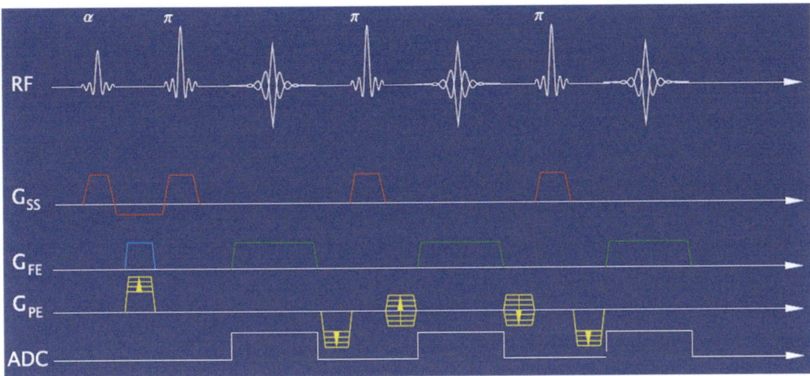

Figure 2.5. Fast Spin-Echo Timing Diagram.

of the multi-echo acquisition scheme, such an arrangement generally is referred to as the fast spin-echo pulse sequence.

In case of such a sequence, a train of echoes is generated after a single excitation pulse by having a manifold of refocusing pulses applied to redirect spin dynamics multiple times. During every formed echo, because the MR signal is sampled along a different line, a distinct phase encoding gradient is needed. The first echo is generated in the same way a single spin-echo is formed. However, at the end of the acquisition period, a rewinder gradient is applied in the phase-encoding direction that cancels the effect of the preceding phase-encoding gradient. Such a manipulation is tantamount to a resetting of the k_{pe} index back to zero. Following the first echo, spin isochromats are allowed to continue to dephase. At some point into the dephasing process, another π-radian pulse is transmitted. The effect of this pulse on spins is exactly the same as that of the original refocusing pulse, namely, it swaps around faster and slower precessing spins. Immediately after the refocusing pulse, another phase-encoding gradient is applied. However, this time its amplitude is set to advance the k_{pe} to a different k-space line. The number of formed echoes, and thus the number of covered k-space lines, is given as the imaging parameter called echo train length (ETL). A number of echoes can be generated following a single RF excitation pulse, and the total acquisition time is reduced as many times as large as the ETL is.

When the entire raw signal matrix is completed for the selected slice, the process is started anew, either to acquire and average more signal for the same slice or to proceed onto another slice.

Contrast Characteristics of Spin-Echo Sequences

Vascular Effects

It was briefly mentioned that although the π-radian pulse refocuses acquired phase offsets by dephasing spin isochromats due to existing inhomogeneities, the phase coherence at the echo time is never restored to the pre-excitation level. Indeed, only in case of a particular spin isochromat seeing a fixed inhomogeneity throughout the acquisition can a phase angle acquired by this spin isochromat before the refocusing pulse be fully balanced out by the phase displacement that the spin isochromat experiences after the refocusing pulse. In other words, in order to fully restore spin coherence, the precessional frequency of a particular spin isochromat has to remain the same throughout the repetition period.

In reality, however, the precessional frequency of spin isochromats constantly experiences tiny aberrations that are largely imparted by the process of diffusion. A diffusing water molecule drifts in a random fashion through inhomogeneity gradients established by various physical factors, including the magnetic susceptibility caused by the BOLD effect. The degree to which the diffusion influences the spin-echo MR signal depends on the spatial range of inhomogeneities in regard to the motion extent a water molecule travels during the acquisition. If inhomogeneities vary significantly only over far larger distances that a wandering water molecule can possibly travel, then it is likely that the spin isochromats experience the same field before and following the refocusing pulse. In this case, the spin-echo is fully refocused and the MR signal does not carry the imprint of inhomogeneities. Conversely, a moving water molecule does change fields if the range of distances it travels is larger than the spatial scale of inhomogeneities. Because water molecules diffuse rather quickly, it is likely that the phase dispersion developed by molecules between two pulses is not refocused by the time of the echo, thus leaving some dephasing to last through the echo and to attenuate the MR signal.

This line of thinking can be used in determining how the vessel size impacts the spin-echo MR signal: Because the spatial extent of inhomogeneities originated from the larger structures such as venulae and arteriola spans further than that of capillaries, the diffusion-related reduction of the MR signal in capillary-rich areas is stronger than in vicinities of larger vessels. Such an argument can be substantiated by assessing the average diffusion-induced displacement a water molecule sustains and comparing it with the average vessel's size.

The average displacement $\langle L \rangle$ over time t of a randomly moving particle can be estimated from the Einstein's diffusion equation:

$$\langle L^2 \rangle = 6\mu kTt = 6Dt, \tag{2.10}$$

where $k \approx 1.38 \cdot 10^{-23}\, \dfrac{m^2 kg}{s^2 K}$ –Boltzmann's constant; T is the temperature in Kelvins; the quantity $D = \mu kT$ is called the diffusion coefficient, and m is the mobility coefficient that can be expressed through the average time between collisions τ_c and molecular mass m:

$$\mu = \frac{\tau_c}{m}. \tag{2.11}$$

Every particle experiences about 10^{14} collisions per second on average, which means that it spends 10^{-14} seconds between collisions.[14(p41–48)] The mass of a water molecule is $3 \cdot 10^{-26}$ kilograms. With these values, the diffusion coefficient is on the order of $D \approx 10^{-9}\left[\dfrac{m^2}{s}\right]$. It is now possible to estimate the average displacement. Because only the in-plane displacement alters relaxation rates, the corrected expression for the average displacement is now

$$\langle L^2 \rangle = 4Dt. \tag{2.12}$$

Taking $t = 100$ milliseconds, a typical echo time in case of the spin-echo pulse sequence, the average displacement is estimated at 20 micrometers.

It is therefore expected that the effect of diffusion in areas of venulae larger than 20 micrometers in diameter gradually diminishes reversely proportional to the venule's size. This is due to the fact that the spin-echo is refocused relatively better because the water molecule spends more time in the same field. Consequently, the MR signal is changed ever so slightly. In the areas of smaller venulae and larger capillaries, their diameter being on the order of 10 to 20 micrometers, the water molecule experiences different fields as it wanders in a near vicinity of vessels; hence, the spin-echo is poorly refocused and the MR signal is relatively weaker. For even smaller vessels, mostly capillaries with the lumen's diameter below 10 micrometers, the phase dispersion at the moment of spin-echo is even stronger as water molecules transgress even a larger number of fields. Therefore, it is tempting to expect relaxation rates to increase and the MR signal to lessen further. However, in this case, the average phase dispersion encountered by all water molecules is very similar, as it is more likely that they cross over the same fields. A similar phase dispersion is tantamount to a very little phase dispersion. Therefore, counterintuitively, the spin-echo MR signal coming from areas of very small vessels, namely less than five micrometers in diameter, is in fact comparable to that acquired near the largest vessels.

Thus, the spin-echo MR signal is strongest in areas of very small and very large vessels and dips to its minimum around vessels that measure about 20 micrometers in diameter. Due to such a bell-shaped dependence of the spin-echo MR signal on the vessel's size, the spin-echo sequences are desirable to use in BOLD experiments, as the spin-echo MR signal is sensitized to the BOLD-related oxy/deoxygenated exchanges that occur in capillaries.

Flow Effects

The contrast produced by the spin-echo sequences is sensitive to inflow effects and becomes apparent on T_2-weighted images. Implications of the inflow effects on the MR signal are caused primarily by spin isochromats that were brought into the region of the excited imaging volume by the blood flow following the $\frac{\pi}{2}$ –radian excitation RF pulse.

It has been discussed earlier that only spin isochromats that initially get excited by the RF excitation pulse can return RF photons and thus contribute to the overall MR signal. Moreover, because the transverse component of the bulk magnetization is solely responsible for production of the MR signal, it is desirable to have initial large longitudinal components of as many spins as possible be transferred to the transverse plane by the excitation RF pulse in order to increase MR signal generation capacity. Finally, the refocusing RF pulse acts to minimize relative phase differences between transverse components of precessing spins and to restore the spin coherence in the transverse plane, thus yielding larger bulk magnetization and a stronger MR signal.

Consider fresh, undisturbed spins moving into already excited imaging volume. Because these spins enter between the excitation and refocusing RF pulses, they are exposed only to the π-radian RF pulse, which is, in effect, an excitation pulse for them, whereas it acts as a refocusing pulse for already excited spins. Unlike the latter, the freshly entered spins are forced into the excited state by the π-radian RF pulse. As the name of the pulse assumes, a bulk magnetization built out of these spins is rotated by 180 degrees, all the way from being oriented colinearly with the B_0 to the opposite direction, thus remaining in the longitudinal plane. Therefore, such a magnetization ends up having a very small transverse component so its contribution to the MR signal generation capacity is greatly reduced. The spins that make up the 180-degree deflected magnetization eventually will return to the unexcited state, contributing little to nothing to the overall MR signal.

In the meantime, a portion of those spins within the blood that were excited along with all other stationary spins were forced to leave the imaging volume by the fresh incoming blood. The spins forced out from the imaging volume before the refocusing pulse was applied to the same imaging volume contribute a negligible amount of the MR signal during the acquisition period because they remained dephased and did not undergo the refocusing. Those excited spins that did experience the refocusing pulse before exiting the imaging volume during the acquisition period do contribute to the MR signal. However, because their space-frequency association is now broken by the blood flow motion, they generate the MR signal that is originated from outside of the selected imaging volume, and therefore can now be regarded as flow artifacts.

The actual number of spins leaving and entering the imaging volume depends on timing characteristics of the sequence, size and position of the excited volume, and the parameters of the flow. If the time between the excitation and refocusing pulses is relatively shorter, a smaller number of excited spins is replaced by fresh ones; therefore, the MR signal would be suppressed to a lesser degree.

From another perspective, the time between the two pulses is equal to $\frac{T_E}{2}$. Therefore, it is optimal to keep the echo time short enough to reduce the inflow suppression, but long enough to collect sufficient amount of the MR signal with BOLD contrast. It was shown that such an optimal echo time is on the order of the T_2 relaxation time of the examined tissue.[15]

Because the echo time is usually much shorter than the repetition time for the spin-echo sequences, the inflow suppression would become significant only for relatively high flow velocities, which typically do not occur in the capillaries and small venulae, the primary source of the BOLD contrast.

Gradient-Echo Formation Mechanism

As has already been shown, the refocusing RF pulse is essential for the spin-echo formation, as it rephases spin isochromats and leads to reappearance of the transverse magnetization. However, the rephasing action and refocusing effect of the RF pulse also can be achieved if gradient fields are employed to modulate spin phase in a controlled fashion. The MR signal is then recovered in the form of a gradient-echo generated only through gradient reversals.

Consider the gradient-echo formation mechanism in an example with a system of four spin isochromats at different locations along the z axis, so that $z_{fs} = -z_{fN}$ and $z_{sS} = -z_{sN}$,[j] as shown in the Figure 2.3. The application of the gradient field makes spins in the North half precess slower than those

---

[j] The subscripts $_f$ and $_s$ stand for fast and slow. The subsubscripts $_S$ and $_N$ stand for South and North.

in the South half. Indeed, because of the additional gradient field, the two South spins experience higher than B_0 field, and they precess slightly faster in regard to the spin unaffected by the gradient field, thus precessing at the angular rate of ω_0. Of these two South spins, the one closer to the center of the field, s_S, precesses at slower rate because the field deviation at the location of this spin is less and its precessing frequency is closer to the ω_0. Similarly, for the North section where the magnetic field is less that B_0, the spins precess generally slower than in the South section, with the one further from the center of the field, s_N, precessing slower than the f_N spin.

Therefore, the main effect of the applied gradient field is an introduced spatially depended precessional frequency that makes spin isochromats precess at rates controlled by the amplitude of the applied gradient field. With such a dependence on the gradient field, the generation of the gradient echo can be explained phenomenologically and graphically, as is illustrated in the top of the Figure 2.6.

An excitation $\frac{\pi}{2}$ –radian RF pulse[k] is applied at the moment of time $t = 0$, putting the longitudinal magnetization into the transverse plane. Immediately at the end of the excitation pulse, all spin isochromats precess at the same rate. However, naturally occurring spatially varying field inhomogeneities and energy-dissipating interactions between spins[l] change precessional rates, causing spin isochromats to become out of phase with each other. The dephasing is a time-dependent process, increasing linearly with time. The

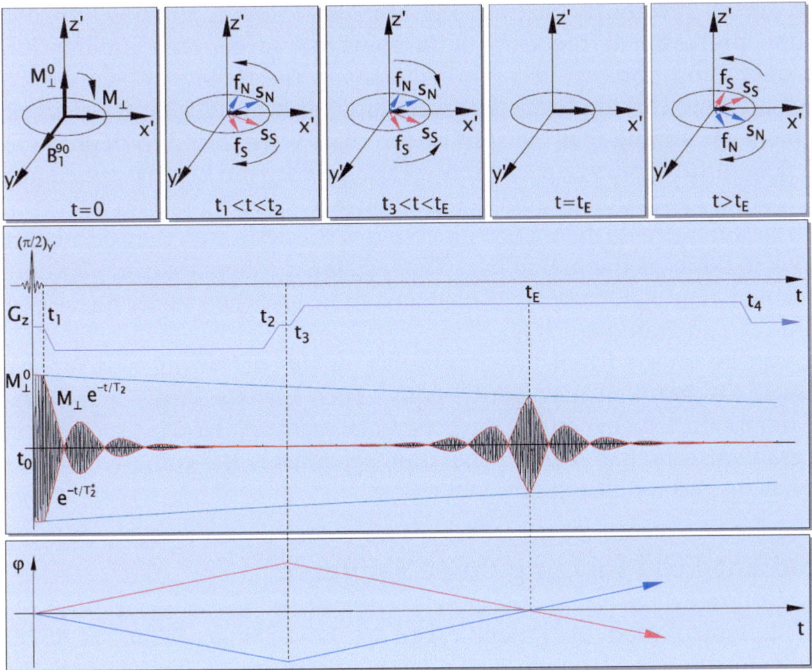

Figure 2.6. Gradient-Echo: Evolution, MR Signal, Spin Phase Dynamics.

---

[k] In the fast imaging applications, a smaller flip angle can be used, anywhere from $\frac{\pi}{6}$ to $\frac{\pi}{2}$.

[l] T_2^* and T_2 types relaxation, respectively.

dephasing among individual spin isochromats ultimately leads to decreased aggregate transverse magnetization; therefore, the recoverable MR signal in the process known as *Free Induction Decay* (FID). The FID connotes the MR signal loss due to naturally occurring phenomena taking place when the excited sample is left on its own after the excitation pulse and no additional external manipulations with spin isochromats are performed. The picture, however, changes when the gradient is turned on at the moment of time $t = t_1$.

Applying an extra gradient field along the z axis further intensifies the spin dephasing. Indeed, under the influence of the gradient field, the spin isochromats that experience stronger than usual field rapidly spring forward whereas those spins that sustain weaker than usual field are held back. Because of the general loss of phase coherence, the rapid decay of the magnetization continues until the gradient is turned off at the moment of $t = t_2$, when the aggregate transverse magnetization is essentially nonexistent. The beat pattern exhibited by the aggregate transverse magnetization is due to transient coherence improvements that occur when individual spin isochromats precessing at common multiple frequencies align in the transverse plane.

At the moment of time t_2, the gradient is turned off so that no additional gradient-induced coherence loss is incurred, and by the moment of time t_3, the South and North spin isochromats have reached their largest values of phase angles, respectively.

At the moment of time t_3, another gradient field of the same magnitude and direction, but opposite polarity, is applied to the sample. This gradient field forces previously fast-moving spin isochromats to slow down and assume precessional frequency of the spins that earlier were trailing during the dephasing portion. In a similar manner, the previously slow-moving spins are now chasing those that were moving faster during the dephasing segment. Assuming that the spin isochromats were forced to dephase from the state of full transverse coherence and ignoring the irrecoverable energy-dissipating losses due to inter-actions between spins[m], the spin isochromats rephase and recreate the transverse coherence exactly after the period of time it took to dephase them, that is, τ. The reinstated coherence is tantamount to a restored aggregate transverse magnetization, and thus newly formed echo; in this case, a gradient-echo.

It can be inferred that the amplitudes of the dephasing and rephasing lobes of the gradient may not be equal, such that the larger amplitude of the rephasing lobe expedites the coherence recovery. However, common to all gradient echo-like signal generation schemes is the combination of the dephasing and rephasing gradient lobes.

Gradient-Echo Imaging Pulse Sequence

An implementation of a simplest—Fast Low Angle SHot (FLASH)[n]—gradient-echo pulse sequence is shown in Figure 2.7. The design of the gradient sequence includes such components common to all imaging pulse sequences such as the excitation structure, comprised of the RF excitation pulse and the slice selection gradient with the following rephasing lobe, and

---

[m]As mentioned earlier, such loses are characterized by T_2 relaxation time.
[n]Here and further in text the Siemens nomenclature is used.

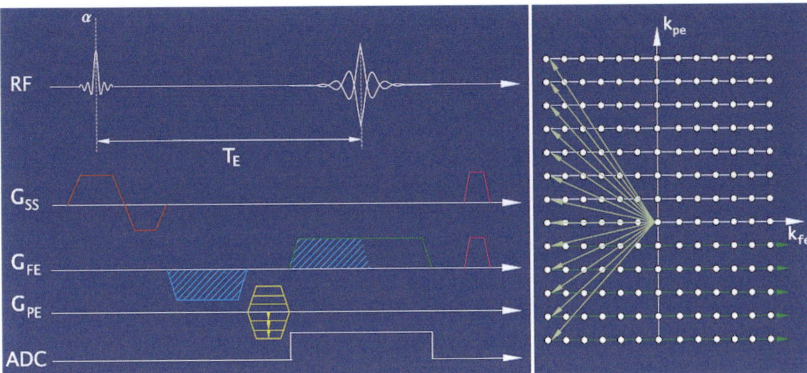

Figure 2.7. Gradient-Echo Timing Diagram.

the data collection segment during which the echo is generated and associated MR signal is received. Moreover, it may include additional gradients called spoilers, which are employed to avoid a transverse steady state.

The spatial encoding in a conventional gradient-echo sequence is achieved in the same manner in which it is accomplished for the spin-echo counterpart. In particular, the spatial encoding in one of the directions is performed by conditioning spin isochromats' precessional frequency (the *frequency-encoding direction*), whereas the spatial information in the other direction is encoded by modulating the phase angle of spin isochromats (the phase-encoding direction). During the frequency-encoding period, the scanner's receiver circuitry is turned on and the MR signal returned by spin isochromats is recorded as the raw MR signal.

In the noticeable difference from the spin-echo implementation, the gradient-echo pulse sequence design does not retain a π-radian refocusing pulse. The lack of thereof is rather consequential. First, in the absence of the refocusing pulse, the RF power released by the coil and thus absorbed by tissues is reduced significantly. This factor makes sequences utilizing the gradient-echo signal recovery mechanism safer and more desirable in general. The reduced-energy deposition in the case of the gradient-echo sequence is especially salient when performed in higher field strength scanners (1.5 Tesla and up) because it requires larger amounts of RF energy to disturb a longitudinal equilibrium magnetization. Moreover, with the overall RF energy emission reduced, it is possible to pack more RF pulses closer together and therefore speed up the signal acquisition without a risk of exceeding Specific Absorbtion Rate (SAR) limits established by the U.S. Food and Drug Administration (FDA).

The absence of the refocusing pulse affects the sensitivity of gradient-echo sequences to magnetic field inhomogeneities and, consequently, the type of image contrast. The main effect of the refocusing pulse used in the spin-echo formation mechanism is achieved by nullifying phase angles of spin isochromats and reversing the direction of the dephasing. Therefore, phase angles developed due to constant field inhomogeneities and magnetic susceptibilities are cancelled by the time of the echo.[o] Therefore, the

---

[o] The field inhomogeneities and magnetic susceptibilities are assumed constant over the single T_R.

spin-echo sequence has an inherent property to suppress MR signal contributions from large fixed inhomogeneities.

On the contrary, because it lacks the refocusing pulse, the gradient-echo sequence is very much sensitive to field inhomogeneities and magnetic susceptibilities. Indeed, instead of an RF refocusing pulse, the gradient-echo imaging pulse sequence employs a structure that contains alternating gradients to re-establish coherence of spin isochromats and generate the echo, as it is shown in the Figure 2.7. The overall phase change introduced by the gradients by the echo time is zero, as the phase change during the rephase segment is offset by the opposite phase change during the following dephasing segment. However, such a gradient reversal can only compensate for the spin phase gained or lost due to the gradient field itself. Any amount of spin phase advanced or retarded due to factors other than gradients fields, such as effects of sample-related magnetic susceptibilities, remain uncompensated at the echo time. In other words, phase angles, neither refocused nor compensated, continue to develop through the entire echo formation period, and thus are non-zero at the time of an echo, effectively reducing the MR signal.

Because the spin coherence is achieved by having reversal gradients to nullify spin phase changes, thus rendering the refocusing pulse unnecessary, the repetition time T_R now can be made shorter. Having been given less time to die down, the spin coherence at the end of the signal detection period turns out to be higher than that in the spin-echo case,[p] leaving a relatively stronger transverse magnetization to linger before the next excitation pulse.

In addition to the increased transverse coherence, the effects of consecutive RF pulses on the magnetization should be mentioned. It is known that a series of several arbitrary RF pulses is capable of producing spin echoes and so called stimulated echoes.[16] Generally, such echoes are not treated as a primary source of the gradient-echo MR signal, and thus are disregarded in the majority of gradient-echo pulse sequences. However, if allowed to propagate freely and undisturbed throughout subsequent repetition periods, the lingering magnetization responsible for the formation of such echoes may affect the gradient echoes formed later, and is likely to cause imaging artifacts. Moreover, coupled with the aforementioned enhanced transverse magnetization, the artifacts may have very consequential ramifications on the MR signal in pulse sequences where either transverse or longitudinal magnetization is maintained in the steady state.

There are two ways to mitigate the effects of unwanted MR signal echoes—to destroy the lingering transverse magnetization with additional gradient fields or RF pulses, or to refocus magnetization components leading to formation of spin and stimulated echoes.

The methods of the first group use either additional gradients alone or coupled with quasi-random flip-angle RF pulses to further and irreversibly[q] dephase spins in the transverse plane, effectively destroying the remnant aggregate transverse magnetization. With the bulk transverse magnetization essentially nonexistent, only longitudinal component of the aggregate

---

[p] It is due to the fact that less transverse magnetization is lost to irreversible T_2 relaxation.

[q] So that the transverse magnetization created in this repetition period does not reform sometime later.

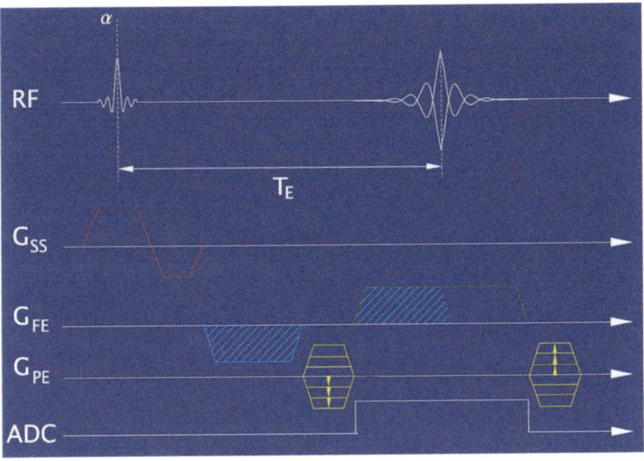

Figure 2.8. FISP Pulse Sequence Timing Diagram.

magnetization contributes to the fresh bulk transverse magnetization at the next RF pulse, which is during the next T_R period.

Alternative to the mechanism of spoiling of the bulk transverse magnetization is the process of refocusing its components, contributing to formation of spin and stimulated echoes. The first sequence to take advantage of the refocusing was fast imaging with steady precession (FISP).[17] In the most trivial way, it is achieved by adding an extra phase-encoding gradient to the existing FLASH-like pulse sequence, as shown in the Figure 2.8. Its function is to compensate for the phase change introduced by the initial phase-encoding gradient step. For that purpose, the new gradient has the same magnitude as the initial phase-encoding gradient field; however, it is applied in the opposite direction. The partial rephasing of the transverse magnetization allowed an additional T_2-weighted signal be recovered from refocused spin and stimulated echoes.

The reversal of gradients just in the direction of the phase encoding does not fully rephase transverse magnetization. Indeed, the phase of spin iso-chromats is changed by any disturbance, leading to the Larmor frequency variation, regardless of directionality of the such. In order to attain a fully refocused transverse magnetization and the largest possible MR signal, the area under gradient lobes has to be zero in all three directions.

This approach is implemented in the pulse sequence known as trueFISP. The design of the trueFISP sequence (Figure 2.9) contains a train of equally spaced RF pulses and gradient structures balancing the phase in all three directions. Having the phase of the transverse magnetization at the end of the repetition period restored to its prepulse value improves overall trans-verse coherence, and thus the SNR while maintaining a relatively short T_R and higher receiver bandwidth. The recent studies showed that the trueFISP sequences are capable of recovering a relatively strong BOLD signal.[18]

Contrast Characteristics of Gradient-Echo Sequences

Vascular Effects

As in the case with the spin-echo pulse sequences, the diffusing motion of water molecules is a crucial and defining factor in the development of the gradient-echo contrast. The nature of diffusion effects is again due to

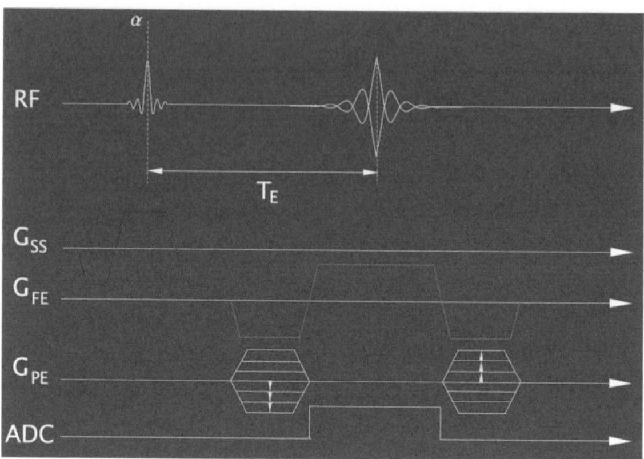

Figure 2.9. trueFISP Pulse Sequence Timing Diagram.

microscopic phase variations that the water molecule experiences as it traverses through magnetic field gradients established by nearby vessels. However, although identical by nature, the diffusion effects are exhibited somewhat differently in case of the gradient-echo pulse sequences.

If the spatial extent of field variations created by larger venule vessels spans over distances larger than a diffusing molecule travels on average, it experiences a very similar field at any point of its trajectory. Without a refocusing pulse, the average phase displacement acquired by molecules due to these offset fields is increased linearly as a function of time and is not compensated at the end of the acquisition period. Consequently, due to the procured dephasing, the relaxation rate increases and the MR signal is weakened to a relatively higher degree.

When water molecules traverse several fields over their trajectory's average length, the phase offsets gained by water molecules are very similar; therefore, the range of phase offsets is minimal, as is the overall dephasing. The T_2 relaxation rate, and thus the MR signal, remain largely unaffected. Such an attenuation regime is identical to that achieved with the spin-echo formation mechanism for vessels up to six micrometers in diameter.

The extent to which the MR signal is attenuated depends on the amount of the phase offset that spin isochromats accumulate during their traversal through field gradients over a specific time, usually the echo time T_E. Therefore, it can be inferred that the relaxation rate increases with the vessel's size.

It is noteworthy to compare the sensitivity of spin- and gradient-echo formation mechanisms to the BOLD-related changes as a function of vessel's size. It has been mentioned previously in this chapter that the spin-echo pulse sequences appears to be most sensitive to diffusion effects occurring in capillaries. In contrast, the sensitivity of the gradient-echo sequence reaches its maximum towards larger structures, like venulae and small veins.

Inflow Effects

The impact that the blood inflow has on the gradient-echo MR signal mechanism is quite different from that on the MR signal recovered in a spin-echo. In the case of the spin-echo sequence, contrary to the MR signal reduction caused by unexcited spins flowing into a region partially saturated after a series of closely following excitation pulses, the inflow of unsaturated spins leads to the increase of the MR signal collected by the gradient-echo sequence.

Consider an imaging slice with a vessel carrying flowing blood surrounded by stationary tissues. Continuous application of RF excitation pulses designed to nutate the longitudinal magnetization into the transverse plane by partial flip angles[r] may cause a condition called saturation. The spin ensemble within stationary tissues becomes saturated after a considerable number of RF pulses are transmitted in a rapid succession, each released before the longitudinal magnetization is allowed to recover fully to its equilibrium value, M_0. During the allotted time, T_R, only so much of the longitudinal magnetization gets restored so that at the end of current T_R period

$$M_z < M_0.$$

This implies that not all spins excited by the last excitation pulse have radiated RF photons and are returned to their stable state, and the next RF excitation pulse acts on the longitudinal magnetization M_z, which is restored only partially. Similarly, at the end of the next repetition interval, the longitudinal magnetization is not given to relax to its pre-pulse value, M_z, so that even less of the fresh longitudinal magnetization is available to be acted upon by the following excitation pulse. Thus, each following RF pulse acts on smaller longitudinal magnetization than the previous one.

On the other hand, each RF pulse brings a magnitude of the longitudinal magnetization to the same value, since the RF pulse's flip angle is kept constant.[s] Because the magnitude of the pre-pulse longitudinal magnetization is falling and its post-pulse magnitude is maintained, it can be inferred that the reduction of the longitudinal magnetization gradually[t] ceases after a certain number of RF pulses. Such dynamics imply that the magnitude of the longitudinal magnetization becomes confined between its pre- and post-pulse values throughout the entire T_R interval. This happens when the number of excited spins returned to their stable state is equal to the number of spins excited by the following RF pulse.

Because few spins get excited by a new RF pulse and consequently return the signal at the end of the T_R interval, the pre-pulse magnitude of the longitudinal magnetization is only slightly different from its post-pulse value; thus, the amount of available MR signal from stationary tissues is reduced. On the other hand, fresh spins contained in the blood entering the imaging slice are not saturated at all because they did not experience all previous excitations. The spins from the flowing blood enter the imaging slice and become slightly saturated as they pass through it. Since less saturated spins are capable of returning higher MR signal than the more saturated, such a dynamic leads to an intense MR signal coming from the blood. The differences between sufficiently saturated stationary tissues and partially saturated moving blood can therefore be identified in the image contrast.

---

[r]Partial is any flip angle which causes less than $\dfrac{\pi}{2}$ –radian nutation.

[s]Of course, variable flip angles are possible,[19] however consideration of such is beyond of this chapter's scope.

[t]As a matter of fact, exponentially, with the exponent's power being negative.[v,p127]

The degree of saturation sustained by the blood spins largely depends on the blood flow velocity, the T_R interval, and the amount of the RF energy transferred to the spins, which is tantamount to the flip angle. The increase of the MR signal occurs when the sufficient number of unsaturated spins enter the imaging slice over several T_R periods. In case of the relatively short T_R or a fast blood flow, the MR signal increases due to the partial desaturation by the fresh spins. However, with the longer T_R period, a larger number of the saturated spins may have sufficient time to return to the equilibrium so that the signal from stationary tissues increases and the contrast with the blood MR signal diminishes. In case of a relatively slower blood flow, for instance capillary flux, it may take a few more T_R intervals for entered spins to pass through the imaging slice. Experiencing more RF pulses, blood spin isochromats become more saturated, which also equalizes the contrast between MR signals from stationary tissues and blood.

In addition to their inflow sensitivity, the gradient-echo methods are likely—more so than those of a spin-echo variety—to produce an MR signal that reflects sample-induced magnetic susceptibilities and scanner-related field inhomogeneities. Generally, the increased sensitivity of the gradient-echo methods to such perturbations originates from uncompensated spin phase contributions developed during an MR signal echo's formation.

Indeed, a spatially dependent field distribution gives rise to a corresponding spatially varying distribution of the Larmor frequency. In this case, even adjacent spin isochromats may happen to precess at slightly different frequencies, leading to the phase dispersion and loss of the aggregate transverse magnetization. As was pointed out in the previous section, it is due to the absence of a refocusing pulse that the phases acquired by spin isochromats due to sustained inhomogeneities other than gradient fields do not get cancelled, but rather continue to develop until the echo time. On top of a distribution of fixed Larmor frequency-affecting factors, there are various effects that further modulate local field: random motion of water molecules (diffusion), varying magnetic properties of blood and tissues (oxygenation/deoxygenation), and eddy currents.

Sample-induced susceptibilities alter local magnetic fields, thus causing inhomogeneities. The effects created by sample-related susceptibilities usually can be seen as signal enhancement/reduction near tissue–tissue and, even to a larger degree, tissue–air interfaces. Furthermore, image distortions may be observed in or near regions with cavities and sinuses, where the inhomogeneities are high.

Only in part does the severity of image distortions depend on the degree of the inhomogeneity. Equally consequential are the imaging parameters, such as receiver bandwidth, direction of phase encoding, image resolution, and others. The imaging parameters have to be changed with caution and with the understanding of the implications of such changes. For instance, raising the receiver bandwidth mitigates image distortions, especially so in the phase-encoding directions. However, it also would decrease the SNR.

Echo Planar Imaging Methods

The generic gradient-echo sequence displayed in the Figure 2.7 acquires n MR signal samples sequentially, one by one, along a single chose k-space line per an excitation period. Therefore, it has to be repeated n times in order to create a $n \times n$-pixel image.[u] The acquisition time is reduced in the steady-state sequences, for their T_R values usually are shorter than that of a conventional FLASH-like gradient-echo methods. Although either of these sequences can be used to detect gross BOLD-related MR signal variations originated in areas that are capable of producing a relatively robust signal, such as visual or motor cortices, they are proved to be unfittingly sluggish to adequately resolve rather fine BOLD effects elicited by swift subtle cognitive and behavioral processes.

The pulse sequence tailored for imaging of physiological markers of transient events and processes would acquire the MR signal needed to reconstruct the entire image in the shortest time possible, at the same time lasting sufficiently long enough for BOLD-inducing factors influencing the MR signal to develop. The demand for higher temporal resolution necessitates more rapid MR signal sampling. Certainly, the shortest acquisition time is attained when the entire k-space is covered after a single excitation pulse. The group of imaging methods that traverse the k-space in a single passing shot, or in a series of multiple shots or segments, make up a class of Echo Planar Imaging (EPI) techniques.

It is noteworthy to mention that although the EPI methods belong to the distinct class of imaging techniques, they are not based on nor do they establish entirely new acquisition principles. As a matter of fact, EPI pulse sequences use the same echo-formation mechanisms as spin- or gradient-echo methods, with an exception that they are very quick to traverse the entire k-space, and thus offer a drastic improvement in acquisition time.

Echo Planar Imaging Pulse Sequences

As implied above, unlike the collection strategy employed in the conventional imaging that repeats excitation-sampling pair over every k-space line, a typical EPI pulse sequence collects and spatially encodes all MR signal samples necessary for a subsequent reconstruction of the entire image in a single acquisition period following an excitation pulse.

The schematics of a generic EPI pulse sequence is shown in Figure 2.10. Initially, a pair of gradients is applied in both the phase- and frequency-encoding directions in order to advance to the first sample point of the first k-space line. Then an oscillatory gradient is applied along the frequency-encoding direction so that the train of echoes is generated, each for every gradient lobe, positive or negative.

Such a waveform of the read-out gradient establishes alternating directions of traversing the read-out lines, whereas brief blip phase-encoding gradient pulses shift the current k-space location from one line to another in the phase-encoding direction. Such waveforms of the phase- and frequency-encoding gradients draw the zig-zag k-space trajectory shown in the right of Figure 2.10. As it can be seen on the k-space diagram, each line comes through the point of $k_x = 0$. This is the moment of time when the line-echo is formed. Each echo is produced in the same fashion as the gradient-echo, that is via an application of the bipolar dephasing–rephasing gradient structure.

---

[u]A trivial case is considered here, as the $n \times n$ pixel image also can be created from the undersampled MR signal pool using various reconstruction tricks.

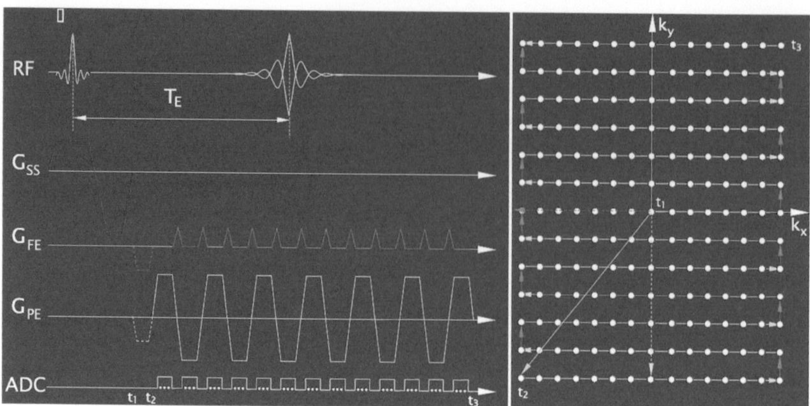

Figure 2.10. EPI Pulse Sequence Timing Diagram.

After every echo, the phase-encoding gradient advances the trajectory to the next line, and so on until the entire k-space is traversed.

It should be taken into account that although every gradient forms its own echo, only the echo that coincides with the k-space center, the so-called primary-echo where the net gradient encoding is zero, is taken to calculate the echo time. Because the effect of gradients on spins during the formation of this echo is minimal so that their precessional frequencies are very near the Larmor frequency established by the main magnetic field B_0, the MR signal gain during this echo is the largest and determines the image contrast.

The implementation of the acquisition mechanism that allows a rapid collection of data to complete an entire image does not come without a few principle obstacles and challenges along the way. The accelerated sampling and shortened acquisition time that becomes comparable with such characteristic relaxation time T_2^* and T_2 put additional demands on the scanner's gradient hardware, and the relaxation effects that influence the collected MR signal become more pronounced. In fact, the greatest challenge in the design of EPI sequences is imposed by the effect of the intrinsic decay owing to the T_2^* relaxation. Such an effect is twofold.

The T_2^* relaxation accounts for the global MR signal dropout across the entire image. Indeed, every k-space sample is attenuated by the signal decay during the acquisition, including the one located at the k-space center $k_x = k_y = 0$. Because this MR signal sample coincides with the primary and the strongest echo, the overall signal dropout is determined by the amount of the MR signal lost to the T_2^* relaxation at the time of passing through the k-space center. Thus, the effective T_E assigned to the time of the primary echo defines the overall loss of the MR signal.

Whereas the extent of the MR signal dropout depends on the position of the primary echo in respect to the T_2^*-relaxation decay profile, the length of the acquisition window determines the amount of the image blurring accounted to the T_2^* relaxation. Because the sampling through the entire k-space is performed within a single acquisition window, the MR signal may experience the T_2^* decay modulation large enough to cause a significant difference between the magnitude of MR signal samples acquired at the beginning and at the end of the acquisition window. In the zig-zag trajectory, it is high spatial frequencies ascribed by the peripheral k-space samples that get covered at the edges of the acquisition window. To this end, the substantial drop of the MR signal's amplitude over the acquisition window amounts to the image blurring.

Both caused by a decay due to the T_2^* relaxation, these effects are related, but somewhat separable. Consider an MR signal collected during a 20-millisecond long acquisition window with its primary echo located around $T_E =$ 100 milliseconds. If the shortest T_2^* is 40 milliseconds, only minimal blurring occurs because the amplitude of k-space samples acquired in the beginning of the window does not differ substantially from that acquired at the window's rear. On the other hand, the signal decays considerably by the time of the primary echo. Therefore, the image reflects the overall attenuation rather than the blurring effects. Alternatively, the blurring in the image made with the acquisition window of 100 milliseconds long and centered around $T_E =$ 50 milliseconds dominates over global attenuation effects.

Therefore, in order to mitigate the blurring, the length of the acquisition window has to be shortened. Usually, it is realized by increasing the reception bandwidth that allows faster MR signal sampling. The contrariety of the raised bandwidth is reduced image SNR. The length of the acquisition window also can be abridged by lowering the image resolution and thus the number of acquired k-space samples, for instance, from the image matrix of 128×128 pixels to one comprised of 64×64 pixels. In this case, in order to preserve the same coverage, the in-plane size of voxels is increased twofold. Having more spins in each voxel provides a larger per-voxel MR signal, and thus the SNR. However, it is more likely for a larger voxel to span intrinsic gradients caused by local inhomogeneities. To that end, the degree of the intravoxel inhomogeneity is also higher because it includes a wider range of frequencies; it inevitably shortens the T_2^* and decreases the SNR. The shorter T_2^* forces the T_E to decrease accordingly in order to maintain sufficient SNR, per global attenuation effect described above. On the other hand, the T_E has to be long enough to let the BOLD effect sufficiently modulate the MR signal.

Another aspect of the sampling process performed by an EPI pulse sequence is associated with characteristics of gradient coils. Implementation of EPI pulse sequences requires rather high gradient strength and switching rates in order to accomplish the rapid sampling. Based on the chosen field-of-view (FoV) and the resolution (image matrix), a size of the k-space grid that must be covered during the acquisition and the spacing between adjacent samples Δk are prescribed. From Equations (2.6–2.8), simplified for the case of a constant gradient, the distance between adjacent k-space samples is:

$$\Delta k = \gamma G \Delta t, \tag{2.13}$$

where Δt is the sampling rate. The FoV and Δk are directly connected as

$$\mathrm{FoV} = \Delta k^{-1}. \tag{2.14}$$

The sampling rate can be found if the resolution N_{fe}, N_{pe} and the duration of the acquisition window T are known:

$$\Delta t \approx \frac{T}{N_{fe} \cdot N_{pe}}. \tag{2.15}$$

In the most favorable case, when the duration of the excitation RF pulse[v] and the gap between its end and the beginning of the gradient waveform are neglected, the duration of the acquisition window is almost equal to the total acquisition time. The sampling rate can be readily found under such approximation conditions. If the pulse sequence is designed so that its primary echo occurs in the center of the acquisition window, then the total time is about twice the echo time, $T = 2T_E$. The estimated gradient amplitude can now be expressed through conventional imaging parameters:

$$G \approx \frac{N_{fe} \cdot N_{pe}}{2\gamma \cdot \text{FoV} \cdot T_E} \qquad (2.16)$$

Therefore, to acquire a 128-square-pixel image with the FoV of 220 millimeters and the echo time of 30 milliseconds, the highest gradient amplitude should be on the order of 30 milliTesla per meter (mT/m). Technically challenging to implement a mere five years ago, gradient fields of such magnitude are now considered typical, and they become increasingly available for research and clinical applications. Following recent FDA approval of operating MR scanners equipped with gradient coils capable of reaching gradient field magnitudes as high as 40mT/m, such imaging techniques as EPI-based diffusion and perfusion and fMRI are now actively employed in clinical studies. Even higher gradient strengths, up to 1000mT/m, are available on experimental human and animal scanners.

Another essential characteristic of gradient field hardware and coil is the slew rate that describes how fast the gradient field can be changed. It is defined as a ratio

$$\text{Slew rate} = \frac{\text{Gradient magnitude}}{\text{Rise time}},$$

where the rise time is the time required to advance the gradient amplitude from 0 to its maximum. Typical for clinical scanners, rise times may vary from 100 to 600 microseconds. The gradient ramping, the period of time during which the gradient's amplitude changes between its extrema is thus twice as long, if the rise time is constant. Therefore, the slew rate is on the order of few hundred Tesla per meter per second, with the most prevalent values being 100 to 200T/m·s.

As the EPI pulse sequences are in essence a special way to traverse k-space and do not introduce fundamentally new echo formation principles, the same contrast mechanisms can be implemented using the EPI spatial encoding scheme.

Gradient Echo-Recalled EPI Sequence

The gradient echo-recalled EPI acquisition is the most commonly used imaging method in functional neuroimaging applications and research due to several reasons. First and foremost, although some amount of the T_2 weighting is inevitably present because of the overall irreversible transverse decay through the acquisition, the MR signal generated by this type of the EPI

---

[v]The duration of the excitation RF pulse ranges from two to five milliseconds.

sequence carries a robust T_2^* contrast. The prevailing T_2^*-weighted contrast component comes from the sensitivity of the sequence's echo-formation mechanism to local field inhomogeneities. Because the nature of the BOLD contrast is exactly rooted in tiny field inhomogeneities imparted by variations in oxy/deoxyhemoglobin-induced blood susceptibility, the gradient-recalled EPI sequences are very appropriate for collection of BOLD-related MR signal changes sought in the functional imaging.

As in generic gradient-echo sequences, a smaller flip angle can be employed in gradient-recalled EPI designs without suffering large MR signal losses. The smaller flip angle makes it possible to decrease the T_R period, as less time is needed to restore the original longitudinal relaxation. Alternatively, a larger number of slices can be covered over the same T_R period. The optimal flip angle at which the gradient-echo–generated MR signal reaches its maximum, the Ernst angle, can be calculated to provide the best possible contrast.[21]

Spin-Echo Recalled EPI Sequence

When the EPI spatial encoding mechanism itself is not a subject of interest but rather is taken as a component of a pulse sequence in whole, it can be considered as a black box that is designed to properly encode recovered MR signal and fill the k-space matrix. In case of a spin-echo pulse sequence, it is positioned following the excitation and refocusing RF pulses and all necessary gradient structures that define the image contrast, as is shown in the Figure 2.11.

The contrast-defining properties of the spin-echo–recalled EPI are similar to those of a regular spin-echo pulse sequence. In particular, although the spin-echo pulse sequence appears to be most susceptible to inhomogeneities imparted by capillaries, overall image contrast generated by this pulse sequence shows relatively little sensitivity to field inhomogeneities.

Somewhat more sensitive to BOLD-related changes in the T_2^* relaxation is the asymmetric spin-echo. As discussed earlier, a key feature that differentiates it from the typical spin-echo pulse sequence is temporal misalignment between the center of the k-space (no spatial encoding condition) and the echo time. Such a mismatch usually is achieved by advancing the refocusing

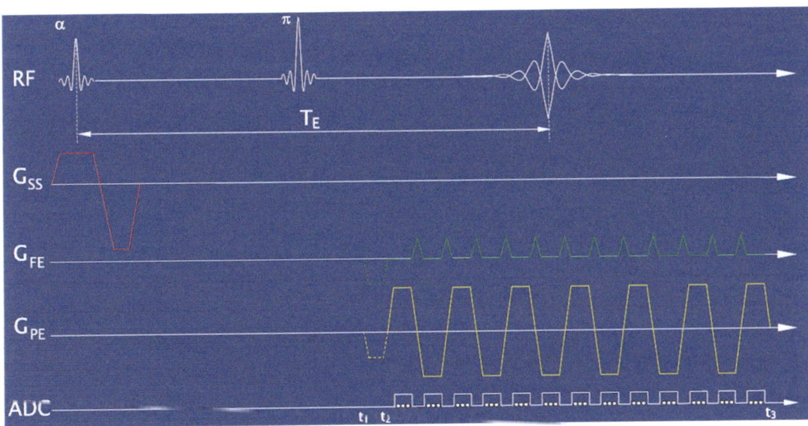

Figure 2.11. Spin-Echo EPI Pulse Sequence Timing Diagram.

pulse and, consequently, the EPI spatial collection module towards the excitation pulse. In this case, there is a certain amount of T_2^* dephasing present at the moment of the contrast-defining central echo of the EPI read-out echo train, thus bringing about the imprint of BOLD-related inhomogeneities.

The benefit from using the ASE pulse sequence may become greater in higher field strengths, where the effects of constant inhomogeneities are amplified, and thus present an increasingly bothersome factor in SNR and overall image quality.

Spiral-Echo Planar Imaging Methods

Because the EPI is just a clever trick to cover the entire k-space fast, there is no restriction on the trajectory along which the k-space is traversed. In fact, it can be quite arbitrary, as suggested by Dale and colleagues.[22] One of trajectories that has been proven effective to implement fast scanning technique while producing relatively high BOLD-related SNR resembles a spiral. Thus, the pulse sequence that utilizes such a trajectory is called spiral EPI pulse sequence. These sequences have been found effective in cardiovascular, renal,[23,24] and multiple functional brain imaging studies.[25,26] The imaging with spiral algorithms excels in these application because of its relatively low sensitivity to motion and flow and an efficient use of the gradient power.[27]

The term spiral refers to the method of the k-space traverse. In particular, the k-space trajectory is indeed a spiral, as shown in Figure 2.12. The spiral sequences do not constitute a whole new class of imaging methods. Rather, they should be considered as a subset of EPI techniques because of many similarities between their designs, including collection of the MR signal corresponding to a large portion of the k-space with time-varying gradients following a single excitation pulse.

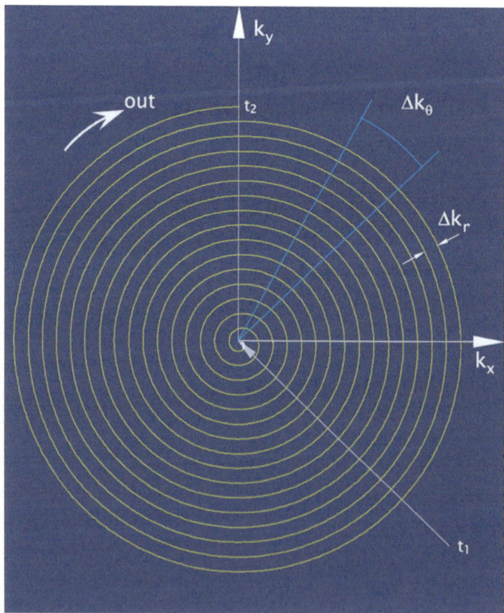

Figure 2.12. k-Space Diagram for Spiral EPI.

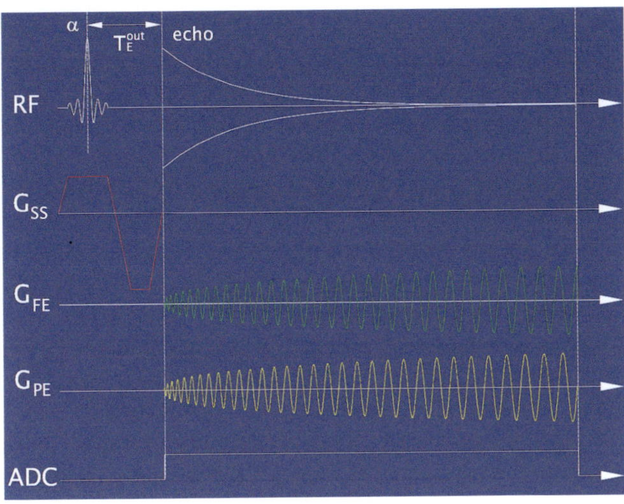

Figure 2.13. Spiral-Out Pulse Sequence Timing Diagram.

The design of a spiral pulse sequence involves two aspects. First, based on the mathematical expressions for a particular spiral trajectory and system-specific hardware characteristics, the gradient waveforms are calculated. The simplest type of the spiral trajectory, a so-called Archimedean spiral, is described by a running angle q as a function of the trajectory radius at a particular point along the spiral, as shown in the right portion of Figure 2.12:

$$k(t) = A\theta(t)e^{i\theta(t)},\tag{2.17}$$

where the azimuthal angle $\theta(t) = \omega_0 t$, with ω_0 being a constant angular velocity. The gradient waveforms that implement the spiral traversal starting in the center and ending on the periphery of the k-space are shown on the pulse sequence diagram in Figure 2.13.

Other shapes of spiral trajectories are possible and widely used. For instance, in order to reduce physiologic noise effects that typically contaminate lower spatial frequencies, the vicinity of the k-space center often is oversampled by making more winds around the k-space's center, thus increasing the coverage density. To achieve an optimal density throughout the k-space and keep acquisition time from growing overly long, the varying sampling density spiral trajectory was proposed by Spielman and colleagues.[28] In this case, the image contrast improves because more MR signal samples are obtained around the center of the k-space and the contribution by physiological noise becomes limited.

Following the signal acquisition, a complementary image-reconstruction algorithm has to be applied to the raw signal data. The need for a gradient-specific reconstruction algorithm implementation is justified by limitations related to fast Fourier transformation (FFT) used to reconstruct the image from the raw MR signal. The regular FFT operation relies on a symmetrical and uniformly sampled rectilinear distribution of k-samples. This is not true for spiral-like traversals—not only do the collected data points not fall on the two-dimensional (2D) grid, but also their distribution is often nonuniform, as in case of the trajectory with the varying sampling density. Therefore, an operation that regrids the distribution of the k-samples into a rectilinear array and approximates the actual trajectory has to be applied before the data is submitted for the FFT.

There are seemingly two key ways to follow the spiral—namely, from the center to the periphery of the k-space and in the opposite direction. The spiral-out pulse sequence traverses the center of the k-space in the beginning of the acquisition period, and therefore obtains the contrast-defining echo immediately following the excitation pulse. In such a design, there is very little time to develop any appreciable T_2^* relaxation; the FID signal is strong and any motion did not have enough time to have an impact on the spatial encoding. On the contrary, the traverse in the opposite direction, from the periphery to the k-space center, leads to accumulation of T_2^*-related phase offsets that sensitizes the image contrast to the field inhomogeneities.

Each of these traversals has benefits and limitations that should be considered in the context of a specific application. In cardiac imaging, where motion and flow artifacts could be severe, the pulse sequence that is capable to limit contributions thereof to the MR signal is advantageous. Therefore, the spiral-out design is more desirable in cardiac and abdominal studies. On the other hand, in order to detect BOLD-related MR signal changes, the inhomogeneities have to be allowed to influence the MR signal. If the contrast-defining echo comes too soon after the excitation pulse, the phase offsets are negligible, thus limiting their effect on the MR signal. Therefore, in BOLD studies, the spiral-in pulse sequence is preferred.

There is, however a significant drawback associated with such a design. Namely, if the entire k-space is sampled over the single trajectory, the overall MR signal may experience a considerable T_2^* decay, leading to the decreased SNR. The solution to this particular predicament is to split the acquisition into several parts, covering the k-space in segments, so that the last echo appears earlier, but still at the end of the acquisition period. This approach reduces nonuniformity effects and eventually increases the SNR. However, the cardiac motion and respiration gives rise to undesirable image-to-image variations.

Several pulse sequence designs were proposed to accommodate the best of two traversals. For instance, one of designs is a two-segment acquisition that includes the spiral-in segment, followed by the spiral-out portion. In this case, both echoes, at the end of the spiral-in segment and at the beginning of the spiral-out portion, occur one after the other. Because the center of the k-space in each segment was acquired virtually at the same time, the two echoes have identical contrast. The MR signal collected during the leading spiral-in section is not severely decayed, which reflects an inhomogeneity modulation. The MR signal recovered in the consecutive spiral-out segment does not experience any substantial inhomogeneity effects and does not suffer from ongoing T_2^* decay. Two k-space samples covered in both segments are later combined into a single k-space and the image is formed through the FFT. As expected, such an image can be sufficiently BOLD-modulated while sustaining sufficient MR signal magnitude and avoiding being degraded by T_2^* relaxation.

By default, the spiral sequences are GE, but they can be turned into SE, and also can be united to produce double-contrast sequences.

In summary, this chapter gives an overview of the various pulse sequences that currently are used today in fMRI BOLD imaging, as well as their characteristics. The appropriate choice of the pulse sequence and its optimal parameters are key factors in maximizing the BOLD signal for every fMRI experiment performed.

References

1. Robitaille PM, Abduljali AM, Kangarlu A. Ultra high resolution imaging of the human head at 8 tesla: 2K × 2K for Y2K. *J Comput Assist Tomogr.* 2000;24(1):2–8.
2. Guinnessy P. Powerful NMR mashines debut in USA. *Physics Today.* 2002;55(3): 30–31.
3. Constans A. NMR hits the big time. *The Scientist.* 2003;17(7):45–47.
4. Clark DD, Sokoloff L. Basic neurochemistry. In: *Circulation and Energy Metabolism of the Brain*, New York: Raven; 1994:645–680.
5. Hasselbalch SG, Knudsen GM, Jakobsen J, Hagenman LP, Holm S, Paulason OB. Brain metabolism during short term starvation in humans. *J Cereb Blood Flow Metab.* 1994;14:125–131.
6. Schwartz WJ, Smith CB, Davidsen L, Savaki H, Sokoloff L, Mata M, Fink DJ, Gainer H. Metabolic mapping of functional activity in the hypothalamo-neuro-hypophysial system of the rat. *Science.* 1979;205:723–725.
7. Hyder F, Rothman DL, Mason GF, Rangarajan A, Shulman KL. Oxidative glucose metabolism in rat brain during single forepaw stimulation: A spatially localized ^{1}H[^{13}C nuclear magnetic resonance study]. *J Cereb Blood Flow Metab.* 1997;17:1040–1047.
8. Gross PM, Sposito NM, Pettersen SE, Panton DG, Fenstermacher JD. Topography of capillary density, glucose metabolism, and microvascular function within the rat inferior colliculus. *J Cereb Blood Flow Metab.* 1987;7:154–160.
9. Klein B, Kuschinsky W, Schrock H, Vetterlein F. Interdependency of local capillary density, blood flow, and metabolism in rat brains. *Am J Physiol.* 1986;251:H1333–H1340.
10. Fox PT, Raichle ME, Mintun MA, Dence C. Nonoxidative glucose consumption during focal physiologic neuronal activity. *Science.* 1988;241:462–464.
11. Davis TL, Kwong KK, Weisskoff RM, Rosen BR. Calibrated functional MRI: Mapping the dynamics of oxidative metabolism. *Proc Nat Acad Sci USA.* 1998;95:1834–1839.
12. Thulborn KR, Waterton JC, Mattews PM, Padda GK. Oxygenation dependence of the transverse relaxation time of water protons in while blood at high field. *Biochem Biophys Acta.* 1982;714:265–270.
13. Turner R, Le Bihan D, Moonen CT, Despres D, Frank D. Echo-planar time course MRI of cat brain oxygenation changes. *Magn Resón Med.* 1991;22:159–166.
14. Feynman RP, Leighton RB, Sands M. *The Feynman Lectures on Physics*, vol. 1. Addison-Wesley Publishing Company; 1964.
15. Bandettini PA, Wong EC, Jesmanowicz A, Hinks RS, Hyde JS. Spin-echo and Gradient-echo EPI of human brain activation using BOLD contrast. A comparative study at 1.5T. *NMR Biomed.* 1994;7:12–20.
16. Hahn EL. Spin echoes. *Physical Rev.* 1950;80:580–594.
17. Oppelt A, Graumann R, Barfuss H. FISP: A new fast MRI sequence. *Electromedica.* 1986;54:15–18.
18. Scheffler K, Seifritz E, Bilecen D, Venkatesan R, Hennig J, Deimling M, Haacke EM. Detection of BOLD changes by means of a frequency-sensitive trueFISP technique: Preliminary results. *NMR Biomed.* 2001;14(7–8):490–496.
19. Scheffler K, Hennig J. TIDE (transition into driven equilibrium)-sequences for brain imaging with improved signal and contrast behaviour. In: *Proceedings of ISMRM. 11thScientific Meeting and Exhibition*. Toronto, Ontario, Canada: 2003:973.
20. Haake EM, Brown RE, Thompson MR, Venkatesan R. *Magnetic Resonance Imaging: Physical Principles and Sequence Design*. New-York: John Wiley & Sons Inc.; 1999.
21. Ernst R, Anderson W. Application of Fourier transform spectroscopy to magnetic resonance. *Rev Sci Instrum.* 1966;37:93–102.
22. Dale B, Wendt M, Duerk JL. A rapid look-up table method for reconstructing MR images from arbitrary *k*-space trajectories. *IEEE Trans Med Imaging.* 2001;20(3):207–217.

23. Meyer C, Hu B, Nishimura DG, Macovshi A. Fast coronary artery imaging. *Magn Reson Imaging*. 1992;28:202–213.
24. Yacoe ME, Li KC, Cheung L, Meyer CH. Spiral spin-echo magnetic resonance imaging of the pelvis with spectrally and spatially selective radiofrequency excitation: Comparison with fat-saturated fast spin-echo imaging. *Can Assoc Radiol J*. 1996;48:247–251.
25. Noll DC, Cohen JD, Meyer CH, Schneider W. Spiral k-space MR imaging of cortical activation. *J Magn Reson Imaging*. 1995;5(1):49–56.
26. Cohen JD, Perlstein WM, Braver TS, Nystrom LE, Noll DC, Jonides J, Smith EE. Temporal dynamics of brain activation during a working memory task. *Nature*. 1997;386:604–608.
27. Nishimura DG, Irarrazabal P, Meyer CH. A velocity k-space analysis of flow effects in echo-planar and spiral imaging. *Magn Reson Med*. 1995;33:549–556.
28. Spielman DM, Pauly JM, Meyer CH. Magnetic resonance fluoroscopy using spirals with variable sampling densities. *Magn Reson Med*. 1995;34:388–394.

3

Experimental Design and Data Analysis for fMRI

Geoffrey K. Aguirre

Introduction

Functional magnetic resonance imaging (fMRI) methods have evolved rapidly over the last decade. Ever more subtle experimental designs have been joined by ever more powerful data analysis methods to detect evoked changes in neural activity. Despite constant developments, there are several core principles of fMRI methodology that can be used as a guide to understand the current state of the field, as well as whatever advances await tomorrow. Here, the primary concern will be with this core understanding, but several specific aspects of fMRI experiments also will be considered. Along the way, some of the specific challenges that face fMRI studies of clinical populations will be noted, although a detailed consideration of these issues is contained in Chapter 5.

Topics will be raised roughly as they present in the course of the conception and completion of an fMRI experiment. This order of presentation will also move us from general issues in neuroimaging inference to more specific aspects of fMRI, and finally to the idiosyncratic properties of blood oxygenation level-dependent (BOLD) fMRI and their implication for experimental design and analysis. To start, three general categories of neuroimaging experiments will be considered, each of which probes a slightly different aspect of the relationship between the brain and behavior. Next, different techniques of isolating and manipulating mental operations that might be used in the service of these experimental designs will be discussed. Rounding out experimental design, the possible temporal ordering of stimuli within an fMRI experiment will be considered, including the paradigmatic blocked and event-related designs. This section will require us to grapple with two critical properties of BOLD fMRI data: the hemodynamic response function and the temporal autocorrelation of the noise. Attention will then be turned to related analysis issues. The steps of data preprocessing that prepare fMRI data for statistical analysis will be reviewed, followed by a consideration of univariate analysis of fMRI data.

This chapter previously appeared in *Functional MRI: Basic Principles and Clinical Applications*, edited by S. Faro and F. Mohamed. New York: Springer Science+Business Media, LCC 2006.

From: *BOLD fMRI: A Guide to Functional Imaging for Neuroscientists*
Edited by: S.H. Faro and F.B. Mohamed, DOI 10.1007/978-1-4419-1329-6_3
© Springer Science+Business Media, LLC 2010

Basic Types of Neuroimaging Inference

Regardless of the particular neuroimaging methodology employed [e.g., fMRI, positron emission tomography (PET), event-related potential (ERP)], there are a few broad categories of experimental question that might be asked. Each category probes a different aspect of the relationship between the brain and behavior, and each makes different assumptions for valid inference. Although not an exhaustive classification, these categories can help organize one's thinking about the assumptions that underlie a particular experiment.

In the past, neuroimaging techniques have been applied mostly to *localization* questions that asked: what are the anatomical neural correlates of a given mental operation? For example, does perception of a face activate a particular area of the brain different from that evoked by perception of other stimuli? Does the cognitive process of working memory evoke neural activity within the frontal lobe or somewhere else? In general, these designs present a subject with a task designed to selectively evoke a particular cognitive state of interest, and the neuroimaging method identifies if and where changes in neural activity accompany that cognitive process. Clearly, this type of experiment requires a way to manipulate the mental state of the subject, isolating the mental operation of interest from the other processes that invariably are present (e.g., button pushing, preparing responses, etc.). In the next section, several methods are considered that might be used to do so.

If successful, a localization study allows one to conclude that a particular area of the brain is activated by a particular cognitive operation. Importantly, neuroimaging methods in general are severely restricted in their ability to make conclusions regarding the necessity of a region for a cognitive operation. In other words, the presence of focal activation for a particular mental operation does not imply that a lesion to that area of the brain would impair the subject's ability to perform that mental operation. The reasons for this are manifold; for example, multiple areas of activity might be found, any one of which (perhaps working in parallel, or one serving as a backup for the other) would be capable of supporting the process of interest. In this case, the region still plays an interesting role in the cognitive process, although it is not strictly necessary. A second challenge is that we do not have perfect control over the mental states of the subject we seek to study. Although stimuli and instructions designed to evoke a particular cognitive process can be presented, there are no guarantees that the subject has entered that cognitive state and no other. The subject may unwittingly engage in confounding cognitive processes in addition to that intended by the experimenter, or alternatively, may fail to differentially engage the process. This is the central challenge of interpretation of most neuroimaging studies of localization—it is difficult to be certain that the experimental variable of interest has been properly manipulated.

Several applications of localization-type neuroimaging studies of patient populations can be conceived. The use of fMRI to identify the eloquent (or otherwise functionally important) cortex for neurosurgical planning is one example. Importantly, the caveats expressed above regarding the conclusion of necessity using a neuroimaging study are particularly relevant for this application (see Chapter 7 for further details). Localization studies also can be used in the study of rehabilitation and brain-damaged patients. Consider a patient with a focal lesion within a cortical area that previously has been demonstrated to be activated by a given mental operation. If the patient can still perform that mental operation despite the lesion, it could be presumed that some other back-up cortical area is now mediating this ability. A localization study could be used to identify the other cortical areas that are involved in the cognitive process.

In contrast, implementation studies ask about the computational mechanisms of a cognitive process within a cortical region. This type of study begins with the assumption that a cortical region engages in computations that support a particular cognitive process. The purpose of the study is then to determine the parameters of neural activity that mediate the area's participation in that process; for example, does an area of the prefrontal cortex change its bulk level of neural activity as a function of increasing working memory load (i.e., remember four items instead of two)? Is speed of motion encoded differently from direction of motion within area MT? As the field of cognitive neuroscience has moved beyond brain mapping, implementation experiments have become more prevalent. Patient studies might apply an implementation design to understand how altered performance in a clinical population is reflected in regional neuro-computational processing; for example, autistic patients are known to have impaired face recognition ability. Within an area of the fusiform gyrus that responds maximally to faces, do autistic patients have a blunted (or exaggerated?) response to changes in some properties of face perception, but not others; for example facial identity, emotional expression, or direction of gaze? Such a study might identify the specific processing impairment in autistics that is manifest clinically as impaired facial perception.

Finally, an evocation design reverses the typical direction of neuro-imaging inference and asks: What cognitive process does a given task evoke? This type of experiment leverages knowledge about the neural correlates of particular mental states to learn something about an imperfectly understood behavior. One begins by assuming that neural activity in a particular area of the brain is a marker of the presence of a particular mental state and no other; for example, neural activity of a certain magnitude at a certain spot in the fusiform gyrus indicates that the subject has the visual perception of a face. The subject then performs a task that may or may not evoke the cognitive process of interest; for example, ambiguous stimuli are presented that can be perceived as a face or a vase. If the specified neural activity is seen, the conclusion is drawn that the subject saw a face at that moment in time. Therefore, this type of design may be used to test hypotheses regarding the engagement of cognitive processes during a behavioral state in which the cognitive processes need not be under experimental control. Within the clinical realm, this type of design could be used, for example, to reveal intact visual pathway responses in patients with functional impairments from the psychiatric diagnosis of conversion disorder. The extent of depression might be inferred from the functional responses of the amygdala to sad stimuli. Alternatively, the level of consciousness or pain perception of a patient who is in a locked-in state might be assessed.

Usually, experiments from these three categories concern changes in the bulk neural activity measured by neuroimaging methods. However, other types of inference are also possible; for example, methods exist to measure the degree of effective connectivity between different cortical regions—the extent that one cortical region influences neural activity in another region.[1]

Such a metric could be used with any of these three categories of inference. One might hypothesize within an implementation framework that retrieval of semantic information about living things increases the effective connectivity between inferior frontal and ventral temporal regions, whereas retrieval of semantic information about tools is associated with similar connections between inferior frontal and premotor cortical areas.

Manipulation of the Cognitive Process

As was discussed previously, many neuroimaging experiments depend upon the isolated manipulation of a cognitive process for study. In particular, localization experiments require that a cognitive process of interest be isolated from other mental operations so that the neural correlates of that solitary process can be observed. In implementation experiments, some aspect of the stimulus or mental operation must be varied so that the neuro-computational correlate of its processing can be studied. Here, several broad classes of experimental manipulation of a cognitive operation are considered. Note that any of these techniques can be coupled with a particular temporal structure of design (e.g., event-related or blocked), which is described in the next section.

Cognitive subtraction is the prototypical method of isolation of a cognitive processes, and it is the most problematic. Typically, one condition of an experiment is designed to engage a particular cognitive process, such as face perception, episodic encoding, or semantic recall. This experimental condition is contrasted with a control condition designed to evoke all of the cognitive processes present in the experimental period except for the cognitive process of interest. Differences in neural activity between the two conditions are attributed to the cognitive process of interest. In essence, a cognitive process is isolated in an all-or-none fashion. As was discussed previously, we do not have direct control over the mental states of the subject, so the danger is always present that the subject might engage in a confounding mental operation in addition to the one of interest. Additionally, cognitive subtraction relies upon the assumption that a cognitive process can be added to a pre-existing set of cognitive processes without affecting them (an assumption termed pure insertion). This might fail if, for example, the act of pressing a button to signal a semantic judgment is different from pressing a button in response to a visual cue. Effects upon the imaging signal that result from this difference would be erroneously attributed to semantic judgment per se.

The cognitive conjunction design[2] has been proposed to reduce reliance upon the assumption of pure insertion. The method uses a set of paired cognitive subtractions, each of which need not completely isolate the cognitive process of interest. The imaging data are then analyzed to find areas that have a significant consistent response across subtractions. The identification of the same region across multiple pairs of subtractions strengthens the conclusion that the area is activated by the cognitive process that is isolated in each of the subtraction pairs.

Parametric designs offer an attractive alternative to cognitive subtraction approaches. In a parametric design, the experimenter presents a range of different levels of some parameter and seeks to identify relationships (linear or otherwise) between imaging signal and the values that the parameter assumes.

This can be done to identify the neural correlates of straightforward changes in stimulus properties or manipulations of a cognitive process. As compared to cognitive subtraction methods, failure of the pure insertion assumption is less plausible for parametric designs as the cognitive process is present during all conditions. This method can be extended further using *factorial* designs, in which multiple parameters are manipulated to identify additive and interactive changes in neural activity.[3]

There are further manipulations of stimuli and mental operations that have seen application in neuroimaging methods. For example, adaptation designs have been used to examine the sensitivity a of cortical area to particular stimulus properties.[4] The approach exploits the well-demonstrated repetition-suppression phenomenon in which a set of neurons have a reduced response to the repeated presentation of a stimulus; for example, one might hypothesize that the fusiform face area encodes a view-point independent representation of a face. Reduced responses from this cortical area to the second presentation of the same face viewed from a different angle would support this assertion.

Properties of the BOLD fMRI System That Impact Experimental Design

The preceding sections have described properties of experimental design that might apply to any neuroimaging method. In the next section, the ordering of experimental conditions in time will be discussed, and specifically, are will contrast blocked- and event-related designs. To understand the consequences of these experimental design choices, the idiosyncratic properties of one particular neuroimaging method will be considered: BOLD fMRI. Two key properties of BOLD fMRI data that fundamentally impact the design of BOLD fMRI experiments will be discussed here: the hemodynamic response function and the presence of low-frequency noise.

As was described in Chapter 1, changes in neural activity give rise to a series of vascular and hemodynamic changes that ultimately result in changes in the BOLD fMRI signal. Whereas many of the details of this relationship between neural activity and hemodynamic change are still under study, much of the messy detail can be side-stepped by noting that the transformation of neural activity to BOLD fMRI signal is nearly *linear*. This implies, for example, that a doubling in the amplitude of neural activity results in a doubling of the amplitude of the BOLD fMRI signal, and so on. One important property of BOLD fMRI as a linear system is that it can be well characterized by the *hemodynamic response function* (HRF). This is the BOLD fMRI signal that results from a brief (less than one second), intense period of neural activity. Given the shape of the HRF, one can predict the BOLD fMRI signal change that would result from any arbitrary pattern of neural activity.

The HRF itself can be measured empirically from human subjects by studying the BOLD fMRI signal that is evoked by experimentally induced brief periods of neural activity in known cortical areas (e.g., neural activity in the primary motor cortex in response to a button press). The shape of the HRF reflects its vascular origin and rises and falls smoothly over a period of about 16 seconds. Whereas the shape of the HRF varies significantly across subjects, it is very consistent within a subject, even across days to months.[5]

The stability of the shape of the HRF proves to be of value in the analysis of fMRI data, as it allows one to predict that pattern of BOLD fMRI signal that might result from an arbitrary pattern of neural activity. One difficulty, however, is that there is some evidence that the shape of the HRF varies from one region of the brain to another (perhaps from variations in neurovascular coupling). This is, however, a difficult notion to test, as it is necessary to create evoked patterns of neural activity in disparate areas of the brain that can be guaranteed to be very similar. A further problem is that the properties of the HRF may differ between elderly and young subjects, perhaps as a consequence of vascular disease.[6] The consequences of misspecification of the shape of the HRF will vary depending upon the experimental design used, as elaborated below.

The temporal dynamics of neural activity are quite rapid, on the order of milliseconds, but changes in blood flow take place over the course of seconds. One consequence of this, as demonstrated by the smooth shape of the HRF, is that rapid changes in neural activity are not well represented in the BOLD fMRI signal. The temporal blurring induced by the HRF leads to many of limitations placed on the types of experiments that can be conducted using BOLD fMRI. Specifically, the smooth shape of the HRF makes it difficult to discriminate closely spaced neural events. Despite this, it is still possible to detect: 1) brief periods of neural activity, 2) differences between neural events in a fixed order, spaced as closely as four seconds apart, 3) differences between neural events, randomly ordered, closely spaced (e.g., every second or less), and 4) neural onset asynchronies on the order of 100 milliseconds. The reason that these seemingly paradoxical experimental designs can work is that some patterns of events that occur rapidly or switch rapidly create a low-frequency envelope—a larger structure of pattern of alternation that can pass through the hemodynamic response function. In the next section, several types of temporal structures for BOLD fMRI experiments will be discussed, and how the shape of the HRF dictates the properties of these designs will be considered.

Another important property of BOLD fMRI data is that greater power is present at some temporal frequencies as compared to others under the null hypothesis (i.e., data collected without any experimental intervention). The power spectrum (a frequency representation) of data composed of independent observations (i.e., white noise), should be flat, with equal power at all frequencies. When calculated for BOLD fMRI, the average power spectrum is found to contain ever-increasing power at ever-lower frequencies, often termed a 1/frequency distribution. This pattern of noise also can be called pink, named for the color of light that would result if the corresponding amounts of red, orange, yellow, etc., of the visible light-frequency spectrum were combined. The presence of noise of this type within BOLD fMRI data has two primary consequences. First, traditional parametric and nonparametric statistical tests are invalid for the analysis of BOLD fMRI data, which is why much of the analysis of BOLD fMRI data is conducted using Keith Worsley and Karl Friston's "modified" general linear model[7] and its heirs, as instantiated in SPM and other statistical packages. The second impact is upon experimental design. Because of the greater noise at lower frequencies, slow changes in neural activity are more difficult to distinguish from noise.

Interestingly, the consequences for experimental design of the shape of the HRF and the noise properties of BOLD fMRI are at odds. Specifically, the shape of the HRF would tend to favor experimental designs that induce slow changes in neural activity, whereas the presence of low-frequency noise would argue for experimental designs that produce more rapid alterations in neural activity. As it happens, knowledge of the shape of the HRF and the distribution of the noise is sufficient to provide a principled answer as to how best balance these two conflicting forces.

It is worth noting that other neuroimaging methods have different data characteristics, with different consequences for experimental design; for example, perfusion fMRI is a relatively new approach that provides a non-invasive, quantifiable measure of local cerebral tissue perfusion.[8] Perfusion data do not suffer from the elevated low-frequency noise present in BOLD; consequently, perfusion fMRI can be used to detect extremely long time-scale changes in neural activity (over minutes to hours to days) that would simply be indistinguishable from noise using BOLD fMRI.[9] This may prove to be very advantageous in studies of clinical populations. Functional changes in patient cognition, either improvement by functional recovery following focal lesions or decline in neurodegenerative disease, evolve over long time scales as well. Perfusion fMRI can be used to obtain stable measurements of evoked neural activity from this dynamic system.

Different Temporal Structures of BOLD fMRI Experiments

As BOLD fMRI experiments by necessity include multiple task conditions (prototypically, an experimental and control period), several ways of ordering the presentation of these conditions exist. Different terms are used to describe the pattern of alternation between experimental conditions over time and include such familiar labels as blocked or event-related. Whereas these often are perceived as rather concrete categories, the distinction between blocked, event-related, and other sorts of designs is fairly arbitrary. These may be better considered as extremes along a continuum of arrangements of stimulus order. Consider every period of time during an experiment as a particular experimental condition. This includes the inter-trial–interval or baseline periods between stimulus presentations. In this setting, blocked and event-related designs are viewed simply as different ways of arranging periods of rest (or no stimulus) with respect to other sorts of conditions. (For a more complete exploration of these concepts, see Friston[10]).

The prototypical fMRI experimental is a blocked approach in which two conditions alternate over the course of a scan. For most hypotheses of interest, these periods of time will not be utterly homogeneous, but will consist of several trials of some kind presented together. For example, a given block might present a series of faces to be passively perceived, a sequence of words to be remembered, or a series of pictures to which the subject must make a living/nonliving judgment and press a button to indicate his response. Blocked designs have the obvious difficulty that the subject can anticipate trial types, which may be undesirable in some settings (e.g., studies of recognition of novel versus previously learned words). On the other hand, blocked designs have superior statistical power compared to all other experimental designs. This is because the fundamental frequency of the boxcar can be positioned at an optimal location with respect to the filtering properties of the hemo-dynamic response function and the low-frequency noise. For typical shapes of the HRF and distributions of temporal noise, this ideal balancing point occurs with epochs of about 20 to 30 seconds in duration.

Event-related designs model signal changes associated with individual trials, as opposed to blocks of trials. This makes it possible to ascribe changes in signal to particular events, allowing one to randomize stimuli, assess relationships between behavior and neural responses, and engage in retrospective assignment of trials. Conceptually, the simplest type of event-related design to consider is one that uses only a single stimulus type and uses sufficient temporal spacing of trials to permit the complete rise and fall of the hemodynamic response to each trial; a briefly presented picture of a face once every sixteen seconds for example. This is frequently termed a sparse event-related design. Importantly, while this prototypical experiment has only one stimulus, it has *two* experimental conditions (the stimulus and the inter-trial–interval). If one is willing to abandon the fixed ordering and spacing of these conditions, more complex designs become possible. For example, randomly ordered picture presentations and rest periods could be presented as rapidly as once a second. The ability to present rapid alternations between conditions initially seems counter-intuitive, given the temporal smoothing effects of the hemodynamic response function. Whereas BOLD fMRI is insensitive to the particular high-frequency alternation between one trial and the next, it is still sensitive to the low-frequency envelope of the design. In effect, with closely spaced, randomly ordered trials, one is detecting the low-frequency consequences of the random assortment of trial types. These rapid event-related designs are fairly sensitive to the accurate specification of the HRF for their success (unless a basis set is used for analysis; see below).

For experimental settings in which one has an unlimited number of trials to present (e.g., flashes of light) but a limited period of scanning time, then rapid randomly ordered designs are more statistically powerful than sparse designs. Alternatively, when the experiment is limited by the number of available trials (e.g., pictures of flightless birds), then maximal statistical power is obtained by presenting the available trials in a sparse manner and stretching the scanning period out as long as possible.

The discussion thus far regarding event-related designs has assumed an ability to randomize perfectly the order of presentation of different event types. There are certain types of behavioral paradigms, however, that do not permit a random ordering of the events. For example, the delay period of a working memory experiment always follows the presentation of a stimulus to be remembered. In this case, the different events of the trial cannot be placed arbitrarily close together without risking the possibility of false-positive results that accrue from the hemodynamic response to one trial event (e.g., the stimulus presentation) being interpreted as resulting from neural activity in response to another event (e.g., the delay period). It turns out that, given the shape typically observed for hemodynamic responses, events within a trial as close together as four seconds can be reliably discriminated.[11] Thus, event-related designs can be used to examine directly, for example, the hypothesis that certain cortical areas increase their activity during the delay period of a working memory paradigm without requiring the problematic assumptions traditionally employed in blocked subtractive designs.

There is a multiplicity of further designs that might be considered that do not fall strictly within blocked or event-related categories. Neural-onset asynchrony designs[12,13] are used to detect differences in the timing of neural activity evoked by different stimuli. Here, a sparse event-related design is used, along with exquisite coupling of the timing of stimulus presentation to image acquisition. A difference in the time of onset of the smooth BOLD hemodynamic response evoked by two different stimuli within a cortical region is sought. Traveling wave stimuli are used to define topographic maps of cortical responses, the most familiar being the retinotopic organization of early visual areas.[14] These designs use stimuli that vary continuously across some sensory space (e.g., retinal eccentricity), and identify for any point within a cortical area what was the optimal position of the stimulus within the sensory space for the evocation of neural activity. These designs often are combined with cortical flat-map techniques for the display of results.[15]

Data Preprocessing

In a perfect world, BOLD fMRI images would be acquired instantaneously from a stationary brain of uniform shape. Unfortunately, this is not the case, and a number of processing steps must be performed prior to the statistical analysis of fMRI data. These steps have two primary goals: 1) to reverse displacements of the data in time or space that may have occurred during acquisition, 2) to enhance the ability to detect spatially extended signals within or across subjects. In this section several preprocessing steps will be discussed that are commonplace in the analysis of BOLD fMRI data.

Distortion Correction

Blood oxygenation level-dependent fMRI data typically are acquired as echoplanar images, and as such are likely to be distorted (stretched and pulled) in space to some extent as a result of static magnetic field inhomogeneities produced by concentration of magnetic field lines at (for example) air tissue interfaces. There are several methods to correct for this spatial distortion; in most cases, they use a map of the magnetic field within the bore of the magnet to correct distortion. Additionally, in most cases, this correction is performed by the scanning system itself prior to writing out image data for analysis and does not enter into the routine preprocessing of fMRI data at most institutions.

Slice Acquisition Correction

A single volume of BOLD fMRI data, collected during one TR, is assembled from multiple planar acquisitions (slices). One slice is collected at a time, either sequentially or in an interleaved fashion, with the result that each slice samples a slightly different point in time. For a repetition time (TR) of two seconds and 20 axial slices, this would mean that one slice of the brain would be obtained 1.8 seconds later than another spatially adjacent slice within the same TR. Consequently, a neural event that occurs simultaneously on multiple slices within the brain will appear as different time-delayed BOLD fMRI responses in the data from different slices. Slice-acquisition correction compensates for this staggered order of slice acquisition. The correction works by calculating (using sinc-interpolation) the BOLD fMRI signal that would have been obtained for a given slice had that slice been acquired instead at the beginning of the TR. While not of great importance for low-temporal-frequency blocked designs, this preprocessing step is quite important for even-related designs.

Motion Correction

A variety of methods are used to minimize head motion during scanning. These include foam padding around the head; bite bars; custom-designed, thermo-plastic face masks; and so on. Despite these efforts, subjects nonetheless move their heads during scanning. Therefore, a common data preprocessing step is to attempt to correct for the effects of this motion. This generally is done by realigning the image of the brain obtained at each point in time back to the first image acquired at the start of the scanning session. Several methods exist to do so, but most use a six-parameter motion correction in which the brain is treated as a rigid body and the six possible movements (three translations and three rotations) are calculated at each point in time to minimize the image difference between the realigned brain and the brain in its original position. Importantly, motion correction of this kind does not completely remove the effects of movement upon the BOLD fMRI signal. This is because movement of the brain within the exquisitely defined magnetic field gradients created during scanning alters the signal obtained at different points in the slice acquisition. As a result, even after realigning the brain to its original position, movement-induced signal artifacts can remain. Consequently, statistical analysis of BOLD data often will include nuisance covariates that are themselves the six movement parameters measured during realignment. These covariates serve to account for changes in the signal within voxels that are correlated with the movement of the head (see below for a further description of nuisance covariates).

Spatial Normalization

If one wishes to test a hypothesis regarding a certain area of the brain within a population, then it is first necessary to identify that same area of the brain across subjects. This is frequently done by computationally warping the anatomical structure of the brain of one subject to match a template brain within a standard defined space. While there are a variety of sophisticated methods available for registering and aligning the brains of different subjects into a standard space, there are theoretical limits to what such an alignment can achieve. First, there may be intersubject variability in anatomy that cannot be overcome by warping brains to a standard space. For example, the arrangement of the sulci may vary between subjects. Thus, while two subjects may have neural responses at the same true cyto-architectonic location, the position of this site with respect to other landmarks in the brain may differ between subjects, leading to spread of these locations when data are converted to a standard space. Second, even given rigid alignment of anatomy across subjects, there may be variability in the structure to function relationships between subjects. For example, two subjects may truly have distinct face-selective neural regions, but these may be located in different sections of a cortical area as a consequence of differences in experience. Again, when normalized to a standard space, this variability in location will obscure functional dissociations. An alternative to anatomical registration is functional identification. The approach here is first to identify a region across subjects by its functional responses. For example, one might identify a region that responds more to pictures of faces than to general objects. Then hypotheses regarding the response of this functionally defined region to other types of stimuli can be tested independently across subjects within this area. This powerful approach allows one to make inferences across subjects regarding the responses of some functional area (e.g., the fusiform face area) at the expense of making statements regarding some particular position in a standardized anatomical space.

Spatial Smoothing

It is a common practice to digitally smooth BOLD fMRI data in space prior to statistical analysis. There are several reasons for this. First, BOLD fMRI data typically are composed of time-series information from many thousands of individual voxels. Statistical analysis of this data involves application of a statistical test (e.g., t test) at each of these voxels. Because there are thousands of individual statistical tests being performed, control of the false-positive rate requires a fairly large t result to exceed the chance that random noise will produce a significant result in one or more of those thousands of voxels. By smoothing the data in space, one reduces the number of independent statistical tests that are being performed, thus allowing less-stringent control over what t value is considered a significant result. Another motivation for smoothing is that, when analyzing data across a population, spatial smoothing helps to overcome residual differences in anatomy between subjects that might otherwise render common areas of activation nonoverlapping. The amount of spatial smoothing to perform can be difficult to determine, as smoothing too much will decrease statistical sensitivity for small focal areas of activation, whereas smoothing too little will have the same deleterious effects upon large areas of signal change. A reasonable balance between these two extremes can be obtained by smoothing data with a filter that has a width roughly equal to the size (in voxels) of predicted areas of activity.

Statistical Analysis

Several methods exist to analyze BOLD fMRI data. Some of these are described as multivariate techniques, in which latent patterns of spatially coherent activity are identified automatically by the method (e.g., Partial Least Squares[16]). The more commonly implemented univariate techniques will be focused upon here, in which a statistical model is applied to each voxel independently within a data set. The discussion concerns in particular the details of the creation of a statistical model for analysis. In many software packages, such as statistical parametric mapping (SPM), some of these details are handled automatically. The purpose of this section is to provide an understanding of what is going on under the hood.

The centerpiece of the analysis of neuroimaging data is the construction of a model that is composed of one or more covariates. In general, covariates are predictions regarding patterns of variability in the data expressed as changes in the BOLD fMRI signal over time within a single voxel. The better the predictions, the more valid and powerful the statistical model becomes. Covariates can be divided broadly into two categories. Covariates of interest describe changes in the signal that typically are the result of experimental manipulations and are the subject of hypothesis testing. Covariates of no interest instead describe changes in the signal that are unintended or undesired; they are not typically the focus of a hypothesis test.

Covariates of interest might be generated in one of two ways. First, covariates might be created to model the expected shape in time of evoked BOLD fMRI signal changes. A principled way to create covariates of this kind is to begin with a prediction regarding the pattern of neural activity that might be evoked by the experiment in a single voxel. For example, a simple blocked experimental design might be predicted to produce a uniformly greater amount of bulk neural activity during an experimental condition as compared to a control condition. The anticipated BOLD fMRI signal under these circumstances can be obtained by applying a model of the HRF to the predicted pattern of neural activity. As was mentioned previously, knowledge of the HRF is sufficient to predict the BOLD fMRI signal that will result from any arbitrary pattern of neural activity through the mathematical process of convolution. This prediction of BOLD fMRI signal change is then suitable for use as a covariate of interest. The model of the HRF that is used might be obtained from the subject himself during a preliminary experiment,[5] or an average representation of an HRF across subjects might be employed, as is the case in the SPM and other analysis packages.

Alternatively, covariates of interest can represent not a specific pattern of BOLD fMRI response, but instead have the property of flexibly fitting a family of possible responses that might occur. This approach uses a basis set, which is a collection of covariates that can be scaled and combined to fit any pattern of BOLD fMRI response that might be evoked within a set period of time by a particular experimental condition. In general, the basis set will be composed of multiple covariates, with as many elements as there are points in time to be modeled. For example, in a sparse event-related experiment in which a stimulus is presented every 8 TRs (16 seconds at a TR of 2), then a basis set of eight covariates will be needed to model, in effect, the average evoked BOLD fMRI response across trials. Typically, there is no clear interpretation of any one element of a basis set. Instead, one interprets the explanatory power of the set en mass using an F test. Basis set approaches provide the advantage of flexibility in that one is sensitive to any pattern of response (or difference between two trial types) that might take place. The price of this flexibility is reduced inferential power. One can no longer say, for example, that a given response was greater in amplitude than another, or longer in duration. Instead, one can only say that some consistent response was present.

As was mentioned earlier, covariates of no interest model changes in the BOLD fMRI signal that are not thought to be the result of experimental influence. For example, if one was aware of an influence of the room temperature upon the BOLD fMRI signal, and if the pattern of fluctuations of the room temperature were known, a representation of temperature could be included as a covariate to explain variations in the signal that are attributable to temperature fluctuations. Note that some covariates that are not of interest model changes in neural activity and some do not. For example, the experiment occasionally may present instruction screens, which would be expected to elicit transient changes in neural activity that are not the subject of any hypothesis. For these types of covariates that model expected neural effects of no interest, one would want to convolve the representation of neural change by the HRF. For other covariates that are not derived from neural activity (e.g., a measure of subject head motion), then convolution is not indicated.

One can further classify covariates of no interest as nuisance covariates or confounds. A nuisance covariate is defined as a covariate, the inclusion of which is expected to alter only the magnitude of the error term, but not the relationship between the data and covariates of interest. When covariates of no interest are correlated with covariates about which one wishes to test a hypothesis, they are termed confounds, and their inclusion will be expected to alter the behavior of the covariates of interest. Under some circumstances, the sign of the relationship between the covariate of interest and the data can be reversed. An example of a covariate that frequently acts as a confound is a global signal covariate. A global signal is average signal change over time across the entire brain, obtained by taking a simple average of the voxel-wise time series. It is common to included a measure of the global signal as a covariate of no interest (or to scale the data prior to analysis by this measure) to remove changes in blood oxygenation that impact the entire brain (resulting from changes in heart rate or respiration) that otherwise would obscure regional changes in neural activity. Because of the way in which it is measured, however, the global signal is expected to have some positive correlation with any experimentally evoked signal changes (as the average of all brain voxels will include those voxels responding to the task). As a result, correction for global signal changes can have a confounding effect upon covariates of interest and greatly change the interpretation of evoked signal changes.[17]

The resulting statistical model, composed of covariates of interest and those of no interest, is then used to evaluate the time-series data from each voxel within the brain. The resulting weights upon the covariates (termed beta values) then can be evaluated alone or in combinations using t and F statistics. The product is a statistical map in which every voxel in the brain contains a corresponding statistical value for the contrast of the covariates of interest. The final step of analysis involves assigning a level of statistical significance to those values. If the data set was composed of a single voxel, then this would be a straightforward enterprise: a t value of greater than 1.96 would be significant at a $p = 0.05$ level (presuming many degrees of freedom and a two-tailed test). Because there are many voxels, however, the likelihood that noise alone might render one t value significant if many are tested must be corrected. Such a correction attempts to control the false-positive rate at a *map-wise* level, meaning that if twenty statistical maps were produced under null-hypothesis conditions (i.e., in the absence of any actual experimental treatment), only one, on average, would be expected to contain even a single false-positive voxel. Solutions to perform this correction in the face of spatial smoothness within the statistical map (which yields statistical test in adjacent voxels that are not fully independent) exist within Gaussian Random Field Theory.[7]

Performing the appropriate map-wise correction to control the false-positive rate frequently can yield a rather stringent statistical value necessary to label any result significant. In turn, this raises concerns about false-negative results in which true experimental effects might be missed because the experiment is underpowered. There are several responses to this concern. Beyond the flippant call for more data, one might choose to relax the p value that will be accepted as significant. Note that stating that the data were evaluated at a $p = 0.1$ level (corrected for multiple comparisons) is more intellectually honest than reporting results at a $p = 0.00023$ level (uncorrected), the latter tending to lull statistically naïve readers into a false sense of security. It also is preferable, whenever possible, to anatomically narrow one's hypothesis test. Using a predefined region of interest within which to test hypotheses can greatly reduce the number of independent statistical tests for which correction is required improves power. In the limit, the number of tests can be reduced to one by taking the average signal within a region and performing the statistical test upon this representative data. Several methods are available for the definition of regions of interest. They might be defined anatomically based upon gyral or cyto-architectonic boundaries, or on the basis of previously reported lesion or functional neuroimaging studies. Regions of interest also might be defined functionally; for example, subjects might participate in an initial scan, the purpose of which is to define a region of cortex that is maximally responsive to faces. Data obtained from this putative face region in subsequent experiments could then be studied with the benefits of having focused the hypothesis test. Finally, regions might be defined using a main effect contrast, with subsequent orthogonal interaction contrasts tested within the region. For example, an experiment might present pictures of upright faces and inverted faces. A region would be defined as the area that responds more to pictures of faces, in either orientation, as compared to a third baseline condition. Within the defined region, the difference in response between upright and inverted faces could be assessed without loss of statistical rigor, as the result of the test used to define the region does not prejudice the result of the subsequent orthogonal test of the effect of orientation of the stimulus. Of course, there are inferential consequences (such as loss of generality) of testing hypotheses only within predefined regions of interest. This might be countered by performing in the same experiment-focused hypothesis tests within regions of interest, followed by more exploratory analyses that evaluate the data from the remainder of the brain using appropriate map-wise correction for the increased number of voxels.

Yet another approach that has gained popularity is the use of a false-discovery rate statistical threshold.[18] Instead of controlling the false-positive rate at a map-wise level (allowing, for example, only one in twenty maps to have a single false-positive voxel), the FDR method controls the proportion of false-positive voxels present within a single map. For example, an FDR threshold of five percent implies that, of the voxels identified as significant within a statistical map, five percent of them are, on average, expected to be false positives. This is neither better nor worse than traditional map-wise control of the statistical significance, but is instead a different stance with regard to inference. FDR methods will likely be of considerable use in clinical applications; for example, it may be desirable to express the confidence of results of functional mapping for surgical planning in terms of the specificity of the population of voxels identified.

Another approach for estimating a collection of unobservable signals from observation of their mixtures uses independent component analysis (ICA). Several researchers have demonstrated that ICA identifies task-related loci of activation with accuracy comparable to that of established techniques (see the Appendix for details on ICA).

References

1. Buchel C, Friston KJ. Assessing interactions among neuronal systems using functional neuroimaging. *Neural Netw.* 2000;13:871–882.
2. Price CJ, Friston KJ. Cognitive conjunctions: a new experimental design for fMRI. *Neuroimage.* 1997;5:261–270.
3. Sternberg S. Separate modifiability, mental modules, and the use of pure and composite measures to reveal them. *Acta Psychol.* 2001;106:147–246.
4. Grill-Spector K, Malach R. fMR-adaptation: a tool for studying the functional properties of human cortical neurons. *Acta Psychol.* 2001;107:293–321.
5. Aguirre GK, Zarahn E, et al. The variability of human BOLD hemodynamic responses. *NeuroImage* 1998;8:360–369.
6. D'Esposito M, Zarahn E, et al. The effect of normal aging on coupling of neural activity to the BOLD hemodynamic response. *Neuroimage.* 1999;10(1):6–14.
7. Worsley KJ, Friston KJ. The analysis of fMRI time-series revisted-again. *Neuroimage.* 1995;2:173–182.
8. Detre JA, Alsop DC. Perfusion fMRI with arterial spin labeling. In: Bandettini PA, Moonen C, eds. *Functional MRI.* Berlin: Springer Verlag; 1999:47–62.
9. Aguirre GK, Detre JA, et al. Experimental design and the relative sensitivity of BOLD and perfusion fMRI. *Neuroimage.* In press.
10. Friston KJ, Zarahn E, et al. Stochastic designs in event-related fMRI. *Neuroimage.* 1999;10:607–619.
11. Zarahn E, Aguirre GK, et al. A trial-based experimental design for fMRI. *Neuroimage.* 1997;6(2):122–138.
12. Menon RS, Luknowsky DC, et al. Mental chronometry using latency-resolved functional MRI. *Proc Nat Acad Science U S A.* 1998;95:10902–10907.
13. Henson RNA, Price CJ, et al. Detecting latency differences in event-related BOLD responses: application to words versus nonwords and initial versus repeated face presentations. *Neuroimage.* 2002;15:83–97.
14. Engel SA, Rumelhart DE, et al. fMRI of human visual cortex [letter] [published erratum appears in Nature 1994 Jul 14;370(6485):106]. *Nature.* 1994;369(6481):525.
15. Sereno MI, Dale AM, et al. Borders of multiple visual areas in humans revealed by functional magnetic resonance imaging [see comments]. *Science.* 1995;268(5212):889–893.
16. McIntosh AR, Bookstein FL, et al. Spatial pattern analysis of functional brain images using partial least squares. *Neuroimage.* 1996;3:143–157.
17. Aguirre GK, Zarahn E, et al. The inferential impact of global signal covariates in functional neuroimaging analyses. *Neuroimage.* 1998;8(3):302–306.
18. Nichols T, Hayasaka K. Controlling the familywise error rate in functional neuroimaging: A comparative review. *Stat Methods Med Res.* 2003;12(5):419–446.

4

Challenges in fMRI and Its Limitations

R. Todd Constable

Introduction

This chapter will explore some of the challenges of functional magnetic resonance imaging (fMRI), particularly the constraints encountered in terms of spatial and temporal resolution, as well as the factors that limit the ability of MRI to detect functional activation. These issues of sensitivity and resolution are intimately related and not easily separable; for example, increasing spatial resolution usually can only be achieved at the expense of temporal resolution and sensitivity loss. In addition to examining the factors limiting the sensitivity and resolution of fMRI, this chapter will explore some of the trade-offs involved in optimizing one or more of these variables.

There are a number of characteristics that the ideal functional MRI experiment would exhibit. Chief among them is the ability to acquire reliable data in a short period of time with high spatial and temporal resolution. It is currently an open question as to what the ultimate spatial and temporal limits should be. Generally, if investigators had the flexibility of choosing from a range of spatial and temporal resolutions, the choice would need to be tailored to the specific application. The challenges in obtaining reduced acquisition times with high spatial and temporal resolution will be discussed in detail in the sections that follow.

As fMRI experiments are performed at higher fields, the limits of temporal and spatial resolution continue to be pushed. Recent experiments have shown that fMRI is capable of sufficient resolution to examine cortical columns in the visual cortex, and that activation maps have been presented demonstrating differential activation across cortical layers. It is unlikely, for reasons explained below, that ultimately all experiments will be performed at very high spatial resolution (at the layer of columns), but continued improvements in fMRI acquisition strategies are bringing this goal closer. Clearly, much more needs to be understood about brain function at the systems level, at the level of the cortical layers, and ultimately

<hr>

This chapter previously appeared in *Functional MRI: Basic Principles and Clinical Applications*, edited by S. Faro and F. Mohamed. New York: Springer Science+Business Media, LCC 2006.

From: *BOLD fMRI: A Guide to Functional Imaging for Neuroscientists*
Edited by: S.H. Faro and F.B. Mohamed, DOI 10.1007/978-1-4419-1329-6_4
© Springer Science+Business Media, LLC 2010

at the neuronal level. Much research is underway examining brain function at all of these levels, and as these systems become better understood, the required spatial and temporal resolution for specific fMRI investigations will become more clear.

Most cognitive and many sensory/motor fMRI experiments are limited in terms of spatial and temporal resolution by a range of factors. Some of the limitations are imposed by the physics of magnetic resonance (MR), some are physiological, and others are neuronal systems based. The sections that follow discuss these issues in detail.

MR Physics-Based Limitations in fMRI

As explained in Chapter 1, the reader should keep in mind that magnetic resonance imaging (MRI) is based primarily on measuring signals from protons (H) on water molecules (H_2O). The local magnetic environment that these protons experience determines in part the signal strength obtained from a given tissue region. The magnetic properties of blood are different depending on the oxygenation state of the hemoglobin (Hb), with deoxy-hemoglobin (diamagnetic) introducing small local field inhomogenenities and oxyhemoglobin (paramagnetic) producing a more uniform microscopic field homogeneity. During the echo time (TE), the protons (water molecules) diffuse in and around these Hb molecules. Protons diffusing near deoxyhe-moglobin will experience a range of local magnetic fields, leading to rapid dephasing of the signal, and hence, signal loss. This state typically represents the baseline or control condition in an fMRI experiment. As deoxygenated blood is replaced by oxygenated blood upon neuronal activation, the amount of dephasing is reduced as the local field inhomogeneities are reduced and the water protons experience a more uniform field as they diffuse. Therefore, the signal in the presence of oxygenated blood decays more slowly, and thus, at the echo time, TE, there will be more signal remaining in the oxygenated state than in the deoxygenated state. Comparing the signal obtained in the activation state with the control state, a small increase in signal intensity is observed of the order of four percent or less (at 1.5T), with the actual amount dependent upon a range of factors. This slight change in signal is the chief mechanism exploited in fMRI and forms the basis of blood oxygenation level-dependent (BOLD) contrast.

Physics-Based Limitations on Spatial Resolution

Two parameters are of interest in determining the optimum spatial resolution of MRI; these are image signal and noise. Signal is the signal intensity recorded by the coil for any given tissue. It is dependent upon the amount of magnetization present at the time of the echo. The amount of magnetization present is dependent upon field strength (higher field strength results in higher spin polarization, leading to greater initial magnetization), relaxation times (signal decays with two different relation times T1, T2, and in the case of gradient echo imaging, a third time, T2*), proton density, and the imaging parameters and magnetization history. Proton density refers to how much water is present in a given volume of tissue.

Holding all other imaging parameters constant, the signal varies in direct proportion to the voxel volume. The voxel volume, of course, is directly related to the spatial resolution, and it is typically changed by changing the spatial encoding gradient strength (and hence the field of view) and/or by increasing the acquisition matrix size. The relationship between spatial resolution and the signal-to-noise ratio (SNR) is given by: $SNR \propto \Delta x \Delta y \Delta z \sqrt{N_x} \sqrt{N_y} \sqrt{N_{ave}} / \sqrt{v}$, where Δx and Δy represent the voxel dimensions in x and y, Δz is the slice thickness, N_x, N_y represent the sampling matrix size in the x and y directions, N_{ave} is the number of averages, and v represents the acquisition bandwidth (one over the sampling rate of the data acquisition).

In general, the noise is unaffected by changes in voxel volume, but the signal intensity is directly proportional to the voxel volume. Voxel volume is determined by the product of slice thickness times the in-plane spatial resolution (volume = $\Delta x \Delta y \Delta z$). The in-plane resolution is determined by dividing the field of view (FOV) in the x- and y-directions by the acquisition matrix size in these directions. Consider some typical imaging parameters—For a 200 × 200 millimeter (mm) FOV and an acquisition matrix of (N_x = 64) × (N_y = 64) the in-plane voxel size is 3.125 × 3.125 millimeter (dividing 200mm/64). A slice thickness of Δz = 5mm will then result in a voxel volume of 3.125 × 3.125 × 5 = 48.8 mm^3. Changing any of these dimensions can have a dramatic effect on SNR. Decreasing the slice thickness by a factor of two will reduce the volume by half; thus, the SNR will be reduced by a factor of two. Similarly, doubling the in-plane resolution in the x and y directions simultaneously (which will reduce the voxel size in the above example to 1.56 × 1.56 mm^2) will reduce the voxel volume, and hence the SNR, by a factor of four. Clearly, the choice of imaging resolution has a significant impact on the SNR of the images.

If sufficient SNR is present in the raw images of an fMRI experiment, the spatial resolution may be increased by increasing the matrix size, or decreasing the FOV, or both. Ultra-high resolution MR images have been obtained with in-plane resolutions of the order of tens of micrometers, which is easily the size of individual neurons. The ultimate constraints on the spatial resolution in MR arise from two phenomena. First, most imaging is performed by collecting an echo, and while this echo is being collected, the signal is decaying across the echo with a relaxation time of T2 in a spin echo sequence, or T2* in a gradient echo sequence. In most fMRI experiments, the effects of this T2 decay across the echo are minimal, but as the resolution becomes very high, the blurring caused by T2 decay can begin to dominate and limit the resolution achievable. At this extreme, tissues with long T2 will be sharper than tissues with shorter T2; thus, the resolution throughout the image may vary as a function of tissue T2. The second limiting factor is the diffusion rate of water. Because MR images rely on the signal obtained from freely diffusing water, if the water molecules move a significant amount during data acquisition, this will lead to a blurring, reducing the ability to localize the signal. The localization of this signal is limited to the mean square diffusion distance of water in the amount of time required to spatially localize the signal. At the extremes of spatial resolution in MR, water diffusion is the ultimate limiting factor (see Callaghan PT, Principles of Nuclear Magnetic Resonance Microscopy, Oxford Science Publications, 1993). To date, MRI experiments are in a regime well removed from this diffusion effect; therefore, this is not a primary limiting factor in fMRI. As will be seen below, there are a number of other considerations—such as the number of slices acquired, temporal resolution, image distortion, and brain coverage— that can influence the choice of spatial resolution. Most studies to date that have used very high spatial resolution tend to focus on one specific cortical area, and studies involving whole brain coverage typically are performed at much more modest spatial resolutions.

SNR and Field Strength

Increasing field strength leads to increased polarization of spin populations, and therefore to a larger initial magnetization vector. This holds true in fMRI with the added benefit that the measured change in BOLD amplitude also is larger at higher field.[1,2] This increase in BOLD signal change, and the increase in image SNR, can allow for imaging at higher spatial resolutions at higher fields, allowing for imaging at higher temporal resolution [repetition time (shorter TR)], and/or allow shorter imaging sessions. T1s are longer at higher field strength; thus, smaller flip angles or longer TRs must be used to ensure maximal signal amplitude. In contrast, T2s, and T2* in particular, are shorter at higher field strength; thus, the optimum TE for BOLD imaging is shorter than at lower field strength.

Noise in MRI is the term given to any unwanted signal, and these unwanted signals may arise from multiple sources. Thermal noise (random fluctuations of spins aligned with the field) is always present in MRI and can only be eliminated by reducing the sample temperature to absolute zero, which usually is not practical in fMRI. Some noise also is generated in the electronics of the MR scanner, and if other electronic equipments, such as projectors for presenting visual stimuli, are present in the room, these devices may emit radiofrequency (rf) radiation at a frequency that the head coil could pick up, also leading to significant noise. If the noise from a projector is at a particular frequency, then a streak artifact, a line of bright intensity, in the phase-encoded direction will be clearly visible, whereas if the rf noise is of a broader bandwidth, it will simply decrease the overall SNR of the images (and thus decrease the significance of any activations) without obvious artifacts.

Static Field Inhomogeneities

Also amplified at higher field strengths are the problems of field inhomogeneities that result in signal loss and image distortion. Thus, without compensation methods for BOLD imaging in the presence of field inhomogeneities, moving to higher field strengths may not always be advantageous. Medial frontal and medial temporal areas are particularly affected by the amplification of susceptibility effects.

A number of methods have been investigated to attempt to reduce the impact of macroscopic field inhomogeneities. These are the local field inhomogeneities that arise at air/tissue junctions and, in particular, in brain regions near sinuses.[3] These are referred to as macroscopic static field inhomogeneities because they alter the main magnetic field in relatively large areas.

The challenge in solving this problem is that the BOLD mechanism relies upon differences in local microscopic field inhomogeneities between paramagnetic oxygenated and diamagnetic deoxygenated blood; therefore, a method that removes the pulse sequence sensitivity to field inhomogeneities will solve the signal-loss problem due to static field effects, but also will remove sensitivity to BOLD signal changes.

Static field effects are more pronounced along the largest dimension of a voxel, and the source of signal loss is dephasing across this dimension. In most cases, the slice thickness (Δz) represents the largest dimension of a voxel, and because the largest dimension is the most sensitive to signal loss through dephasing, all the methods developed to date have focused on reducing this through-plane dephasing. It should be noted, however, that most of the methods developed are general and can be applied in any direction. Decreasing the voxel size in any dimension (Δx, Δy, Δz) will reduce the dephasing across that dimension. The simplest approach to reducing macroscopic susceptibility loss is to move to thinner slices and higher spatial resolution.[4,5] This involves a significant cost, however, in terms of absolute number of images collected and the necessarily longer TR required to accommodate the additional slices need to cover the same brain region. Increasing the TR to accommodate these additional slices leads to a decrease in statistical power[6] and decreases temporal resolution.

Other approaches to solving this problem include z-shimming[7–9,73,74] based on original work by Frahm,[10] in which multiple acquisitions are collected with different z-refocusing gradient lobes, wherein these gradients are designed to cancel the gradients created by macroscopic susceptibility effects in the body. A minimum of two acquisitions are required (thereby effectively doubling TR), with more acquisitions leading to better compensation. An alternative approach is to design tailored rf pulses[11,12] such that the rf imposes a phase gradient across the slice, which compensates the phase shifts introduced by the local field gradients. Theoretically, such pulses can be designed, but in practice it is very difficult to play out these pulses in a reasonable amount of time, and the rf power deposition can be a limiting factor.

Many of these approaches are multi-shot approaches, requiring 2 or more acquisitions, and thus incur penalties in temporal resolution and statistical power. Two single-shot z-shimming approaches have been presented. Song and colleagues[13] showed results in which two gradient echo images were collected with different z-shim gradients on each side of a 180-degree rf pulse. More recently, Yang[14] published a single-shot approach in which the even echoes in an echo train had one z-shim value, whereas the odd k-space line acquisitions had a second z-shim value and the phase-encoded gradient was only incremented on every other echo rather than on each echo. Such an approach produces two exactly registered (except for distortion effects in the x-direction) z-shim images with equal T2* weighting in a single shot, and therefore without the usual penalty in TR. This approach, however, doubles the width of the acquisition window, which in turn increases the geometric image distortion in the y direction by a factor of two. Because these single-shot approaches also at least double the acquisition window width, fewer slices may be obtained within a given TR, or increased TR is required to collect the same number of slices as a conventional single-shot acquisition. Thus, the ideal solution remains to be found for compensating for these field inhomogeneities while maintaining BOLD sensitivity and temporal resolution.

Moving to higher field strengths, such as 3T or greater, provides sufficient BOLD contrast using spin echo techniques or asymmetric spin-echo methods wherein microscopic field effects are not refocused by the spin echo, but macroscopic effects are refocused. Spin echo–based BOLD imaging has been shown at 1.5T[15], but the sensitivity at this relatively low field strength is insufficient for most fMRI applications. Sensitivity increases with field strength, and using an asymmetric spin echo echo planar imaging (EPI) acquisition, it is possible to tune the sensitivity to field inhomogeneities at different scales.[16–18]

Effect of Acquisition TR

If functional imaging is to be performed in a small, localized brain region, and if subject motion is minimal, then scanning with short TR of the order of one second or less provides excellent statistical power relative to the same study performed with a much longer TR.[6] In the limit of decreasing TR, the temporal correlations in the data leads to redundant data collection, and thus the gain in statistical power as TR is decreased diminishes at very short TR. However, if subject motion is a problem, moving to a longer TR with maximal spatial coverage and very high resolution (both in-plane and through-plane) maximizes the ability of motion-correction algorithms to re-register the brain volumes collected over time. In this case then, moving to a longer TR and increasing through-plane resolution and coverage can improve the statistical power in the data. The reader is clearly learning at this point that there are no easy trade-offs in fMRI and many factors must be considered in designing a study and choosing the imaging pulse sequence and parameters. While the discussion above has focused primarily on MR physics-based challenges in fMRI, the next section discusses a number of physiological phenomena that tend to be the dominant factors limiting the resolution of fMRI.

Physiological Factors Influencing Spatial Resolution

In addition to the standard physics-based factors of signal and noise influencing the spatial resolution of the underlying MR images, a number of physiological factors also impact the resolution that can be obtained with functional MRI.

Physiological-Based Limitations/Constraints in fMRI

Physiological noise refers to the introduction of unwanted signal changes to the fMRI time-course data as a function of various physiological processes not directly associated with the functional region of the brain that is of interest. The two dominant sources of this noise include signal changes as a function of pulsatile flow through the brain associated with the cardiac cycle and signal changes associated with respiration. These two primary sources of noise contribute substantially to the need for collecting multiple images per task condition in order to reliably detect brain activation. In the case of the cardiac cycle, the entire brain pulsates with each beat of the heart, introducing both very small motions and variable vessel flow conditions that must be averaged out of the data. Respiration changes the susceptibility in the chest as deoxygenated air in the chest is replaced with oxygenated air, and while the chest is obviously some distance from the brain, these changes in susceptibility are detectable in the brain.[19]

Blood Oxygenation Changes and Localization

A local change in blood oxygenation in the capillaries does not simply produce a local change in the magnetic field in the capillary. Magnetic field changes are always locally smooth (there are never discontinuities in magnetic field gradients); thus, the field inhomogeneity produced by deoxyhemoglobin extends beyond the wall of the capillary containing the blood. Furthermore, the water, which, as was seen above, produces the signal that is recorded, diffuses some distance past these inhomogeneities and also can broaden the effective spatial extent of the field perturbation. Together these factors tend to increase the area in which the signal changes are detectable and lead to signal changes in the cortical tissue, not just the individual capillaries.

The density of the local vasculature also may impact the amplitude of the signal change detected. A change in oxygenation of blood in a capillary-dense region (high blood volume) will have a bigger impact on the BOLD signal intensity than the same relative change in oxygenated blood in a region with a sparse capillary network. Work in animal models has demonstrated variable cortical and subcortical capillary densities in several brain regions.[20]

The change in blood oxygenation that occurs with activation is over and above the increase in demand for oxygenated blood, and the extent of the region in which a vasculature response is initiated may be larger than the local region where function is increased. This also may contribute to an over estimation of the functional area under investigation. It is currently unclear as to what is the exact relationship between the spatial extent of the cortical tissue activated (and the number or fraction of neurons in that region that are activated) and the spatial extent of the region experiencing a blood-flow response.

Functional Spatial Limitations

The question of maximal resolution obtainable with fMRI may be turned around, and the question might be posed in terms of the minimum functional unit that can cause a blood-flow response upon activation. In fMRI, typically hundreds of thousands of neurons are included in a voxel, and it is the mean activity of some part of those neurons that leads to a blood-flow response. The relationship between the number of neurons that fire and the BOLD response associated with that number is unclear. However, it is clear that there is a tight coupling between glucose utilization and neuronal spike activity, at least in the sensory/motor cortex. It is not currently feasible to measure by independent methods a significant fraction of the neurons involved in a particular task; thus, to date, investigators have either examined gross EEG-based signals or recorded single neuron spike activity and related magnitude changes in these measures (using either the change in power at a particular frequency in the case of EEG, or the spike rate in the case of single unit recordings) to the BOLD signal change detected.[21–25] Better spike recording methods must be developed before the relationship between the fraction of neurons firing in a voxel can be directly related to a change in oxygenation and/or blood-flow.

Brain System Dependent Limitations

As cognitive tasks become more sophisticated in design and more subtle cognitive functions are examined, it will be important to relate the BOLD activation signal to specific networks involved in a task; for example, in a region such as the primary motor cortex wherein the neurons for the digits in the hand are highly interleaved, it is not currently possible to distinguish activation patterns for the individual digits. There may be many other brain systems that are wired in this interleaved fashion, in which case it could be very difficult to distinguish between different functional roles for these interleave neurons. Clearly, if neurons are highly interleaved in the cortex, then different groups of neurons may be activated by different tasks within a single voxel, but if the same number are activated by different tasks, no difference in activation will be detectable. This also is related to the issue of the modularity of the brain. To what extent can brain functions be divided into separate modules and what are the neuronal components that make up these modules? Higher resolution fMRI studies may someday answer such questions, and this issue will ultimately determine the spatial resolution required for fMRI.

Draining Vein Problem

A problem that has been discussed since the advent of fMRI is the potential spatial misregistration of functional activity that may occur as a function of the microvasculature. The capillaries, in which the small changes in oxygenation take place upon activation, drain into larger veins downstream from the activation site. Because the amount of blood in a draining vein may be larger than in the upstream capillaries, and because the small changes that occur in each capillary may add up to larger BOLD signal changes in the draining veins, this effect could contribute to spatial misregistration of the activation some distance downstream from the true area of cortical activity. A recent study by Turner[26] used a quantitative analysis of the geometry of the venous vasculature together with hydrodynamic considerations to calculate upper bounds on the extent of this problem. These calculations revealed that an activated cortical area of 100 square millimeters could generate an oxygenation change in venous blood that extends no more than 4.2 millimeters beyond the edge of the activated area. While the venous blood obviously drains much greater distances beyond this limit, the oxygenation effect is sufficiently diluted as to be undetectable.

In an attempt to reduce the draining-vein problem and produce highly localized functional maps, Menon and Goodyear[27] used the initial increase in the BOLD signal intensity to image ocular dominance columns in the human visual cortex and demonstrated that this use of the initial slope of the BOLD signal increase was effective.

Field strength also influences the relative signal change with changes in oxygenation for both tissue and vessels. It has been shown, for example[28], that increasing field strength increases the BOLD sensitivity to tissue changes in oxygenation faster than the increase in vessels. Thus, moving to higher field strengths reduces the relative contribution of the venous signal changes compared to the true tissue signal changes.

The reader should keep in mind that the draining-vein problem does not preclude true BOLD activation in the cortical region activated, but can produce additional, potentially stronger activations further down-stream. The fact that the BOLD response in draining veins can be large allows them to be identified by the large percent signal change measured. Excluding signal changes above a certain threshold (in terms of percent signal change), it is possible to produce high-resolution maps of cortical function free of this draining-vein problem. Cheng and colleagues,[29] for example, produced maps of the cortical columns in the visual cortex adapting this approach to sustained stimulus presentations. But caution is required with this activation amplitude threshold approach because the signal in draining veins does not necessarily have to be large and the signal does gradually decrease with distance from the activation site so at some point the threshold approach will fail—and this point is unfortunately at maximal distance from the activation site.

Spin-echo imaging is sensitive to microscopic but not macroscopic susceptibility effects.[16–18] At high field strengths (3T and greater), this approach can achieve sufficient sensitivity for fMRI experiments and can mostly eliminate the draining-vein problem. It is well known that spin echo sequences are much less sensitive to the draining-vein problem. While most investigators do not like to admit it, the additional relatively large signal changes associated with larger veins can aid in detecting activation. The sensitivity of gradient echo and spin echo sequences to microscopic susceptibility changes is essentially equal; thus, the choice of gradient echo imaging over spin echo imaging is made to allow the contribution of larger vessels to the BOLD signal change to get an added boost from the bigger signal changes associated with these vessels.

Diffusion gradients also can be applied to BOLD imaging sequences to reduce contributions from large vessels[30,31]; in fact, it is possible to use maps of apparent diffusion coefficients to detect activation.[32–34]

Initial Dip

Another method to eliminate the draining-vein problem and to possibly provide more precise spatial localization of fMRI activity is to localize activation based on finding regions that exhibit an initial dip in BOLD signal intensity prior to the main signal-intensity increase. Following the presentation of a stimulation event, the blood-flow response in the cortical region involved in detecting or responding to the event often leads to a complicated pattern of signal changes. Some experiments have shown that there is first a decrease in signal intensity prior to the increased signal intensity typically observed in BOLD experiments. The initial dip was first observed using optical measures of oxy- and deoxyhemoglobin[35,36] and has more recently been demonstrated using BOLD-sensitive fMRI methods in the visual[37–40] and in the sensory/motor cortex.[75,76] Because the increased oxygen consumption occurs before the blood-flow response has had a chance to compensate, there is a brief decrease in the ratio of oxygenated to deoxygenated blood, leading to an initial dip in signal intensity. This initial dip is followed by a signal-intensity increase as the blood-flow response kicks in and overcompensates for the increased oxygen consumption, leading to an increase in the ratio of oxyhemoglobin to deoxyhemoglobin in the blood and the increase in BOLD contrast that most fMRI experiments typically rely upon. As the blood flow returns to baseline levels after these events, an under-shoot of the signal intensity is also often observed before the intensity finally returns to pre-stimulus levels.

Theoretically, the initial dip could provide extremely good localization of the activated regions because there is no draining-vein problem with this phenomenon, and it directly reflects increased oxygen consumption.[40] Kim and colleagues[41] exploited this phenomenon to map iso-orientation columns in the rat visual cortex. The initial dip also may be important in understanding the link between changes in cerebral blood flow (CBF), cerebral blood volume (CBV), partial pressure of oxygen (PO_2), and oxygen metabolism under dynamic conditions. However, there are two difficulties associated with the initial dip phenomenon. First, it is controversial in that it is not always observed. As Buxton[42] pointed out in a commentary on this issue, two recent studies using optical imaging techniques and whisker barrel stimulation paradigms in a rat model came to opposite conclusions regarding this phenomenon. Lindauer and colleagues[43] found no evidence for this initial decrease in tissue oxygenation, whereas Jones and colleagues[44] did find a reproducible initial increase in deoxyhemoglobin. Many fMRI experiments have failed to detect the initial dip. However, when dealing with such a small signal change in the presence of significant physiological noise, a negative result does not necessarily mean the phenomena does not exist. Secondly, the BOLD signal change associated with the initial dip is approximately one-tenth that observed with the later BOLD signal increases; thus, it is very difficult to measure with fMRI and not practical with current methods for the majority fMRI studies. Thus, while the initial dip may have the potential to provide excellent localization, it has so far proved elusive and the signal changes are much too small to yield reliable results.

Subject Movement

Subject movement is also a constant problem in fMRI experiments, and if human experiments are to move to considerably higher spatial resolution, improved motion-correction methods and motion-limiting devices will need to be developed. The trade-off in limiting subject motion is the tension between subject comfort and ability to move. It is possible to position a subject with sufficient padding, tape, and bite bars, such that they cannot move—however, it is not possible to keep such a subject in the magnet for very long time due to the discomfort associated with these restraints. Systems designed to track motion and algorithms that allow image registration incorporating geometric distortion-correction methods may ultimately improve the ability to correct for any motion, thereby eliminating the need for uncomfortable constraints to be placed on the subjects. Moving to higher field strengths may allow for reductions in the overall study time, and therefore may also allow more restraining devices to be used, particularly if the subject is made aware of the fact that the discomfort is only for a brief period of time. In most cases, however, the gain in SNR in moving to higher field strengths is used to increase the spatial resolution or add more tasks, both of which are good choices, but with the result that study time remains fixed.

Other Physiological Changes Associated with Brain Activation

As discussed above, if cerebral metabolic rate of oxygen consumption ($CMRO_2$) could be directly measured, or if a BOLD measure of the initial dip does indeed reflect the initial consumption of oxygen, then these approaches would likely provide the maximal spatial resolution. It is unlikely that other MR measures of neural activity, such as changes in CBV and CBF, will provide higher spatial resolution than the BOLD effect, as these changes also represent rather gross brain responses to increased oxygen demand.

Threshold Effects and Localization

All functional maps are statistical maps of some sort and therefore involve the use of a statistical threshold to be chosen in order to classify some tissue(s) as activated and some tissue(s) as unactivated. However, the actual threshold chosen is arbitrary and the spatial extent of activation varies significantly as a function of this arbitrary statistical threshold. In order to reduce the multiple comparisons problem and reduce the occurrence of spurious single voxel activations arising by chance alone, spatial filtering is also often preformed in the form of a median or cluster filter of some sort. The definition of the size of these filters is also arbitrary and can significantly influence the extent of the activation measured. Thus, spatial resolution of the final activation maps can be significantly influenced by the statistical parameters chosen in the analysis/display software.

Temporal Resolution of the BOLD Response

The above sections have focused on the issue of spatial resolution in fMRI, but in some cases it may be important to examine the time-course of activation for individual events. Action potentials are recorded as electrical spike activity, and these spikes fire over the course of milliseconds. Electrical recordings of ensembles of firing neurons record characteristic peaks and troughs in the form of evoked response potentials in time-scales of the order of hundreds of milliseconds. Functional MR imaging relies on the blood-flow response to such neuronal activity, which itself is much, much slower than the activity of individual neurons. From a single event, say, for example, a flash of a bright light lasting only 100 milliseconds, the blood-flow response in the primary visual cortex may start to increase some two seconds after the event, it may peak between six to eight seconds and return to baseline by 16 to 20 seconds after this single 100-millisecond flash of light. Because fMRI usually is focused on measuring the response of ensembles of neurons to particular stimuli, it may not be necessary to measure activity with extremely high temporal resolution. However, many interesting questions may be probed by examining even this slow blood-flow response with high temporal resolution, and recent work by Qgawa et al.[77] demonstrates BOLD sensitivity to neuronal system interaction that occur on the millisecond timescale.

There is little evidence to date that within the gross blood-flow response typically measured in fMRI there is detailed information reflecting evoked response potential patterns or specific spike timings. To investigate this further, fMRI experiments will need to be performed with very high temporal resolutions of the order of tens of milliseconds, and such acquisitions are possible—albeit with a very limited number of slices—with the current technology. The mechanism prompting the blood-flow response in the brain is not well understood, nor is the spatial extent of this mechanism clear relative to the actual neuronal activity, and it remains to be seen if there is a meaningful fine-grained modulation of this response with neuronal activity.

Most early fMRI experiments relied upon block designs wherein an activation condition was presented for 30 seconds or more at a time, and this was alternated with a control condition of equal duration many times over the course of a study. In such experimental designs, many images could be collected over the course of a condition and high temporal resolution was not all that important. (Although, as discussed above, shorter TR acquisitions can have significant benefits in terms of statistical power in the activation maps.) Many experiments are still performed using block-designed paradigms because these studies do not require precise timing between the image acquisition and the stimulus presentation, and because the statistical power in such studies is maximized and usually considerably greater than that obtained in event-related designs. Cognitively, however, block-design experiments can be of limited value if habituation effects or changes in strategy occur over the course of a long block of similar stimuli, or if the goal is to separate responses to individual stimuli according to some behavioral measure.

To make for much more natural stimulus presentations and to examine the blood-flow response to specific stimuli, many experimental designs have moved towards event-related studies. Despite the slow blood-flow and oxygenation responses to neuronal activity, many interesting phenomena can be investigated with event-related experimental designs; for example, it is possible to examine the temporal response in a specific region to a wide range of stimuli and quantitatively assess parameters such as time-to-peak, width of response, peak height, and other such factors. For a given brain region, it is possible to examine the linearity of the response as stimulus presentation rate is modified; such studies can provide insight into the coupling of blood-flow, oxygenation, and neuronal activity changes.

To properly sample this blood-flow response function, short TR acquisitions should be used. The TR should be of the order of two seconds or less, with shorter TR again being better, or a technique whereby the time-lock between stimuli presentation and image acquisition is varied such that over the course of many events, the blood-flow response is sampled with high temporal resolution.[78] Increasing the temporal resolution by decreasing the TR necessitates reducing the flip angle of the rf excitation pulse in order to maintain optimum signal. This reduced flip angle in turn leads to decreased SNR in the individual images, but the gain in statistical power associated with more of these noisier images being collected in a fixed imaging time, more than compensates for the slight decrease in SNR of the individual images.

It is very difficult, however, to compare the blood-flow responses across different brain regions, as local differences in the structure of the microvasculature may account for differences in the time-courses observed. It would be desirable to observe temporal progression of activation patterns moving from one region of the brain to another, thereby obtaining a sense of the communication between different brain areas. This is not possible, however, without first characterizing the local variations in the structure of the microvasculature in different cortical regions. Thus, while it is difficult to make claims about the progression of activation from region A to B to C as a single task progresses, it is possible to observe differences in the order of this progression across two or more different tasks, assuming the plumbing remains constant and independent of the task. Event-related paradigms combined with high temporal resolution fMRI acquisition techniques are still in their infancy, and much more will be learned from such studies as the field progresses. A detailed review of such experimental designs for use in fMRI is given in the previous chapter.

Temporal resolution as defined by TR also impacts the ability to filter out or remove periodic noise such as that arising from the cardiac or respiratory cycle. Most acquisition strategies sample at a high enough rate to remove some noise from respiratory effects, but a close look at the noise power spectrum in fMRI revealed that components associated with the cardiac cycle aliased at many different (lower) frequencies due to the relatively low sampling rate of the fMRI data. By low sampling rate, it is meant that a slice acquisition is repeated say every second or more, rather than the required sampling rate of at least 500 milliseconds relative to the cardiac cycle, which has a period of approximately 1,000 milliseconds. Sampling at rates that are at least double the periodicity avoids aliasing of noise components to lower frequencies and makes removal of these components much easier in postprocessing.

Pulse Sequences for fMRI: Spatial/Temporal Resolution

The most common pulse sequences used in fMRI, EPI, and spiral imaging are discussed in detail in Chapter 2. This section will discuss briefly some aspects of these two sequences and alternative strategies that have been investigated to date. If high temporal resolution is desired, most MR imagers are now equipped with the gradient hardware to provide this information with image acquisition times of the order of 40 milliseconds or less. Echo planar imaging and single-shot spiral methods acquire the entire data set for an image from a single excitation pulse, and thus within a single TR. In conventional MRI, a separate excitation pulse is used for each line of data acquired, allowing a time, TR, to elapse for the magnetization to recover before the next excitation pulse. Thus, in conventional scanning, an image with 64 phase-encoding steps would require $64 \times$ TR seconds to acquire the entire dataset. With a TR of 1.5 seconds, this represents an acquisition time of over one minute. Echo planar imaging methods, on the other hand, can collect the data for an entire image in as little as 40 milliseconds. Collecting the data in such a rapid manner does have drawbacks. There is a significant decrease in SNR due to the high bandwidth of the data acquisition, which is needed to collect the data rapidly, and there are also significant distortion effects arising from the accumulation of phase errors over the sampling window. These distortion effects arise in the phase-encoded direction in EPI, and they are projected in all directions in spiral scanning. This distortion is not present in the conventionally acquired anatomic scans, upon which the activation is usually highlighted. Thus, caution must be used in high-resolution work to ensure that the distorted functional image is registered appropriately to the undistorted anatomic image. This is a difficult problem, as the distortion in the functional images is locally variable; thus, simple rigid body fitting of the two different acquisitions is not sufficient to avoid this problem.[45]

Methods for reducing the image distortion include moving to multi-shot methods, which of course involves a penalty in temporal resolution. Another approach is to measure in vivo the image distortion, and then use a map of the distortion to correct the final image. Two approaches have been devised to perform this measure; these are field mapping (the image distortion is directly proportional to the distortion in the static magnetic B-field)[46–48] and point spread function mapping (PSF).[49,50] The field map approach can provide a relatively simple method for correcting image distortions, but it contains no knowledge of the initial distribution of image intensities. This limitation makes it difficult to assign the correct image intensity—and hence functional activation—to the undistorted voxels. The PSF approach can correctly assign the appropriate image intensities to each voxel in addition to correctly locating each voxel in space.

A field map can be obtained using EPI with only two EPI data acquisitions. However, because the field map is calculated from the phase difference between these two images, phase wrap can be a problem. This problem can be reduced by collecting several acquisitions with different phase-offsets, thereby making unwrapping of the phase errors much easier. Point spread function maps require a minimum of 16 acquisitions to obtain the PSF in a single direction, but more acquisitions yield higher-resolution PSF maps, and thus better correction of the image distortion. In summary, with acquisition times of one minute or less, field maps or PSF maps can be obtained at some point in an fMRI study, allowing correction of the geometric image distortion.

Despite this problem of image distortion, the gain in statistical power in collecting multiple images in a short period of time and the need for activation/control intervals to be short for cognitive reasons necessitates the use of EPI or spiral pulses sequences. Echo planar imaging scans the data space using a raster scan approach and requires state-of-the-art gradients in order to produce high-quality images with minimal image distortion. Spiral scanning, as the name implies, spirals, either in- or out-, from the center of the data space and can be less demanding on the gradient hardware. Most modern magnets now have gradients, which easily ramp as fast as allowed by the United States Food and Drug Administration (US-FDA). The limitations currently encountered are not hardware limitations, but are based on subject safety issues. The US-FDA mandates limitations in dB/dt (the rate at which the gradient can be ramped) because ramping gradients can very rapidly induce current loops in the body that could result in stimulation of muscle groups such as the heart. Small gradient insert coils have been developed that may allow even faster ramping of the gradients, as the active length of the gradients may be short enough to minimize the current loops. These gradient insert systems, however, can be physically restricting, limited in terms of FOV, and are not easily moved in and out of the magnet due to the heavy weight of the combined gradients and cooling system. Manufacturers have been reluctant to develop such gradient inserts because the coils are awkward to move, weighing several hundred pounds, and they must be properly fastened down each time they are moved lest they torque in the magnet and seriously injure the subject. Going faster also requires faster sampling along the readout gradient, which increases the bandwidth of the data acquisition and negatively impacts the SNR, but with the advantage of decreased geometric distortion.

While EPI and spiral gradient echo acquisitions in their many forms are by far the most commonly used approaches, these sequences are sometimes implemented in three-dimensional (3D) acquisition mode,[1,9] and besides EPI and spiral scanning, there are many other acquisition strategies that can be adapted to fMRI. Other pulse sequences include asymmetric spin echo imaging[51], which combines some gradient echo (T2*) contrast with spin echo (T2) contrast in order to reduce the signal-loss problem associated with static field inhomogeneities and to reduce the contribution of large vessels while maintaining sensitivity to the BOLD affect. Inversion recovery asymmetric spin echo[52] has been used to reduce the contribution of CSF to the functional images, reducing the chance of spurious activations arising from pulsatile movement of the CSF.

Fast spin echo imaging[15] has been used in MRI, but its sensitivity at 1.5T is too low for most cognitive studies. Variations on the fast spin echo imaging approach include techniques such as GRASE imaging[79] and ultra-fast low-angle RARE imaging (UFLARE),[80] both of which have similar performance to FSE, but with reduced power deposition that can be particularly important as one moves to higher field strength. These sequences can be applied with or without inversion recovery pulses to reduce the contribution of CSF. FSE, GRASE and UFLARE can all be applied in single-shot mode, but because of the large number of additional rf pulses included in these sequences relative to EPI or spiral imaging, the acquisition window can be long. Longer acquisition windows mean fewer slices can be acquired in a TR interval.

A novel technique by Scheffler and colleagues[53] uses true fast imaging with steady precession (FISP) imaging and detects signal changes that occur upon activation due to a slight frequency shift associated with local changes in tissue oxygenation. However, this approach requires long TR and a highly uniform static field to be useful.

Single-shot techniques by definition are fast, but there are also methods for accelerating multi-shot techniques. Multi-shot acquisitions are particularly amenable to multi-coil acquisition strategies and the use of sensitivity-encoded (SENSE) reconstruction techniques. In this approach, fewer phase-encoded lines are collected (thereby saving time), but in order to maintain resolution, the FOV is reduced in direct proportion with the number of phase-encoded lines. Reducing the FOV below approximately 20 centimeters when imaging the brain usually results in FOV wrap artifacts wherein the structures that extend beyond the FOV are folded back over into the image. With multi-coil imaging and SENSE reconstruction, however, the sensitivity profiles of the individual coils making up the multi-coil array are used to unwrap the fold-over artifacts and yield high-quality images in reduced imaging times. Some decrease in SNR occurs, and as the reduction in the number of phase-encoded steps increases, the reconstruction begins to deteriorate, limiting the reductions to factors of two or three. Collecting fewer phase-encoded steps with this approach can be used reduce the imaging time, or it may allow for more slices to be collected within the TR window, thereby increasing spatial coverage without a sacrifice in temporal resolution.

As described above in the discussion on geometric image distortion, increasing the acquisition bandwidth also can allow an extra slice or two to be acquired within a given TR because increased bandwidth leads to shorter acquisition windows. However, this shorter readout time will reduce image distortion and SNR; for example, an acquisition with a bandwidth of 64 kilohertz may have a SNR of 50. Doubling the acquisition bandwidth to 128 kilohertz will reduce the image distortion by a factor of two and reduce the SNR by $\sqrt{2}$ and allow a few more slices to be squeezed into the TR interval.

Imaging Approaches to Other Physiological Measurements

Rather than measuring changes in signal intensity related to relative changes in blood oxygenation as the BOLD contrast mechanism does, it is possible to directly measure changes in cerebral blood flow with neuronal activity. As pointed out by Calamante and colleagues[54] in a review of cerebral blood flow (CBF) methods, the sensitivity of MRI to moving spins was noted in the earliest days of nuclear magnetic resonance (NMR).[55] Today, this approach is exploited in imaging applications using both single-slice and multi-slice acquisition strategies. It is now possible using these MRI approaches to measure absolute CBF, or, more simply, relative changes in CBF with activation. The techniques for performing such measurements generally are referred to as arterial spin labeling methods.

Arterial Spin Labeling

Arterial spin labeling (ASL) incorporates magnetic labeling of blood flowing into the imaging slice in order to obtain quantitative information on CBF. The basic strategy of ASL is to acquire two acquisitions, one with and one without labeling of flowing blood, such that subtraction of these acquisitions can yield quantitative perfusion information. This approach makes use of the properties of spins in flowing blood and does not require an exogenous contrast agent. Several studies have been published describing the application of ASL techniques in functional brain imaging.[56–61] For an excellent review, see Yang.[62]

There are two categories of methods for approaching spin labeling, and these include continuous ASL and pulsed ASL. Continuous ASL uses a train of rf pulses to continuously saturate protons in the blood upstream from the imaging slice.[63,64] The saturated spins flow into the imaging slice and establish a steady-state exchange of magnetization with the brain-tissue water such that the magnetization measured can be related to the CBF. Pulsed ASL applies a single inversion pulse prior to image acquisition and varies the selectivity of the inversion pulse in successive acquisitions. In pulsed ASL, the inversion pulse is placed upstream of the imaging slice and difference images are obtained from acquisitions with and without this labeling pulse.

In both approaches, there are many factors that can influence the quantification of the CBF. These include slice profile effects, wherein a blurred slice profile can make determination of the arrival time of the tagged spins more difficult to determine. These effects can be minimized with well-designed inversion pulses, which produce very sharp slice profiles, such as some of the longer adiabatic FOCI inversion pulses.[65] Transit time or path-length effects also can introduce quantification difficulties.[66] Most CBF analysis approaches assume a straight-line trajectory from the tagging plane to the imaging plane; however, this is not necessarily true. Tagged spins can flow obliquely between the two planes and the spins likely will not flow along a straight line, thereby increasing the path length and transit time to the imaging slice. Knowledge of these pathways for all slices and all locations is usually very limited, making it difficult to take this issue into account in quantifying the CBF. Minimizing the distance between the labeling slice and the imaging slice can reduce these path-length effects simply by reducing the path-length, and therefore the time allowed for these errors to accumulate. Magnetization transfer (MT) effects also can cause changes in signal intensity in the imaging slice, leading to spurious CBF measures. The MT effect leads to direct signal changes in the imaging slice, even in the absence of perfusion. Magnetization transfer effects also can lead to decreases in the apparent T1, which must be taken into account if absolute CBF is to be determined.[67] To avoid such effects, labeling pulses can be applied in a second acquisition, on the opposite downstream side of the slice equidistant from where these pulses were applied on the upstream side. Both acquisitions then will have the same MT effect, and thus, subtraction will eliminate this as a variable.

A final complicating issue in the application of ASL in fMRI is the need for multi-slice acquisitions. Because all the slices cannot be obtained simultaneously, different slices will have different transit times and different distances from the labeling pool. This can lead to erroneous differences in the apparent CBF between slices, when in fact there may be none. Applying ASL techniques with very fast imaging approaches, and taking the different transit time and path-length effects into consideration, can make multi-slice imaging more practical.[68,69]

Most ASL approaches used in fMRI have used fast imaging pulse sequences such as EPI[37,70] or spiral imaging, although modified single-shot RARE and GRASE pulse sequences have been adapted to ASL for fMRI.[61] The advantage of these multi-shot approaches lies in their reduced sensitivity to field inhomogeneities and, in particular, to the image-distortion effect, which can be large in EPI and lead to significant blurring in spiral scanning and in increased SNR due to the short effective TEs that can be used (although it should be noted that spiral out sequences also can have very short TEs). These sequences, however, require multiple shots, which increases imaging time, and the imaging time can only be reduced by increasing the echo train length and decreasing the number of slices acquired. As in BOLD imaging, these CBF imaging sequences may be combined with the parallel imaging approaches (multi-coil SENSE), but to date, that has not been done. Other approaches have been designed to measure both BOLD and CBF in an interleaved fashion in order to better characterize the activation observed.[14,60,71] Finally, just as in BOLD imaging, moving to higher fields with ASL techniques also has its advantages. The SNR is generally higher, and because T1 is longer at high field labeling, it is better and transit time effects are less significant.[14]

Sensitivity

By far the most commonly used measure of neuronal activation is the BOLD contrast mechanism. There are, however, other contrast mechanisms that can be exploited. Changes in both cerebral blood volume (CBV) and CBF can be measured with MR using a contrast agent for the former measure and a technique such as arterial spin labeling as described above for the latter. The change in CBV with activation can be quite large and has been reported to be of the order of 30%. In fact, one of the first functional studies in humans was performed using CBV as the measure of activation.[72] Cerebral blood volume typically is not measured in most experiments, however, as it requires the injection intravenously of a contrast agent that entails a small risk and some discomfort on the subjects part.

As discussed above, CBF can be measured using arterial spin labeling, but this requires extra hardware and/or pulse sequences that usually are not found as standard equipment on most imagers. This approach is most effective in cases where only a very limited number of slices need to be acquired (one) and in cases where it is acceptable to define the slice orientation based on the anatomy of the arterial vasculature. The sensitivity of this approach, however, can be high, as the change in CBF as a function of activation is of the order of 20% or more, with some investigators reporting changes in CBF as high as 100% in animal experiments.

Summary

It is hoped that this chapter has shed some light on the issues associated with defining the spatial and temporal resolution limits and the sensitivity in fMRI. New pulse sequences and new imaging hardware are being developed constantly and, combined with a better understanding of the physiological changes that occur with brain activation, the ability to obtain high resolution fMRI studies in short exam times will continue to improve. There are many trade-offs to be made in deciding on the imaging sequence and parameters to use, and it is hoped that this brief overview will shed some light on the issues involved. Clearly, because many trade-offs must be made, an understanding of these issues will help the investigator to tailor some of these parameters to the specific brain region or study design of interest.

References

1. Yang Y, Wen H, Mattay VS, Balaban RS, Frank JA, Duyn JH. Comparison of 3D BOLD functional MRI with spiral acquisition at 1.5T and 4.0T. *Neuroimage.* 1999;9:446–451.

2. Yacoub E, Shmuel A, Pfeuffer J, Van De Moortele PF, Adriany G, Andersen P, Vaughan JT, Merkle H, Ugurbil K, Hu X. Imaging brain function in humans at 7 Tesla. *Magn Reson Med*. 2001;45(4):588–594.
3. Ojemann JG, Akbudak E, Snyder AZ, McKinstry RC, Raichle ME, Conturo TE. Anatomic localization and quantitative analysis of gradient refocused echo-planar fMRI susceptibility artifacts. *Neuroimage*. 1997;6:156–167.
4. Merboldt KD, Finsterbusch J, Frahm J. Reducing inhomogeneity artifacts in functional MRI of human brain activation—thin sections versus gradient compensation. *J Magn Reson*. 2000;145(2):184–191.
5. Wadghiri YZ, Johnson G, Turnbull DH. Sensitivity and performance time in MRI dephasing artifact reduction methods. *Magn Reson Med*. 2001;45:470–476.
6. Constable RT, Spencer DD. Repetition time in echo planar functional MR imaging. *Magn Reson Med*. 2001;46(4):748–755.
7. Constable RT. Functional MR imaging using gradient echo EPI in the presence of large static field inhomogeneities. *J Magn Reson Imaging*. 1995;5(6):746–752.
8. Yang QX, Dardzinski BJ, Li S, Smith MB. Multi-gradient echo with susceptibility inhomogeneity compensation (MGESIC): demonstration of fMRI in the olfactory cortex at 3.0T. *Magn Reson Med*. 1997;37:331–335.
9. Glover GH. 3D z-shim method for reduction of susceptibility effects in BOLD fMRI. *Magn Reson Med*. 1999;42(2):290–299.
10. Frahm J, Merboldt JD, Hanicke W. Direct flash MR imaging of magnetic field inhomogeneities by gradient compensation. *Magn Reson Med*. 1988;6:474–480.
11. Cho ZH, Ro YM. Reduction of susceptibility artifact in gradient-echo imaging, *Magn Reson Med*. 1992;23:193–200.
12. Stenger VA, Boada FE, Noll DC. Multishot 3D slice-select tailored RF pulses for MRI. *Magn Reson Med*. 2002;48(1):157–165.
13. Song AW. Single-shot EPI with signal recovery from susceptibility induced losses. *Magn Reson Med*. 2001;46:407–411.
14. Yang Y. Perfusion MR Imaging with pulsed arterial spin-labeling: Basic principles and applications in functional brain imaging. *Concepts Magn Reson*. 2002;14:347–357.
15. Constable RT, Kennan RP, Puce A, McCarthy G, Gore JC. Functional MR imaging using fast spin echo at 1.5T. *Magn Reson Med*. 1994;31:686–690.
16. Boxerman JL, Hamberg LM, Rosen BR, Weisskoff RM. MR contrast due to intravascular magnetic-susceptibility perturbations. *Magn Reson Med*. 1995;34:555–566.
17. Weisskoff RM, Zuo CS, Boxerman JL, Rosen BR. Microscopic susceptibility variation and transverse relaxation: theory and experiment. *Magn Reson Med*. 1994;31:601–610.
18. Kennan RP, Zhong JH, Gore JC. Intravascular susceptibility contrast mechanisms in tissues. *Magn Reson Med*. 1994;31:9–21.
19. Raj D, Anderson AW, Gore JC. Respiratory effects in human functional magnetic resonance imaging due to bulk susceptibility changes. *Phys Med Biol*. 2001;46(12):3331–3340.
20. Cavaglia M, Dombrowski SM, Drazba J, Vasanji A, Bokesch PM, Janigro D. Regional variation in brain capillary density and vascular response to ischemia. *Brain Res*. 2001;910(1–2):81–93.
21. Heeger DJ, Huk AC, Geisler WS, Albrecht DG. Spike versus BOLD: What does neuroimaging tell us about neuronal activity? *Nat Neurosci*. 2000;3(7):631–633.
22. Rees G, Friston K, Koch C. A direct quantitative relationship between functional properties of human and macaque V5. *Nat Neurosci*. 2000;3:716–723.
23. Logothetis NK, Guggenberger H, Peled S, Pauls J. Neurophysiological investigation of the basis of the fMRI signal change. *Nat Neurosci*. 1999;2:555–562.
24. Hyder F, Rothman DL, Shulman RG. Total neuroenergetics support localized brain activity: implications for the interpretation of fMRI. *Proc Natl Acad Sci USA*. 2002;99(16):10771–10776.

25. Smith AJ, Blumenfeld H, Behar KL, Rothman DL, Shulman RG, Hyder F. Cerebrla energetics and spiking frequency: the neurophysiological basis of fMRI. *Proc Natl Acad Sci USA*. 2002;99(16):10765–19770.

26. Turner R. How much cortex can a vein drain? Downstream dilution of activation-related cerebral blood oxygenation changes. *Neuroimage*. 2002;16:1062–1067.

27. Menon RS, Goodyear BG. Submillimeter functional localization in human striate cortex using BOLD contrast at 4 Tesla: Implications for the vascular point spread function. *Magn Reson Med*. 1999;41:230–235.

28. Gati JS, Menon RS, Ugurbil K, Rutt BK. Experimental determination of the BOLD field strength dependence in vessels and tissue. *Magn Reson Med*. 1997;38:296–302.

29. Cheng K, Waggoner RA, Tanaka K. Mapping human ocular dominance columns with high field (4T) functional magnetic resonance imaging. Proc Intl Soc *Magn Reson Med*. 2000;8:978.

30. Song AW, Wong EC, Tan SG, Hyde JS. Diffusion weighted fMRI at 1.5T. *Magn Reson Med*. 1996;35:155–158.

31. Andersson L, Bolling M, Wirestam R, Holtas S, Stahlberg F. Combined diffusion weighting and CSF suppression in functional MRI. *NMR Biomed*. 2002;15:235–240.

32. Zhong J, Kennan RP, Gore JC. Effects of susceptibility variations on NMR measurements of diffusion. *J Magn Reson*. 1991;95:267–280.

33. Lee SP, Silva AC, Ugurbil K, Kim SG. Diffusion-weighted spin-echo fMRI at 9.4T: microvascular/tissue contribution to BOLD signal changes. *Magn Reson Med*. 1999;42(5):919–928.

34. Song AW, Woldorff MG, Gangstead S, Mangun GR, McCarthy G. Enhanced spatial localization of neuronal activation using simultaneous apparent-diffusion-coefficient and blood-oxygenation functional magnetic resonance imaging. *Neuroimage*. 2002;17:742–750.

35. Frostig RD, Lieke EE, Ts'o DY, Grinvald A. Cortical functional architecture and local coupling between neuronal activity and the microcirculation revealed by in vivo high-resolution imaging of intrinsic signals. *Proc Natl Acad Sci USA*. 1990;87:6082–6086.

36. Malonek D, Grinvald A. Interactions between electrical activity and cortical microcirculation revealed by imaging spectroscopy: Implications for functional brain mapping. *Science*. 1996;272:551–554.

37. Ernst T, Hennig J. Observation of a fast response in functional MR. *Magn Reson Med*. 1994;32:146–149.

38. Menon RS, Ogawa S, Strupp JP, Anderson P, Ugurbil K. BOLD based functional MRI at 4 Tesla includes capillary bed contribution: Echo-planar imaging correlates with previous optical imaging using intrinsic signals. *Magn Reson Med*. 1995;33:453–459.

39. Hu X, Le TH, Ugurbil K. Evaluation of the early response in fMRI in individual subjects using short stimulus duration. *Magn Reson Med*. 1997;37:877–884.

40. Duong TQ, Kim DS, Ugurbil K, Kim SG. Spatiotemporal dynamics of the BOLD fMRI signals: towards mapping submillimeter cortical columns using the early negative response. *Magn Reson Med*. 2000;44(2):231–242.

41. Kim DS, Duong DQ, Kim S-G. High resolution mapping of iso-orientation columns by fMRI. *Nat Neurosci*. 2000;3:164–169.

42. Buxton RB. The elusive initial dip. *Neuroimage*. 2001;13:953–958.

43. Lindauer U, Royl G, Leithner C, Kuhl M, Gold L, Gethmann J, Kohl-Bareis M, Villringer A, Diirnagl U. No evidence for early decrease in blood oxygenation in rat whisker cortex in response to functional activation. *Neuroimage*. 2001;13:986–999.

44. Jones M, Berwick J, Johnston D, Mayhew J. Concurrent optical imaging spectroscopy and laser-doppler flowmetry: The relationship between blood flow, oxygenation, and volume in rodent barrel cortex. *Neuroimage*. 2001;13:1000–1013.

45. Studholme C, Constable RT, Duncan JS. Accurate alignment of functional EPI data to anatomical MRI physics based distortion model. *IEEE Trans Med Imaging*. 2001;19(11):1115–1127.

46. Jezzard P, Balaban RS. Correction for geometric distortion in EPI from Bo variations. *Magn Reson Med*. 1995;34:65–73.
47. Jezzard P, Clare S. Sources of distortion in functional MRI data. *Hum Brain Mapp*. 1999;8(2–3):80–85.
48. Reber PJ, Wong EC, Buxton RB, Frank LR. Correction of off resonance related distortion in echo planar images from Bo field variations. *Magn Reson Med*. 1995;34:65–73.
49. Robson MD, Gore JC, Constable RT. Measurement of the point spread function in MRI using constant time imaging. *Magn Reson Med*. 1997;38(5):733–740.
50. Zeng H, Constable RT. Image distortion correction in EPI: Comparison of field mapping with point spread function mapping. *Magn Reson Med*. 2002;48:137–146.
51. Houston GC, Papadakis NG, Carpenter A, Hall LD, Mukherjee B, James MF, Huang CLH. Mapping of the cerebral response to hypoxia measured using graded asymmetric spin echo. *Magn Reson Imag*. 2000;18:1043–1054.
52. Zheng J, Ehrhardt JC, Cizadlo T, Yuh WTC. Comparison of inversion-recovery asymmetric spin-echo EPI and gradient-echo EPI for brain motor activation study. *J Magn Reson Imaging*. 1997;7:843–847.
53. Scheffler K, Seifritz E, Bilecen D, Venkatesan R, Hennig J, Deimling M, Haacke EM. Detection of BOLD changes by means of a frequency-sensitive trueFISP technique: preliminary results. *NMR Biomed*. 2001;14:490–496.
54. Calamante F, Thomas DL, Pell GS, Wiersma J, Turner R. Measuring cerebral blood flow using magnetic resonance imaging techniques. *J Cereb Blood Flow Metab*. 1999;19: 701–735.
55. Singer JR. Blood flow rates by nuclear magnetic resonance measurements. *Science*. 1959;130;1652–1653.
56. Edelman RR, Siewert B, Darby DG, Thangaraj V, Nobre AC, Mesulam MM, Warrash S. Quantitative mapping of cerebral blood flow and functional localization with echo-planar MR imaging and signal targeting with alternating radio frequency. *Radiology*. 1994;192:513–520.
57. Edelman RR, Chen Q. EPISTAR MRI: Multislice mapping of cerebral blood flow. *Magn Reson Med*. 1998;40:800–805.
58. Kim SG. Quantification of relative cerebral blood flow change by flow-sensitive alternating inversion recovery (FAIR) technique: application to functional mapping. *Magn Reson Med*. 1995;34:293–301.
59. Yang Y, Frank JA, Hou L, Ye FQ, McLaughlin AC, Duyn JH. Multislice imaging of quantitative cerebral perfusion with pulsed arterial spin-labeling. *Magn Reson Med*. 1998;39:825–832.
60. Hoge RD, Atkinson J, Gill B, Crelier GR, Marrett S, Pike GB. Investigation of BOLD signal dependence on cerebral blood flow and oxygen consumption: the deoxyhemoglobin dilution model. *Magn Reson Med*. 1999;42:849–863.
61. Crelier GR, Hoge RD, Munger P, Pike GB. Perfusion based functional magnetic resonance imaging with single shot RARE and GRASE acquisitions. *Magn Reson Med*. 1999;41:132–136.
62. Yang Y, Gu H, Zhan W, Xu S, Silbersweig DA, Stern E. Simultaneous perfusion and BOLD imaging using reverse spiral scanning at 3T: characterization of functional contrast and susceptibility artifacts. *Magn Reson Med*. 2002;48(2):278–289.
63. Detre JA, Leigh JS, Williams DS, Koretsky AP. Perfusion imaging. *Magn Reson Med*. 1992;23:37–45.
64. Gonzalez-At JB, Alsop DC, Detre JA. Cerebral perfusion and arterial transit time changes during task activation determined with continuous arterial spin labeling. *Magn Reson Med*. 2000;43:739–746.
65. Yongbi MN, Yang Y, Frank JA, Duyn JH. Multislice perfusion imaging in human brain using the C-FOCI inversion pulse: comparison with hyperbolic secant. *Magn Reson Med*. 1999;42:1098–1105.
66. Alsop DC, Detre JA. Reduced transit-time sensitivity in noninvasive magnetic resonance imaging of human cerebral blood flow. *J Cereb Blood Flow Metab*. 1996;16: 1236–1249.

67. Zhang W, Williams DS, Koretsky AP. Measurement of brain perfusion by volume-localized NMR spectroscopy using inversion of arterial water spins: accounting for transit time and cross-relaxation. *Magn Reson Med.* 1992;25:362–371.
68. Wong EC, Buxton RB, Frank LR. Implementation of quantitative perfusion imaging techniques for functional brain mapping using pulsed arterial spin labeling. *NMR Biomed.* 1997;10(4–5):237–249.
69. Ye FQ, Yang Y, Duyn J, Mattay VS, Frank JA, Weinberger DR, McLaughlin AC. Quantitation of regional cerebral blood flow increases during motor activation: A multislice, steady-state, arterial spin tagging study. *Magn Reson Med.* 1999;42:404–407.
70. Darby DG, Nobre AC, Thangaraj V, Edelman R, Mesulam MM, Warach S. Cortical activation in the human brain during lateral saccades using EPISTAR functional magnetic resonance imaging. *Neuroimage.* 1996;3:53–62.
71. Lai S, Wang J, Jahng G-H. FAIR exempting separate T1 measurement (FAIREST): a novel technique for online quantitative perfusion imaging and multi-contrast fMRI. *NMR Biomed.* 2001;14:507–516.
72. Belliveau JW, Kennedy DN, McKinstry RC, Buchbinder BR. Weisskoff RM, Cohen MS, Vevea JM, Brady TJ, Rosen BR. Functional mapping of the human visual cortex by magnetic resonance imaging. *Science.* 1991;254(4):716.
73. Constable RT, Carpentier A, Pugh K, Westerveld M, Oszunar Y, Spencer DD. Investigation of the human hippocampal formation using a randomized-event-related paradigm and z-shimmed functional MRI. *Neuroimage.* 2000;12:55–62.
74. Constable RT, Spencer DD. Composite image formation in z-shimmed functional MR imaging. *Magn Reson Med.* 1999;42(1):110–117.
75. Yacoub E, Shmuel A, Pfeuffer J, Van De Moortele PF, Adriany G, Ugurbil K, Hu X. Investigation of the initial dip in fMRI at 7 Tesla. *NMR Biomed.* 2001;14(7–8):408–412.
76. Yacoub E, Hu X. Detection of the early decrease in fMRI signal in the motorarea. *Magn Reson Med.* 2001;45:184–190.
77. Ogawa S, Lee T-M, Stepnoski R, Chen W, Zhu X-H, Ugurbil K. An approach to probes some neural systems interaction by functional MRI at neural timescale down to milliseconds. *Proc Natl Acad Sci USA.* 2000;97(20):11026–11031.
78. Miezin FM, Maccotta L, Ollinger JM, Petersen SE, Buckner RL. Characterizing the hemodynamic response: effects of presentation rate, sampling procedure, and the possibility of ordering brain activity based on relative timing. *Neuroimage.* 2000;11:735–759.
79. Jovicich J, Norris DG. Functional MRI of the human brain with GRASE-basedBOLD contrast. *Magn Reson Med.* 1999;41:871–876.
80. Niendorf T. On the application of susceptibility-weighted ultra-fast low-angle RARE experiments in functional MR imaging, *Magn Reson Med.* 1999;41:1189–1198.

5

Clinical Challenges of fMRI

Nader Pouratian and Susan Y. Bookheimer

Introduction

Functional magnetic resonance imaging (fMRI) has revolutionized clinical brain mapping and has become the predominant functional neuroimaging technique since its original report by Belliveau and colleagues.[1] The appeal of fMRI is attributable to several advantages that it offers over other functional neuroimaging techniques. Functional MRI is noninvasive; it is a rapid technique that offers the opportunity for repeated measurements of the same task to investigate response consistency, to compare activations across tasks, and to measure change over time.

Despite its advantages, fMRI presents several unique challenges, especially in the clinical setting (Table 5.1). Many of these challenges arise from the fact that fMRI does not directly measure neuronal activity. Instead, fMRI detects perfusion-related signals that are coupled to neuronal activity. Many studies make assumptions about the characteristics of neurovascular coupling, and therefore the significance of fMRI activations; these assumptions are more suspect in a clinical setting when pathology may alter normal coupling mechanisms; for example, the presence of intracerebral pathologies [e.g., arteriovenous malformations (AVMs)] can induce field inhomogeneities and also may alter neurovascular coupling mechanisms, both of which may hamper measurement of reliable hemodynamic-based fMRI signals. Another challenge of clinical fMRI includes the inability of patients to comply with imaging protocols. One study[2] showed that nearly 30% of subjects with intracranial masses were excluded from the final analysis due to gross motion artifact. This may be a particularly difficult problem if one wishes to study patients with known movement disorders. Impairments in cognition also may alter patients abilities to complete tasks, both with respect to motivation and task difficulty.

Finally, clinical brain mapping emphasizes results for an individual rather than for a group, impacting strongly on choice of analysis methods.

This chapter previously appeared in *Functional MRI: Basic Principles and Clinical Applications*, edited by S. Faro and F. Mohamed. New York: Springer Science+Business Media, LCC 2006.

From: *BOLD fMRI: A Guide to Functional Imaging for Neuroscientists*
Edited by: S.H. Faro and F.B. Mohamed, DOI 10.1007/978-1-4419-1329-6_5
© Springer Science+Business Media, LLC 2010

Table 5.1. Potential Limitations of fMRI in Clinical Populations

Field inhomogeneities in ROI
Movement artifacts
Altered baseline intelligence
Impaired task compliance
Impaired motivation
Sensitivity to certain stimuli (e.g., flickering lights)

Moreover, altered anatomy due to intracerebral lesions may prohibit spatial registration and normalization tools commonly used in group statistics, making it difficult to directly compare results from patients with those from a normative sample.[3] This chapter will elaborate on the challenges of fMRI in clinical populations, including issues of field strength and sequence selection, study and task design, and data analysis.

A Brief History of Clinical Brain Mapping

Until the advent of fMRI and other perfusion-based brain mapping techniques, such as positron emission tomography (PET),[4] optical imaging of intrinsic signals (OIS),[5] and near-infrared spectroscopy (NIRS),[6] our understanding of the functional organization of the brain largely stemmed from studying the effects of brain lesions. Although brain lesions initially were limited to strokes and other accidents of nature. Penfield recognized in 1937 that temporary brain lesions also could be induced to study brain function by applying electrical stimulations directly on the cortex.[7] Most recently, transcranial magnetic stimulation (TMS) has been introduced as a means of inducing temporary lesions non-invasiveley.[8] By mapping the effects of lesions, these disruption-based techniques identify parts of the brain that are essential and critical for executing a given task. These disruption-based techniques of mapping the brain have emerged as the gold standard of clinical brain mapping, especially in the neurosurgical arena.

Functional MRI differs fundamentally from the classic lesion-based approach to clinical brain mapping in that, instead of only identifying areas of the brain that are essential for performing a task, fMRI indicates all brain areas that demonstrate activity-related changes during a given task, regardless of whether a given brain area is, in fact, critical for task performance (i.e., both essential and supplementary cortical areas). Because of the differences in methodology, fMRI maps and lesion maps will inevitably differ. Both maps are probably clinically relevant, but one must be aware of the different data produced, their implications, and the types of conclusions that can be drawn from each.

Hemodynamic Basis of fMRI Maps

As discussed in earlier chapters, fMRI offers an indirect measure of brain function: instead of directly measuring neuronal activity, fMRI maps the brain by detecting functional hemodynamic responses that are coupled to neuronal activity. The clinical challenges of fMRI stem, in part, from the fact that the fMRI map is an indirect measure of brain activity. To establish clini-

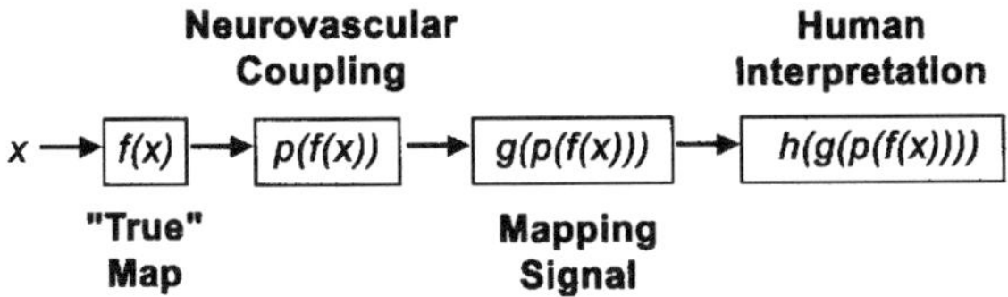

Figure 5.1. Cascade of functional brain mapping functions. The mapping signal observed and reported is actually not a true map of neuronal activity. Rather, it is a product of a series of complex functions, including, for example, the coupling of neuronal activity and local cerebral perfusion, or neurovascular coupling (p). In order to better understand how functional brain maps relate to underlying true maps it is critical to characterize the robustness of neurovascular coupling under different stimulus conditions, in different cortices, and in the presence of different pathologies.

cal validity of the instrument assumes both that MRI signal changes reflect underlying neural activity, and assuming we accept this relationship, that a particular patient has a normal fMRI response (e.g., the blood-flow response is unaffected by their clinical condition). This complexity can be illustrated by conceptualizing brain mapping as a series of mathematical functions (Figure 5.1).[9]

Given a stimuluxs x, there is a given neuronal response $f(x)$, which represents the true brain map. The neuronal response is coupled to a functional hemodynamic response by a neurovascular coupling function, p. The uncertainty of this neurovascular coupling function introduces one of the biggest challenges and one of the most significant sources of error in interpreting clinical fMRI studies. What ultimately matters about the neurovascular relationship is the degree and precision of spatial coupling between neuronal activity. As discussed below, the spatial coupling between fMRI activation signals and electrophysiologically active cortices may not be as precise as most would like.

Several recent studies have indicated that hemodynamic responses can be significantly different across brain regions, especially when adjacent to major pathology. In a study of 98 patients, Krings and colleagues showed that the distance of a central mass from the motor region significantly influenced the magnitude of activation, even within patients without paresis.[10] Other studies have found similar suppression of the hemodynamic response adjacent to pathology.[11,12] Conversely, in a study of 14 patients, Schlosser and colleagues suggested that fMRI activation patterns within patients with frontal lobe tumors, when mapped using a verbal fluency paradigm, were comparable to signals in normal controls.[13] Similarly, Righini and colleagues studied 17 patients with frontoparietal masses and found little difference in motor activations between the affected and unaffected hemispheres.[2] The contradiction in these studies highlight the need to be aware of the possibility that adjacent pathologies may alter cerebral hemodynamics, but that this alteration is most likely pathology and location dependent and, possibly, task dependent. Finally, different physiological states (e.g., hypercapnia, hypoxia, hypertension) and different disease states (e.g., vasculitis, angiopathies) can impact differentially the relationship between neuronal activity and functional perfusion. Schmidt and colleagues have shown in a rodent model that brief exposure to hypercapnia may potentiate the hemodynamic response without affecting the underlying electrophysiological response.[14,15] In fact, highlighting the effect that hypercapnia may have on signals in normal subjects, hypercapnia can be used in normal subject as a means of contrast enhancement.[16] The age of the subject also may affect the magnitude of the hemodynamic response and the coupling mechanism itself.[10] Understanding the underlying coupling dynamics is essential to interpreting fMRI results. It is this uncertainty that continues to motivate continued investigation of neurovascular coupling dynamics.

Assuming neurovascular coupling is intact, several more functions are still applied before arriving at any conclusions from fMRI data. The functional perfusion response produces a brain mapping signal, g: g (p $(f(x))$). The function g is determined not only by the physics behind fMRI signals sources (i.e., field strengths, scan sequences), but also by the recording capabilities of the particular scanner. This includes, but is not limited to, resolution limitations, data filtering, and artifacts that may be introduced by different disease processes or medical interventions (e.g., coils, clips, arteriovenous malformations, air cavities after neurosurgical resections).

Finally, yet another function is introduced into the formula, h, for the introduction of human study design, human interpretation, and statistics. Human interpretation of mapping signals, when not quantitative, is always susceptible to bias. The bias may be inadvertent and may be as subtle as in selecting an inappropriate control for comparison or measuring inappropriate signal parameters from which to draw conclusions. The statistics commonly used in fMRI also introduce error and misinterpretations, presenting yet another challenge to clinical interpretation scans.

Although many studies compare blobs across groups, there are a number of assumptions that underlie those blobs. To better understand the underlying map, or $f(x)$, this complex function must be deconvolved by characterizing the factors that influence all of these functions. Alternatively, the investigator can pay special attention to study design and analysis in order to minimize assumptions and to strengthen their conclusions. Many of these issues of study design and analysis are discussed below.

Technical Considerations

Field Strength

Magnetic field strength is an important consideration in clinical fMRI study design. Increasing field strength provides a greater dynamic range of data collection and, ultimately, a greater signal-to-noise ratio (SNR) and contrast-to-noise ratio (CNR).[17] Increased SNR and CNR improve study power and decrease Type II errors. Presumably, increased CNR can reduce the scanning time needed to obtain significant results, or make it possible to scan in multiple paradigms in the same amount of time.

Another advantage of increased field strength is the potential for increased spatial resolution (smaller voxel size) with greater SNR given the same acquisition time than at lower fields. Increasing spatial resolution can enhance the sensitivity of the mapping technique, particularly where small differences in localization of function are crucial to the clinical decision or outcome. Large voxel size limits fMRI sensitivity because functional changes at cortical capillaries, which are orders of magnitude smaller than voxel size and represent only a small fraction of total voxel size, are drowned out at the level of the voxel.

This partial-volume effect is reduced with smaller voxel sizes. Ultimately, if voxel sizes are too large, a lack of difference between subjects or groups may not actually mean there is no difference. Rather, this may represent a sensitivity limitation of the technique.

However, higher field strengths also pose problems that, in some brain regions or in some clinical conditions, may prove insurmountable. The most difficult complication arising from increased field strength is the associated increase in susceptibility artifact, especially near air–tissue interfaces. This is a particular problem in the inferior temporal lobes and the inferior medial frontal lobes, which are adjacent to the air-filled sinuses. These areas of susceptibility artifact produce both spatial distortion and MR signal loss, which make it difficult or impossible to identify activity-related changes in fMR images. This is of particular importance for language mapping, in which investigators expect to find several temporal lobe language areas.[18] Lack of signal in these regions does not indicate lack of activity, but may be due to lack of sensitivity to identify appropriate signals. Devlin and colleagues have proposed alternate strategies when imaging these regions of high susceptibility, but they also acknowledge that these artifacts can only be partially overcome and that alternative data acquisition paradigms are necessary to address this issue.[19] In some cases, appropriate selection of scan sequence may help overcome some susceptibility artifacts, especially when imaging adjacent to pathology.

Scan Sequence and Susceptibility

The most commonly used fMRI pulse sequence is the gradient echo echo planar imaging (EPI) sequence. Echo planar imaging is the fast scanning technique that acquires all slice locations with a single response time (TR), and which has made fMRI practical.[20] The gradient echo sequence is optimized to maximize susceptibility due to blood oxygenation level-dependent (BOLD) contrast. An unfortunate but necessary side effect is that it also maximizes unwanted susceptibility artifacts at tissue interfaces, especially at high field. In certain brain regions—particularly the amygdala, basal temporal region, and orbitofrontal cortex—the susceptibility artifacts may make imaging these regions impossible.

Clinical fMRI within patients who have had prior brain surgery may be complicated by the presence of implanted devices, such as plates and screws. Whereas most of these devices are considered magnet compatible, that is, they are not ferromagnetic and do not pose a safety concern, susceptibility artifacts can generate profound distortions around these objects that include massive signal loss and spatial distortion. It also should be noted that many of these devices have not been tested at high field and could pose a safety risk that does not exist at lower field strength. Typically, these objects will be implanted close to or on top of the precise regions the clinician would like to have mapped.

There are a variety of simple approaches to reducing susceptibility artifacts at air–tissue interfaces and around objects during functional imaging. Reducing voxel size is one. In the amygdala, for instance, Merboldt and colleagues[21] calculated that voxel sizes of 4 to 8 microliters or less are necessary to recover sufficient signal. Fransson and colleague[22] used a high-resolution acquisition method to receive signal in the hippocampus using coronal acquisitions and in-plane resolution of two square millimeters and slice thickness of one millimeter. For most centers, this approach is impractical, both to a lack of non-standard sequences on clinically oriented machines and because for many systems the associated reduction on field of view (FOV) is not acceptable. However, for patients with a focal lesion in which a small FOV is all that is necessary, small voxel studies may be appropriate. The loss of CNR within small voxels also may prohibit the practical use of this approach.

To some extent, use of alternative pulse sequences can improve, but not wholly overcome these artifacts. Port and colleagues[23] performed a series of imaging studies on titanium screws embedded in gel to determine parameters that would decrease susceptibility artifacts in echo planar (EPI) images. They reported three factors that can reduce artifacts: reducing the echo time (TE), increasing the frequency matrix, and reducing slice thickness. The latter two approaches are identical to those reported by Merboldt and colleagues[21] for imaging at air–tissue boundaries. However, the effect of reducing TE on susceptibility is controversial. Susceptibility artifacts due to signal loss at air–tissue interfaces are greater with longer TEs. One approach to reducing susceptibility artifact is to reduce the TE. Gorno-Tempini and colleagues[24] used a double echo EPI sequence to compare susceptibility artifacts and BOLD signal changes at tissue interfaces, comparing TEs of 27 and 40 milliseconds. They used a face-processing task, which is known to activate the fusiform gyrus in the base of the temporal lobe, an area likely to suffer from susceptibility-induced signal loss. Whereas the lower TE did not reduce their ability to detect BOLD signal in those regions unaffected by susceptibility artifacts, the lower TE was not sufficient to recover the BOLD signal.

Various pulse sequences have differential effects on susceptibility artifacts. One alternative to the commonly used gradient echo EPI scan is the asymmetric spin echo. Both spin echo and gradient echo sequences base their signal on magnetic susceptibility contrast as described above, as well as in the previous chapters. The spin echo sequence, however, refocuses the spin dephasing caused by field inhomogeneity. The consequence is that a spin echo sequence reduces susceptibility artifacts at air–tissue boundaries, but also will result in CNR loss due to reduced BOLD contrast. At high field, this loss may be an acceptable trade-off. Spin echo sequences tend to recover signal from larger, rather than smaller, boundaries, and thus have been thought to affect unwanted susceptibility artifacts preferentially, including effects in larger blood vessels, while preserving signal changes in the capillaries. The asymmetric spin echo sequence shifts the time differential between the image acquisition and readout, allowing the signal to decay; thus, the amount of reversible dephasing that occurs can be varied by adjusting the length of this shift. The longer the asymmetry, the more the spin echo images resemble a gradient echo image. Stables and colleagues[25] have demonstrated that varying these parameters can optimize for a particular perturbation size (i.e., a small or large blood vessel). Several fMRI studies have used a spin echo sequence effectively in high susceptibility areas such as hippocampus and amygdala.[26–28] Figure 5.2 shows examples of a gradient echo and asymmetric spin echo EPI images using otherwise identical parameters in the same subject. The recovery of signal in high susceptibility areas, especially around a lesion, is quite apparent, although not complete.

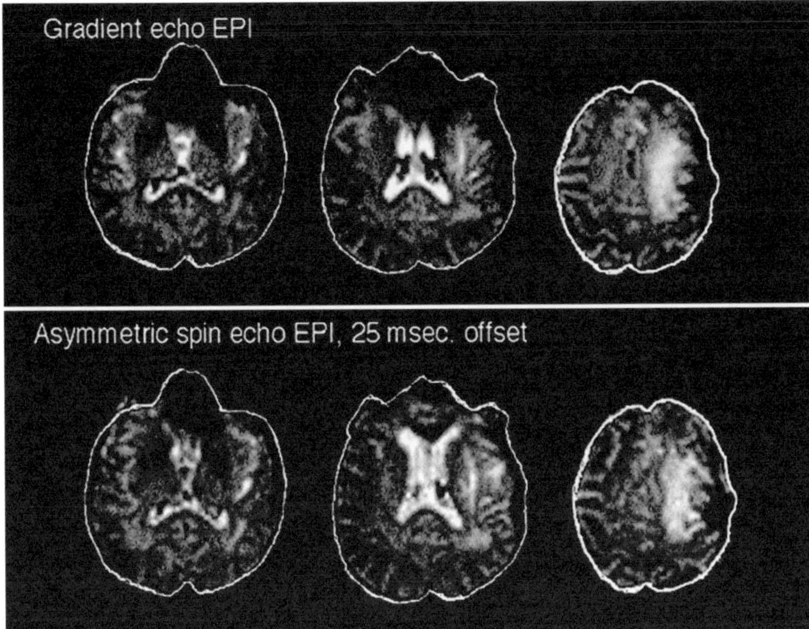

Figure 5.2. Gradient echo versus asymmetric spin echo (ASE) EPI. Gradient echo (TR = 2.5, TE = 45, 64 × 64 matrix, FOV = 20, 1 NEX) and asymmetric spin echo (TR = 2.5, TE = 45, offset = 25msec, 64 × 64 matrix, FOV = 20, 1 NEX) EPI scans in two areas of high susceptibility (left) at air–tissue interfaces in basal temporal and orbitofrontal cortex (right) near the lesion with prior resection. The outlines are derived from a high-resolution spin echo EPI (TR = 4000; TE = 54, 128 × 128 matrix, 20-mm FOV, 5-mm thick, 4 NEX). Note reduced susceptibility in ASE scans in both regions of high susceptibility.

Other modifications to the EPI sequence may reduce susceptibility artifacts. Cordes and colleagues[29] advocated using a second refocusing gradient in the slice-selection orientation to reduce susceptibility artifacts. A more complicated approach offered by Stenger and colleagues[30] used three-dimensional (3D) tailored radiofrequency (RF) pulses to refocus regions where the susceptibility is greatest, using a modified spiral k-space trajectory.

In spiral scanning, k-space is traversed in a spiral pattern emanating either from the center to the exterior (spiral-in), the reverse (spiral-out), or in some combination (e.g., dual-echo in-out). Glover and Law[31] reported that a spiral-in trajectory or combinations of in–out trajectories can both increase SNR while reducing susceptibility. Yang and colleagues[32] developed a reverse spiral scanning technique simultaneous with perfusion imaging with arterial spin labeling. Comparisons of susceptibility artifacts between forward and reverse spiral scanning suggested less susceptibility in the reverse sequence, with adequate BOLD signal in high-susceptibility regions. Other techniques to reduce susceptibility artifacts in spiral scans include a sensitivity-encoded (SENSE) sequencing[33] that shortens the readout duration, thus minimizing signal loss. However, the effects of BOLD signal recovery were less dramatic.

Mapping the Oxy/Deoxyhemoglobin Signal

The choice of mapping signal has become an interesting debate. Although the debate has not yet entered the clinical arena, it deserves brief mention here. Following functional activation, cerebral blood flow (CBF) increases in excess of the cerebral metabolic rate of oxygen ($CMRO_2$), thereby causing a decrease in deoxyhemoglobin (due to an overperfusion of oxyhemoglobin).[34] This functional change in the relative abundance of the different hemoglobin moieties is responsible for the increased BOLD MR signal observed with functional activation. This theory is consistent with several studies that have documented that functional CBF increases exceed that of $CMRO_2$ using multiple modalities, including: positron emission tomography (PET),[35] optical imaging of intrinsic signals (OIS);[5,36] and optical imaging of fluorescent dyes.[37] Recently, an initial decrease in BOLD signal, or initial dip, has been reported that precedes the increased BOLD signal described above. The initial dip is thought to represent an initial burst in oxidative metabolism, which increases local deoxyhemoglobin concentrations before any perfusion changes occur.[37,38] It has been proposed that if this initial negative signal does in fact represent an initial burst in oxidative metabolism, it may be more highly spatially correlated with electrophysiological activity than the later positive BOLD signal.[39] Accordingly, Kim and colleagues[40] was able to use the initial dip signal in cats to map ocular dominance columns in cats using BOLD techniques.

Study and Task Design

Issues in task design—particularly choice of activation and control tasks, as well as difficulty level—are important considerations in all fMRI studies; however, in the clinical arena, these difficulties take on special significance, as errors in task design can lead to false conclusions that may harm patients. Here, three issues of particular importance in clinical fMRI will be discussed: choice of control conditions, the effect of practice on observed fMRI activations, and the appropriate level of difficulty given the population to be studied.

Task Selection

Functional MRI activations represent a contrast between two conditions; in the earliest fMRI studies, this contrast was identified by simple subtracting rest or control condition images from those acquired during a task.[41,42] This simple subtraction approach assumes (1) a hierarchical organization of brain function, (2) that the investigator can accurately decompose a complex task, and (3) cognitive activity and brain function are insignificant during rest conditions.

The assumption that an investigator can accurately decompose a task into its components is a challenge in itself. Not all subjects will repeatedly use the same strategy to perform a task, nor can all the cognitive processes that are required to complete a given task function be deduced easily. This challenge is even more difficult in a clinical population in which there may be subclinical or overt cognitive deficits that may alter the strategies used to perform a task. Tasks that are suitable for brain mapping in the general healthy population may not be appropriate in an impaired population. Finally, this approach assumes that cognitive functions linearly summate to produce the observed fMRI signals, and that there is no interaction between cognitive functions that may produce a unique output based on the combination of tasks.

To test the assumptions of linearity of hierarchical structure, Sidtis and colleagues compared activation maps using simple subtraction (maps were generated by subtracting a rest condition from a task condition) and complex subtractions (maps were generated by subtracting two tasks that were presumed to only differ with respect to a single parameter).[43] The three tasks used were syllable repetition, phonation, and lip closure. Syllable repetition was assumed to be a combination of phonation and lip closure for the purposes of this study. Lip closure maps were generated by simple subtraction of the rest condition from the lip closure condition, and complex subtraction maps were generated by subtracting the phonation condition from the syllable repetition condition. The simple and complex subtraction maps were different both with respect to signal intensities and distribution, suggesting that the condition of additivity necessary to decompose complex tasks by subtraction was not present in the data, calling into question subtraction methodology and the assumption that tasks can accurately decompose.

Stark and Squire examined activation patterns associated with rest conditions (used as a baseline) to determine if rest is necessarily an appropriate control or baseline, with particular attention to memory tasks looking at the medial temporal lobe.[44] The authors measured fMRI signals during seven different tasks: novel pictures, familiar pictures, noise detection, odd/even discrimination, arrow discrimination, moving fixation, and rest. The first two tasks were considered memory tasks, whereas the last five were considered to be various controls. Not surprisingly, the authors demonstrated that identifying activity in the medial temporal lobe (including hippocampal and parahippocampal structures) varied depending on the control condition used. In fact, the authors reported that activity within these structures was higher during the rest condition than during other control conditions. Consequently, identifying activity in the ROI intimately depended on the control condition used. This study highlights two important points. First, rest does not mean that the brain is quiescent; the brain is cognitively active even during rest. Second, fMRI activations represent contrasts between two conditions and do not indicate whether a part of the brain was active. Rather, it means there was not a significant enough change in neuronal activity relative to baseline to evoke a functional hemodynamic response. This highlights the need for careful selection of baseline tasks and even more careful interpretation of observed activation patterns.

Gusnard and Raichle[45] reviewed the concept of a physiological baseline, suggesting that in fact the brain has a high level of activity at baseline, and that this must be considered when using rest as a control condition and when interpreting functional activation studies. Importantly, they provided a thorough discussion of task-related decreases in activation and argued that while some of these decreases may represent a task-dependent decrease in cerebral activity, many decreases seem to be task-independent, representing an organized mode of brain function, which is attenuated during various goal-directed behaviors.[45]

Practice Effects

Paradigm design is not only important with respect to selection of tasks, but also with respect to task timing. Several studies now indicate that practicing a task can significantly alter activation patterns, revealing different maps that may represent alternative strategies for performing the given task, such as automatization.[46–49] Raichle and associates were the first to report that functional activation patterns can be altered by relatively brief periods of practice.[46] Comparing a novel verbal-response selection task with reading visually presented nouns, they found a practice-related decrease in cortical activation of those regions mediating performance at the beginning of the task after only 15 minutes of practice. Moreover, other brain regions increased activity, such that, with practice, the verbal-response task more resembled the reading task. This practice effect was reversed by introducing a novel list of words, allowing the authors to conclude that the activation patterns associated with practice represented an automatization of the task that was reversible. Van Mier and colleagues[48] and Petersen and colleagues[47] reported similar findings of shifts in activation patterns, or changes in functional neuroanatomy, from one part of the brain to another with practice. This is thought to represent an activity dependent shift in effortful task performance to skilled, automatic task performance.

Similarly, Madden and colleagues[49] reported a decrease in functional activation with practice in the two populations they studied: young adults (20–29 years) and older adults (62–79 years). Using a verbal-recognition memory task, this group characterized activation patterns during encoding, baseline, and retrieval and found that activation patterns were different (both increased magnitude and different spatial distribution) between these populations for each task. Interestingly, despite differences both groups initially demonstrated practice-related effects, showing decreased activation magnitude, although the practice effects were greater in the younger population than in the elderly. The authors concluded that older adults required a more distributive network of brain activation in order to perform the given task and, whereas task performance improved with practice, the smaller practice effect observed in the older group represents a continual recruitment of cognitive processes and attention to support task execution. This is not required in the younger population, who can learn and automate more quickly and effectively.

Not all groups, however, have reported activation of additional areas with practice. Garavan and associates argued that if the core task is unchanged by practice, then practice may cause a decreased magnitude of activation, but will not necessarily recruit additional areas of the brain.[50] Using a visuospatial working memory (VSWM) task, they reported decreased fMRI activations in the four areas of interest with activation, but did not report seeing additional areas of activation with practice. They suggested that their observations are consistent with the fact that the task used continues to tax the VSWM system and could not be automated completely, regardless of amount of practice. This raises an interesting consideration that not all cognitive tasks are equally susceptible to practice effects.

The existence of practice effects and relatively rapidity of onset are important technical considerations in implementing a functional brain-mapping study, especially if one wishes to identify those brain regions that are actively involved in and essential to task performance. Most fMRI studies take approximately one hour to complete, during which time brain-activation patterns may be modified secondary to practice. Therefore, it is critical to plan experiments efficiently and to continually provide novel stimuli and tasks in order to assure that practice-related changes do not taint the results (unless, of course, practice-related effects are under investigation.)

Task Difficulty

Another important consideration that is intimately related to the concept of practice is task difficulty. It is hypothesized that the changes seen due to practice are largely due to decreases in task difficulty with practice, and therefore automatization of task performance. If a task is too easy, the task may activate brain areas involved with performing automatic activities without taxing the appropriate cognitively critical areas of interest. In contrast, if a task is too difficult, it may recruit additional attentional areas and supplementary areas (areas that a task may not normally activate) to help execute a task.

The paradigm of mapping a paretic or plegic patient offers an excellent means of discussing task difficulty and its effects on fMRI activations. For these patients, the effort and difficulty to complete a motor task is undoubtedly greater than for a healthy volunteer. The source of the paresis (i.e., intracerebral versus spinal) will influence the fMRI activation pattern. In a study of patients with central masses near the motor strip, fMRI activations of primary motor cortex decreased with increasing paresis, independent of the distance of the central mass from the motor strip, although the degree of paresis did not correlate with the magnitude of the observed fMRI signal.[3,10] The observed decrease in primary motor activation cannot be unambiguously attributed do decreased number of functional neurons in the motor strip compression due to mass effect (although the observation was independent of distance of the mass from the central strip), tumor-mediated changes in local cerebral hemodynamics, changes in global perfusion due to the presence of a neoplasm, or a combination of these factors.[3] It is critically important from the perspective of clinical brain mapping to consider if a better primary motor strip mapping signal could have been obtained by changing the level of difficulty of the given motor task. Could a more significant signal be elicited from the primary motor strip if the motor task was made more complex and drove the remaining primary motor neurons harder? What if the motor task was made simpler? Could a simpler task induce greater activation by giving the remaining primary motor neurons a task they are fully capable of executing? These may be important points of consideration in interpreting clinical data.

In the same study, the investigators reported larger secondary motor activations within patients with paresis than without paresis. This is most likely attributable to the difficulty of the task for the paretic patients.[3] Similar to the case of elderly patients recruiting a broader network of neurons than younger controls in order to execute a memory task,[49] the paretic patients may be recruiting additional cortical areas in order to execute a task that is relatively difficult for them given their current medical condition. Krings and colleagues therefore concluded, With increasing task complexity (or with decreasing motor skills), this network must increase its excitatory output, resulting in a higher neuronal activity, more pronounced regional cerebral blood flow changes.[3]

In tasks of higher cognitive functioning, the problem of task difficulty may be even more complex. For example, in our work with patients who have a genetic risk for Alzheimer's disease (AD), older volunteers with normal memory, but who carried the APO-4 allele (which conveys a strong risk of AD), had an increase in the magnitude and spatial extent of brain activation on fMRI in comparison to age- and memory-matched controls.[51] This increase in activation correlated with functional decline after two years. However, among subjects who have mild AD, the same memory paradigms produced the opposite effect; there was a significant decrease in magnitude, spatial extent, and total number of regions showing activation in those subjects who had great difficulty performing the task.

Patients with aphasia due to brain lesions showed similar alterations in brain activity. For instance, Sonty and colleagues[52] showed that patients with primary progressive aphasia had activation like normal patients in primary language areas, but also had additional language activation in regions outside language cortices, suggesting the use of compensatory strategies. Kim and collegues[40] found that the pattern of reorganization within patients with focal lesions varied across individuals and appeared related to whether the lesions were cortical or subcortical. Calvert and colleagues[53] found that patterns of fMRI activation during language tasks in a frontal lobe cerebrovascular accident (CVA) patient depended upon the task; increased right-hemisphere Broca's analog was activated during the most difficult task, whereas the left-hemisphere Broca's was active for a matched control subject.

Together, the existing data suggest that patients with deficits tend to utilize compensatory strategies that engage additional brain regions to accomplish the task. The pattern of fMRI activation during compensation may give a false impression about localization of function; for instance, increased compensatory RH, activation may incorrectly suggest the patient has right-hemisphere speech dominance. Thus, clinical use of fMRI for localization of function must take into account the patient's level of cognitive performance. Impaired performance can easily lead to false conclusions about functional localization, particularly in language tasks.

Ultimately, it is important to consider whether differences in activation patterns across conditions or groups represent differences in brain organization and function or an artifact of differential capability to cope with task difficulty. It is suggested that investigators pay close attention to task difficulty in designing, interpreting, and drawing conclusions from their clinical studies, especially when the general medical condition of one group is significantly different than the comparison group.

Analysis

Adequate study and task design is not sufficient to be able to draw strong conclusions from a clinical fMRI study. Careful selection of analysis techniques and attention to the particular challenges of analysis limitations is necessary in order to accurately interpret the results of the study. Analysis in the clinical studies differs from other studies most significantly with respect to the type of analysis done: within subject versus group analysis. Attention also must be paid to the technique used to quantify fMRI activations and techniques used to minimize false–positive and false–negative results.

Within Subject Versus Group Analysis

The vast corpus of data in functional imaging relies almost exclusively on group-averaged data. Early efforts in PET, and later fMRI research, focused on developing superior tools for registering and ultimately warping brains from different subjects into a common space in order to increase SNR through subject averaging. While these efforts have been extremely useful in making it possible to answer broad questions about human cognition, these approaches add little to the clinical utility of these skills. Here, we differentiate between clinical research studies, which have and will continue to use group averaging procedures, from true clinical fMRI, in which a clinician will attempt to make a diagnosis or decision for a single individual based on their fMRI results. First, the broad nature of the question to be answered will be considered.

Why will patients be referred for fMRI? Common current applications are to make a decision relevant to surgical intervention, such as, in what hemisphere is language located? Or where within a hemisphere does a particular functional reside? Future applications may include diagnosis: does a particular pattern of activation indicate a diagnosis of dyslexia, autism, obsessive compulsive disorder, or even malingering, to name a few. The optimal analysis technique will depend upon the question asked. In general, the former category of questions will be answered best by within-subject analysis, and in these cases, there will be a strong emphasis on reliability, reproducibility, and signal magnitude and on accounting for factors that may alter one of these variables. In the latter case, approaches may contrast a particular brain against a databank of brains with and without the disorder in question, calculating the degree of difference for the normative sample and similarity to a diagnostic group probabilistically. While this approach is not currently available, new attempts to find functional landmarks such as the International Consortium for Human Brain Mapping should further such efforts. Here, we will focus on reliability of methods for within-subject analysis in the common current applications.

Given an experimental design that includes at least one activation and *control* condition, several approaches to analysis may reveal active brain regions. Statistical approaches, including correlation coefficients between MR signal and a predicted response curve, *t*-tests comparing activation versus control pixel intensities, on Komogorov–Smirnov tests that show differences not only in mean, but also in variance, all produce a statistical value that the investigator must threshold and display in some way. Current controversies include how to threshold data and whether to use a statistical value or magnitude measure (percent change) or to count volume of activation—that is, the number of pixels exceeding a statistical threshold as a dependent variable. Each technique has its advantages and disadvantages, but few studies have carefully examined the reliability and validity of various approaches.

Dependent Measures

Functional MRI activations can be quantified broadly into two dimensions: spatial extent and magnitude of activation. Calculating activation size by means of pixel counting has become the most common approach to quantifying fMRI activity, especially in the clinical arena. This approach to activity quantification has several limitations that are discussed below. As an example, the application of pixel counting to studies of language lateralization will be reviewed.

Binder and colleagues[54] compared language lateralization using both fMRI and the intracarotid amobarbital procedure (IAP, the Wada test). For fMRI activations, they studied the contrast between semantic word categorization and a perceptual discrimination task, observing variable amounts of right and left hemisphere activation. The variable activation was quantified using a laterality index (LI), defined as $[V_L - V_R]/[V_L + V_R] \times 100$, where V_L and V_R are activation volumes for the left and right hemispheres, respectively, such that a LI of -100 indicates complete left-sided dominance and a score of $+100$ would indicate complete right-sided dominance. Volume of activation was defined as the number of pixels exceeding a statistical threshold of correlation with a derived hemodynamic function. A similar index was calculated for errors made during Wada testing using the error rates for each hemisphere injected. Statistical comparisons between the two different measures of laterality, or asymmetry, indicated a strong correlation between the two procedures. This led the authors to suggest a model of relative laterality, which was not completely novel because studies had already indicated by that time that the nondominant hemisphere had participated in language processing.[54]

These results are striking considering the methodology used. As discussed earlier in this chapter, disruption-based mapping (i.e., Wada testing) and activation-based mapping (i.e., fMRI) may map very different processes. Whereas Wada testing will identify those areas that are essential for language function, fMRI identifies all areas that are involved, essential or not, with language processing. For example, activation paradigms used in fMRI mapping may engage a number of brain systems not specifically related to language, including, including, motor, sensory, and attentional systems that may not be essential and therefore may not cause language disturbance by Wada testing. The high-correlation of the two methods is therefore impressive. The authors proposed that their use of a control paradigm (perceptual discrimination task), in part, controls for these factors, which is probably, in fact, true, but it cannot account for all the methodological differences that seemingly are unimportant in the analysis. They proposed that this be accounted for by the control task.

Beyond differences in methodology between the two techniques, the use of pixel counting to compare relative activity between the two hemispheres may not be valid under all circumstances. Pixel counting has been shown to be remarkably susceptible to noise, and therefore may not be an accurate or precise way of quantifying relative fMRI activation.[55,56] Moreover, this methodology does not account for differences in the magnitude of activation at activated pixels. What if the LI were 0 (indicating equal number of active pixels in both hemispheres), but the average magnitude of activation were three times greater in the left hemisphere? Should one conclude that there is no hemispheric asymmetry? The reliability of language lateralization studies is limited by the preponderance of left-hemisphere–dominant subjects included in the studies and the concomitant lack of right-hemisphere–dominant individual individuals. Therefore, it is not possible to conclude, with confidence, that fMRI using pixels counting is, in fact, a reliable method of identifying hemispheric dominance.

The limitations of using fMRI for language lateralization is demonstrated by Springer and colleagues, who studied 100 normal subjects and 50 epilepsy patients to compare laterality in the two populations.[57] Methods were similar to that of Binder and colleagues[54] except that Wada testing was not used to confirm results. Despite reports in the literature that approximately four percent of the general population is right-hemisphere dominant,[57] the authors did not identify any right-dominant individual in their normal population of 100 (expected number should have been four). Amongst their epilepsy population, four percent demonstrated right-hemisphere dominance, allowing the authors to conclude that laterality is differentially affected in early onset epilepsy patients than in normal populations. The low base rate of right-hemisphere speech makes it very difficult to compare populations accurately. Moreover, without a gold standard against which to validate results, there is no objective means to conclude that the data are valid.

A study by Lehericy and associates, in which they studied 10 patients for temporal surgery, compared fMRI activity with WADA testing, looking at LI in direct lobes using different language tasks: semantic verbal fluency, covert sentence repetition, and story listening.[59] This group also used LI as a measure of fMRI activity, counting pixels that exceeded a statistical threshold. The only statistically significant relationships identified were between the asymmetry of frontal-lobe fMRI activations for semantic verbal fluency and covert sentence repetition and Wada asymmetry indices. Functional MRI asymmetry in the temporal lobes (regardless of language task) did not correlate with Wada asymmetries. Moreover, story listening did not correlate with any Wada asymmetry indices in any lobe. It would be interesting to re-analyze this data to determine if better correlation could be identified across tasks and lobes if signal magnitude where considered instead of only the number of pixels exceeding the statistical threshold. This study highlights that fMRI is not completely reliable for assessing asymmetries and that measures of asymmetry may be task and lobe dependent.

Conjunction Analysis

Considering the intrinsic noise associated with fMRI data acquisition (both physiological and equipment related), alternative strategies have been devised in order to extract significant mapping signals that are consistent across tasks (see Figure 5.3).[60,61] Conjunction analysis identifies all voxels in the brain that exceed statistical threshold for two or more independent, yet related, tasks. By Bayes theorem, the probability of observing significant pixels by chance on multiple scans is equal to the product of the prior probability of chance activation on each. For example, if two separate tasks are used, using a Pearson's correlation coefficient threshold of 0.2, the probability of correlation by chance for each individual task is 0.063, and the joint probability is less than 0.004. By using a low statistical threshold for each

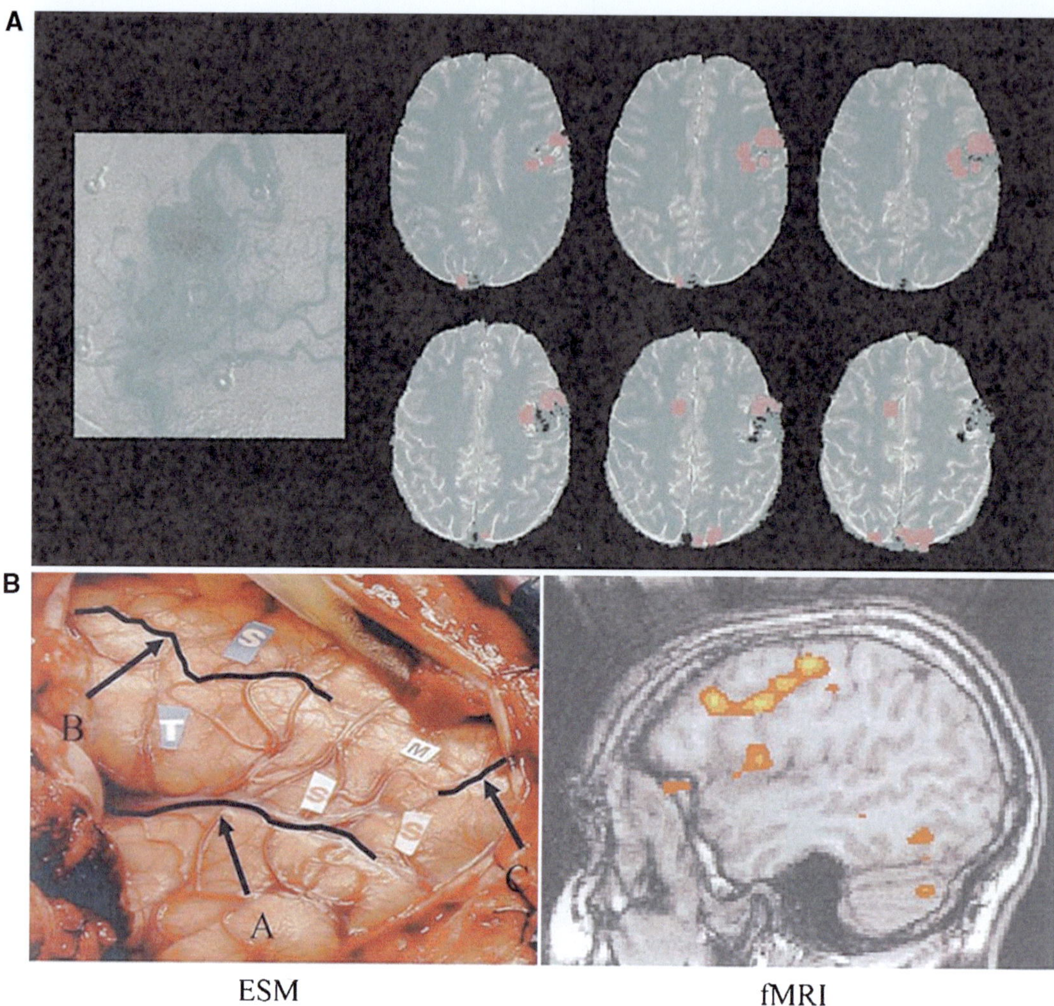

Figure 5.3. (A,B) Functional MRI activations adjacent to AVM. Significant fMRI activations are commonly identified adjacent to a left frontal lobe AVM. In this image, fMRI activations of language expression (created by conjunction analysis) are seen adjacent to a frontal AVM, identifying Broca's Area. Note that activations are not identified within the vascular malformation. Functional MRI activations were both qualitatively and quantitatively similar to the intraoperative electrocortical stimulation maps (B). Adapted with permission from Pouratian N, Bookheimer SY, Rex DE, Martin NA, Toga AW. Utility of pre-operative functional magnetic resonance imaging for identifying language cortices in patients with vascular malformations. *J Neurosurg.* 2002(a);97:21–32.

individual scan, conjunction analysis minimizes the probability of eliminating functionally significant voxels due to noise, which effectively reduces false–negative results. However, by requiring that the same voxel must be active across multiple tasks, this analysis minimizes false–positive results by ensuring that only functionally significant voxels are considered in the final analysis.

The power of this technique was recently demonstrated by Pouratian and colleagues in a study comparing language-related fMRI activations with intraoperative electrocortical stimulation map (ESM).[61] The authors created conjunction fMRI maps of expressive language (conjunction of two of three expressive language tasks: visual object naming, word generation, and auditory response naming) and receptive language (conjunction of visual responsive naming and sentence comprehension) and compared these fMRI activations with intraoperative ESM (Figure 5.3A, B). For the population studied, the authors reported sensitivity and specificity values of expression fMRI activations of up to 100% and 66.7%, respectively, in the frontal lobe, and of comprehension fMRI activations of up to 96.2% and 69.8%, respectively, in the parietal/temporal lobes.

Based on the differences between ESM and fMRI methodology, false–positives consistent with an imperfect specificity should be expected. Whereas ESM is a disruption-based technique that will identify only those areas that are essential to language processing, fMRI is an activation-based technique that will identify all regions of the brain that demonstrate activity-related changes, whether those areas are essential or supplementary. Consequently, areas that are negative for language by ESM may still demonstrate fMRI activations, producing false–positives. The use of the conjunction analysis, however, minimizes this false–positive rate by only identifying those areas that are consistently activated across language tasks. Nonetheless, there clearly are still supplementary and non-essential language areas that are not identified by ESM, but that are consistently active across fMRI activations.

Reproducibility

Reproducibility of fMRI activations, either within subjects or across studies, is rarely addressed. Nonetheless, it is an important consideration, especially now that functional brain mapping is being used increasingly for quantification of brain activity and clinical decision making.[54,61]

Cohen and DuBois reported the most extensive and quantitative study to date of fMRI signal reproducibility, with surprising results with respect to signal stability.[55] Studying both visual and motor cortex, they reported that counting pixels exceeding statistical significance is remarkably unstable, with values varying by 750% across trials. This large degree of variability is attributed to differences in noise levels across trials although the actual activation magnitude is likely the same across trials. (Noise may be composed of a variety of artifacts and physiological factors.) The noise variance propagates through to statistical calculations and produces a widely varying number of pixels that exceed statistical threshold. In contrast, the slope of the regression line, which is essentially the percent signal change, is much more stable across trials and subjects, with less than 20% variability across trials. Monte Carlo simulations support the assertion that even in very poor contrast-to-noise ratio (CNR) conditions, the percent signal change can be determined with relatively good accuracy and precision.[55]

Huetell and McCarthy[56] arrived at a similar conclusion regarding the value of activation size: Group or condition differences may result from differences in voxelwise noise exacerbated by averaging small numbers of trials. By progressively averaging an increasing number of trials to determine activation size, they found that activation size increases exponentially, reaching a plateau at approximately 150 trials averaged a number that is far less than most conventional fMRI studies. This uncertainty in activation size is attributed to noise, high-lighting how intrinsic fMRI noise sources can significantly alter activation sizes.

These studies argue strongly for the lack of reliability of activation size as a measure of response magnitude. Instead, measuring the percent signal change or the slope of the regression line is a much more reliable measure of response magnitude. The latter method of measuring percent signal change is also preferable because it can detect changes in response magnitude across tasks in voxels that are already activated in the original task. Investigators should not only be interested in areas of additional activity, but also in changes in response magnitude of already activated regions.[62] Even if pixel counting were a reliable method, it would not be able to account for such differences. Due to the limited reliability of merely counting pixels, we recommend comparing percent signal change within a statistically defined ROI across trials or tasks in order to compare reliable measures.

Applying fMRI to Clinical Planning

Significance of Signal Localization

Earlier, the concept that the fMRI activation is intimately related to and depends upon the characteristics of neurovascular coupling was introduced. The uncertainty and imprecision of neurovascular coupling introduces one of the biggest challenges and one of the most significant sources of error in interpreting clinical fMRI studies. It is well accepted that the time courses of electrophysiological and hemodynamic responses are different by orders of magnitude. Most investigators also assume tight spatial coupling between electrophysiologically active cortex and the observed hemodynamic response. This, in fact, is probably not as robust a relationship as most assume, limited by neurovascular mechanisms and fMRI physics.

Depending on the scan sequence used, the BOLD fMRI signals often center in adjacent sulci[39,63,64] and can be up to one centimeter away from electrophysiologically active cortex.[39] The sulcal localization suggests that the positive BOLD fMRI signal may not be a very specific mapping signal. Offering relatively poor spatial colocalization with electrophysiological maps and emphasizing changes occurring in vasculature rather than within the cortex.[34,63–65] Alternative mapping signals have been suggested, like the initial dip that may offer a more precise colocalization with electrophysiologically active cortex.[37,38]

Despite the imprecision of spatial localization, fMRI mapping signals are still useful and have been shown to spatially correlate with electrophysiologically active.[66] However, in most cases, in order to achieve spatial colocalization, a sphere of influence of fMRI activity often is assumed to be approximately 0.5–1.0 centimeters in order to achieve high correlation rates.[61,66–69] Because of the spatial imprecision of fMRI, especially when doing whole head imaging, it is important not to over interpret small differences in spatial extent or lack of difference in spatial extent as representing a clear difference in activation patterns or a lack of difference in activation patterns, respectively.

Reliability of Signal Adjacent to Pathology

The reliability of fMRI signals has been called into question both with respect to susceptibility artifact induced by intracerebral pathologies and surgical interventions (e.g., atertiovenous malformations, cavernous angiomas, surgical clips), and with respect to the mass effect and possible physiological disturbance induced by the presence of pathology.

With respect to susceptibility artifact, it is clearly impossible to obtain a signal from within a pathology with significant susceptibility artifact. The question remains as to whether reliable signals can be obtained from adjacent to the pathologies. In a study of 14 patients, Schlosser and colleagues reported that fMRI signals within patients with frontal-lobe tumors were comparable to signals in normal controls.[13] Similarly, Righini and colleagues found little difference in motor activations between the affected and unaffected hemispheres in 17 patients with frontoparietal masses.[2] Pouratian and colleagues also recently reported that functional activations, which correlate with intraoperative cortical stimulation mapping, can consistently and reliably be measured adjacent to vascular malformations (i.e., AVMs and cavernous hemangiomas).[61] These reports are consistent with our findings at UCLA, in which we regularly and successfully map motor and language cortices within patients scheduled for neurosurgical intervention near eloquent cortices (see Figure 5.4).

Reports of abnormal fMRI activations adjacent to pathology like represent cases in which the pathology has infiltrated the cortex of interest, and therefore altered normal cortical function, cerebral hemodynamic, or both. Because of the importance of preserving eloquent function, if fMRI maps are being used for neurosurgical guidance, it is imperative to verify preoperative fMRI maps intraoperatively with intraoperative direct cortical stimulation mapping in order to ensure preservation of eloquent function.

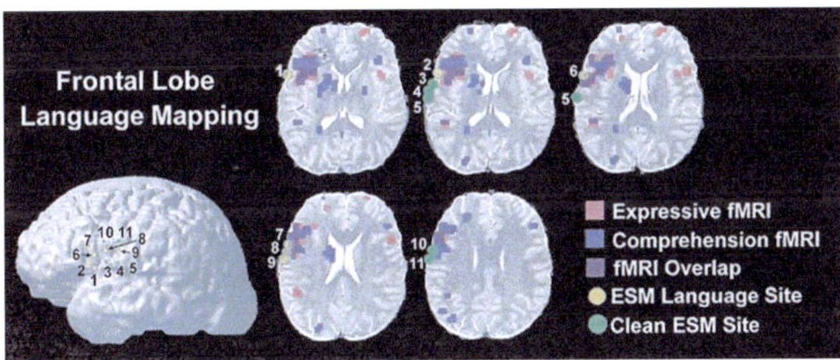

Figure 5.4. Frontal lobe language mapping using fMRI with conjunction analysis. Yellow circles are areas essential for language as determined by ESM. Green circle s are areas that, when stimulated, did not disrupt language function. Red activations are conjunction fMRI maps of language expression. Blue activations are conjunction fMRI maps of language comprehension. Electrocortical stimulation map sites are shown with a five-millimeter radius (determined to produce the highest sensitivity with the least cost to specificity) and parietal/temporal. Red (expression) activations tend to overlap with, or are adjacent to, essential (yellow) ESM sites, but avoid non-essential (green) ESM sites. Blue activations in the frontal lobe also appear predictive, but with lower specificity in this subject than the expression fMRI activations. Adapted with permission from Pouratian N, Bookheimer SY, Sex DE, Martin NA, Toga AW. Utility of pre-operative functional magetic resonance imaging for identifying language cortices in patients with vascular malformations. *J Neurosurg.* 2002(a);97:21–32.

Relationship to Outcomes

Although many studies have investigated the relationship between fMRI and electrophysiological maps,[67–72] very few studies have quantified the sensitivity and specificity of fMRI activations relative to electrophysiological maps or determined the relationship between fMRI maps and clinical outcomes. These are ultimately the most important factors to be determined with respect to the utility of fMRI as a clinical tool. As fMRI analysis techniques are improved, fMRI will surely play an increasing role in identifying clinically relevant motor and language areas, as well as other eloquent cortices.

As long-term outcomes are ultimately the most important variable in clinical neurosurgery, outcomes studies like that of Haglund and colleagues,[73] which characterized clinical outcomes postoperatively relative to distance of resection from essential language sites as defined by ESM, need to be done across different tasks and cortices to determine the best approach to clinical fMRI mapping.

Conclusions

Functional MRI is a powerful brain-mapping tool whose use has grown exponentially over the last decade. Unfortunately, our understanding of signal etiology, neurovascular coupling, and physiological baselines have not evolved at the same rate. As with most other imaging modalities, fMRI will rapidly enter the clinical arena as a commonly used and accepted modality. Before then, it is important to acknowledge and address many of the limitations that continue to challenge this modality. Moreover, as with any clinical test, it will be important to quantify its sensitivity, specificity, and relationship to outcomes in the future. Different clinical applications, experimental paradigms, analysis approach, and even equipment can produce different results; valid application of fMRI to clinical cases will have to demonstrate reliability and validity for each application separately. The field should move rapidly towards developing uniform approaches to clinical fMRI that are valid, reliable, and replicable across centers. We believe that for most applications, clinical decisions should not rest solely on fMRI results. Rather, fMRI may augment existing clinical tools as validation of the techniques continues.

References

1. Belliveau JW, Kennedy DN Jr, McKinstry RC, Buchbinder BR, Weisskoff RM, Cohen MS, Vevea JM, Brady TJ. Functional mapping of the human visual cortex by magnetic resonance imaging. *Science*. 1991;254(5032):716–719.
2. Righini A, de Divitiis O, Prinster A, Spagnoli D, Appollonio I, Bello L, Scifo P, Tomei G, Villani R, Fazio F, Leonardi M. Functional MRI: primary motor cortex localization in patients with brain tumors. *J Comput Assist Tomogr*. 1996;20:702.
3. Krings T, Topper R, Willmes K, Reinges MHT, Gilsbach JM, Thron A. Activation in primary and secondary motor areas in patients with CNS neoplasms and weakness. *Neurology*. 2002(a);58.
4. Mazziotta JC, Huang SC, Phelps ME, Carson RE, MacDonald NS, Mahoney K. A noninvasive positron computed tomography technique using oxygen-15–labeled water for the evaluation of neurobehavioral task batteries. *J Cereb Blood Flow Metab*. 1985;5(1):70–78.

5. Frostig RD, Lieke EE, Ts'o DY, Grinvald A. Cortical functional architecture and local coupling between neuronal activity and the microcirculation revealed by in vivo high-resolution optical imaging of intrinsic signals. *Proc Natl Acad Sci USA*. 1990;87:6082–6086.
6. Villringer A, Planck J, Hock C, Schleinkofer L, Dirnagl U. Near infrared spectroscopy (NIRS): a new tool to study hemodynamic changes during activation of brain function in human adults. *Neurosci Lett*. 1993;154:101–104.
7. Penfield W, Boldrey E. Somatic motor and sensory representation in the cerebral cortex of man as studied by electrical stimulation. *Brain*. 1937;60:389–443.
8. Jahanshahi M, Rothwell J. Transcranial magnetic stimulation studies of cognition: an emerging field. *Exp Brain Res*. 2000;131:1–9.
9. Villringer A, Dirnagl U. Coupling of brain activity and cerebral blood flow: basis of functional neuroimaging. *Cerebrovasc Brain Metab Rev*. 1995;7(3):240–276.
10. Krings T, Reinges MHT, Willmes K, Nuerk HC, Meister IG, Gilsbach JM, Thron A. Factors related to the magnitude of T2* MR signal changes during functional imaging. *Neuroradiology*. 2002(b);44:459–466.
11. Holodny AI, Schulder M, Liu WC, Wolko J, Maldjian JA, Kalnin AJ. The effect of brain tumors on BOLD functional MR imaging activation in the adjacent motor cortex: implications for image-guided Neurosurgery. *Am J Neuroradiol*. 2000;21:1415–1422.
12. Schreiber A, Hubbe U, Ziyeh S, Hennig J. The influence of gliomas and nonglial space-occupying lesions on blood-oxygen-level-dependent contrast enhancement. *Am J Neuroradiol*. 2000;21:1055–1063.
13. Schlosser R, Husche S, Gawehn J, Grunert P, Vucurevic G, Geserich T, Kaufmann B, Rossbach W, Stoeter P. Characterization of BOLD-fMRI signal during a verbal fluency paradigm in patients with intracerebral tumors affecting the frontal lobe. *Magn Reson Imaging*. 2002;20:7–16.
14. Schmitz B, Bettiger BW, Hossmann KA. Brief hypercapnia enhances somatosensory activation of blood flow in rat. *J Cereb Blood Flow Metab*. 1996;16:1307–1311.
15. Bock C, Schmitz B, Kerskens CM, Gyngell ML, Hossmann KA, Hoehn-Berlage M. Functional MRI of somatosensory activation in rat: effect of hypercapnic up-regulation on perfusion and BOLD-imaging. *Magn Reson Med*. 1998;39:457–461.
16. Bandetti PA, Wong EC. A hypercapnia-based normalization method for improved spatial localization of human brain activation with fMRI. *NMR Biomed*. 1997;10:197–203.
17. Kruger G, Kastrup A, Glover GH. Neuroimaging at 1.5T and 3.0T: comparison of oxygenation-sensitive magnetic resonance imaging. *Magn Reson Med*. 2001;45(4):595–604.
18. Ojemann G, Ojemann J, Lettich E, Berger M. Cortical language localization in left, dominant hemisphere. An electrical stimulation mapping investigation in 117 patients. *J Neurosurg*. 1989;71:316–326.
19. Devlin JT, Russell RP, Davis MH, Price CJ, Wilson J, Moss HE, Matthews PM, Tyler LK. Susceptibility-induced loss of signal: Comparing PET and fMRI on a semantic task. *Neuroimage*. 2000;11:589–600.
20. Cohen MS, Weisskoff RM. Ultra-fast imaging. *Magn Reson Imaging*. 1991;9:1–37.
21. Merboldt KD, Fransson P, Bruhn H, Frahm J. Functional MRI of the human amygdala? *Neuroimage*. 2001;14(2):253–257.
22. Fransson P, Merboldt KD, Ingvar M, Petersson KM, Frahm J. Functional MRI with reduced susceptibility artifact: high-resolution mapping of episodic memory encoding. *Neuroreport*. 2001;12(7):1415–1420.
23. Port JD, Pomper MG. Quantification and minimization of magnetic susceptibility artifacts on GRE images. *J Comput Assist Tomogr*. 2000;24(6):958–964.
24. Gorno-Tempini ML, Hutton C, Josephs O, Deichmann R, Price C, Turner R. Echo time dependence of BOLD contrast and susceptibility artifacts. *Neuroimage*. 2002;15(1):136–142.

25. Stables LA, Kennan RP, Gore JC. Asymmetric spin-echo imaging of magnetically inhomogeneous systems: theory, experiment, and numerical studies *Magn Reson Med*. 1998;40(3):432–442.

26. Stern CE, Corkin S, Gonzalez RG, Guimaraes AR, Baker JR, Jennings PJ, Carr CA, Sugiura RM, Vedantham V, Rosen BR. The hippocampal formation participates in novel picture encoding: evidence from functional magnetic resonance imaging. *Proc Natl Acad Sci USA*. 1996;93(16):8660–8665.

27. Hariri A, Bookheimer SY, Mazziotta J. A neural network for modulating the emotional response to faces. *Neuroreport*. 2000;11(1):43–48.

28. LaBar KS, Gatenby JC, Gore JC, LeDoux JE, Phelps EA. Human amygdala activation during conditioned fear acquisition and extinction: a mixed-trial fMRI study. *Neuron*. 1998;20(5):937–945.

29. Cordes D, Turski PA, Sorenson JA. Compensation of susceptibility-induced signal loss in echo-planar imaging for functional applications. *Magn Reson Imaging*. 2000;18(9):1055–1068.

30. Stenger VA, Boada FE, Noll DC. Three-dimensional tailored RF pulses for the reduction of susceptibility artifacts in T(*)(2)-weighted functional MRI. *Magn Reson Med*. 2000;44(4):525–531.

31. Glover GH, Law CS. Spiral-in/out BOLD fMRI for increased SNR and reduced susceptibility artifacts. *Magn Reson Med*. 2001;46(3):515–522.

32. Yang Y, Gu H, Zhan W, Xu S, Silbersweig DA, Stern E. Simultaneous perfusion and BOLD imaging using reverse spiral scanning at 3T: characterization of functional contrast and susceptibility artifacts. *Magn Reson Med*. 2002;48(2):278–289.

33. Weiger M, Pruessmann KP, Osterbauer R, Bornert P, Boesiger P, Jezzard P. Sensitivity-encoded single-shot spiral imaging for reduced susceptibility artifacts in BOLD fMRI. *Magn Reson Med*. 2002;48(5):860–866.

34. Cohen MS, Bookheimer SY. Localization of brain function using magnetic resonance imaging. *Trends Neurosci*. 1994;17:268–277.

35. Fox PT, Raichle ME. Focal physiological uncoupling of cerebral blood flow and oxidative metabolism during somatosensory stimulation in human subjects. *Proc Nat Acad Sci USA*. 1986;83:1140–1144.

36. Malonek D, Grinvald A. Interactions between electrical activity and cortical microcirculation revealed by imaging spectroscopy: implications for functional brain mapping. *Science*. 1996;272:551–554.

37. Vanzetta I, Grinvald A. Increased cortical oxidative metabolism due to sensory stimulation: implications for functional brain imaging. *Science*. 1999;286:1555–1558.

38. Menon RS, Ogawa S, Hu X, Strupp JP, Anderson P, Ugurbil K. BOLD based functional MRI at 4 Tesla includes a capillary bed contribution: echo-planar imaging correlates with previous optical imaging using intrinsic signals. *Magn Reson Med*. 1995;33:453–459.

39. Cannestra AF, Pouratian N, Bookheimer SY, Martin NA, Becker D, Toga AW. Temporal spatial differences observed by functional MRI and human intraoperative optical imaging. *Cereb Cortex*. 2001;11:773–782.

40. Kim DS, Duong TQ, Kim SG. High-resolution mapping of iso-orientation columns by fMRI [see comments]. *Nat Neurosci*. 2000;3:164–169.

41. Kwong KK, Belliveau JW, Chesler DA, Goldberg IE, Weisskoff RM, Poncelet BP, Kennedy DN, Hoppel BE, Cohen MS, Turner R, et al. Dynamic magnetic resonance imaging of human brain activity during primary sensory stimulation. *Proc Natl Acad Sci USA*. 1992;89:5675–5679.

42. Ogawa S, Tank DW, Menon R, Ellermann JM, Kim SG, Merkle H, Ugurbil K. Intrinsic signal changes accompanying sensory stimulation: functional brain mapping with magnetic resonance imaging. *Proc Natl Acad Sci USA*. 1992;89:5951–5955.

43. Sidtis JJ, Strother SC, Anderson JR, Rottenberg DA. Are brain functions really additive? *Neuroimage*. 1999;9:490–496.

44. Stark CEL, Squire LR. When zero is not zero: The problem of ambiguous baseline conditions in fMRI. *Proc Natl Acad Sci USA.* 2001;98:12760–12765.

45. Gusnard DA, Raichle ME. Searching for a baseline: Functional imaging and the resting human brain. *Nat Rev Neurosci.* 2001;2:685–694.

46. Raichle ME, Fiez JA, Videen TO, MacLeod AK, Pardo JV, Fox PT, Petersen SE. Practice-related changes in human brain functional anatomy during nonmotor learning. *Cereb Cortex.* 1994;4:8–26.

47. Petersen SE, van Mier H, Fiez JA, Raichle ME. The effects of practice on the functional anatomy of task performance. *Proc Natl Acad Sci USA.* 1998;95:853–860.

48. Van Mier H, Tempel LW, Perlmutter JS, Raichle ME, Petersen SE. Changes in brain activity during motor learning measured with PET: effects of hand of performance and practice. *J Neurophysiol.* 1998;80:2177–2199.

49. Madden DJ, Turkington TG, Provenzale JM, Denny LL, Hawk TC, Gottlob LR, Coleman RE. Adult age differences in the functional neuroanatomy of verbal recognition memory. *Hum Brain Map.* 1999;7:115–135.

50. Garavan H, Kelley D, Rosen A, Rao SR, Stein EA. Practice-related functional activation changes in a working memory task. *Microsc Res Tech.* 2000;51:54–63.

51. Bookheimer SY, Strojwas MH, Cohen MS, Saunders AM, Pericak-Vance MA, Mazziotta JC, Small GW. Patterns of brain activation in people at risk for Alzheimer's disease. *N Engl J Med.* 2000;343(7):450–456.

52. Sonty SP, Mesulam MM, Thompson CK, Johnson NA, Weintraub S, Parrish TB, Gitelman DR. Primary progressive aphasia: PPA and the language network. *Ann Neurol.* 2003;53(1):35–49.

53. Calvert GA, Brammer MJ, Morris RG, Williams SC, King N, Matthews PM. Using fMRI to study recovery from acquired dysphasia. *Brain Lang.* 2000;71(3):391–399.

54. Binder JR, Swanson SJ, Hammeke TA, Morris GL, Mueller WM, Fischer M. Determination of language dominance using functional MRI: a comparison with the Wada test. *Neurology.* 1996;46:978–984.

55. Cohen MS, DuBois RM. Stability, repeatability, and the expression of signal magnitude in functional magnetic resonance imaging. *J Magn Reson Imaging.* 1999;10:33–40.

56. Huettel SA, McCarthy G. The effects of single-trial averaging upon the spatial extent of fMRI activation. *Neuroreport.* 2001;12:2411–2416.

57. Springer JA, Binder JR, Hammeke TA, Swanson SJ, Frost JA, Bellgowan PSF, Brewer CC, Perry HM, Morris GL, Mueller WM. Language dominance in neurologically normal and epilepsy subject: A functional MRI study. *Brain.* 1999;122:2033–2045.

58. Rasmussen T, Milner B. The role of early left-brain injury in determining lateralization of cerebral speech functions. *Ann NY Acad Sci.* 1977;299:355–369.

59. Leh Rich S, Cohen L, Bazin B, Samson S, Giacomini E, Rougetet R, Hertz-Pannier L, Le Bihan D, Marsault C, Baulac M. Functional MR evaluation of temporal and frontal language dominance compared with the Wada test. *Neurology.* 2000;54.

60. Bookheimer SY, Zeffiro TA, Blaxton T, Malow BA, Gaillard WD, Sato S, Kufta C, Fedio P, Theodore WH. A direct comparison of PET activation and electrocortical stimulation mapping for language localization. *Neurology.* 1997;48:1056–1065.

61. Pouratian N, Bookheimer SY, Rex DE, Martin NA, Toga AW. Utility of pre-operative functional magnetic resonance imaging for identifying language cortices in patients with vascular malformations. *J Neurosurg.* 2002(a);97:21–32.

62. Price C, Wise R, Ramsay S, Friston K, Howard D, Patterson K, Frackowiak R. Regional response differences within the human auditory cortex when listening to words. *Neurosci Lett.* 1992;146:179–182.

63. Lai S, Hopkins AL, Haacke EM, Li D, Wasserman BA, Buckley P, Friedman L, Meltzer H, Hedera P, Friedland R. Identification of vascular structures as a major source of signal contrast in high resolution 2D and 3D functional activation imaging of the motor cortex at 1.5T: preliminary results. *Magn Reson Med.* 1993;30: 387–392.

64. Pouratian N, Bookheimer SY, O'Farrell AM, Sicotte NL, Cannestra AF, Becker D, Toga AW. Optical imaging of bilingual cortical representations: Case report. *J Neurosurg.* 2000;93:686–691.

65. Duong TQ, Kim DS, Ugurbil K, Kim SG. Spatiotemporal dynamics of the BOLD fMRI signals: toward mapping submillimeter cortical columns using the early negative response [in process citation]. *Magn Reson Med.* 2000;44:231–242.

66. Pouratian N, Sicotte N, Rex D, Martin NA, Becker D, Cannestra AF, Toga AW. Spatial/temporal correlation of BOLD and optical intrinsic signals in humans. *Magn Reson Med.* 2002b;47:766–776.

67. Roux FE, Boulanouar K, Ranjeva JP, Manelfe C, Tremoulet M, Sabatier J, Berry I. Cortical intraoperative stimulation in brain tumors as a tool to evaluate spatial data from motor functional MRI. *Invest Radiol.* 1999a;34:225–229.

68. Corina DP, Poliakov A, Steury K, Martin R, Mulligan K, Maravilla K, Brinkly JF, Ojemann GA. Correspondences between language cortex identified by cortical stimulation mapping and fMRI. *Neuroimage.* 2000;11:S295.

69. Lurito JT, Lowe MJ, Sartorius C, Mathews VP. Comparison of fMRI and intra-operative direct cortical stimulation in localization of receptive language areas. *J Comput Assist Tomogr.* 2000;24:99–105.

70. Mueller WM, Yetkin FZ, Hammeke TA, Morris GL 3rd, Swanson SJ, Reichert K, Cox R, Haughton VM. Functional magnetic resonance imaging mapping of the motor cortex in patients with cerebral tumors. *Neurosurgery.* 1996;39:515–520; discussion 520–511.

71. Roux FE, Boulanouar K, Ranjeva JP, Tremoulet M, Henry P, Manelfe C, Sabatier J, Berry I. Usefulness of motor functional MRI correlated to cortical mapping in Rolandic low-grade astrocytomas. *Acta Neurochir.* 1999b;141:71–79.

72. Rutten GJ, van Rijen PC, van Veelen CW, Ramsey NF. Language area localization with three-dimensional functional magnetic resonance imaging matches intrasulcal electrostimulation in Broca's area. *Ann Neurol.* 1999;46:405–408.

73. Haglund MM, Berger MS, Shamseldin M, Lettich E, Ojemann GA. Cortical localization of temporal lobe language sites in patients with gliomas. *Neurosurgery.* 1994;34:567–576; discussion 576.

Part II

fMRI Clinical Applications

6

Brain Mapping for Neurosurgery and Cognitive Neuroscience

Joy Hirsch

Historical Milestones That Enable Imaging of Cortical Processes That Underlie Mental Events Using MRI

One of the primary goals of neural science is to understand the biological underpinnings of cognition. This goal is based on the assumption that cognitive events emerge from brain events and that behavior can be explained in terms of neural processes. Francis Crick referred to this as "the Astonishing Hypothesis."[1] According to this view, the biological principles that underlie cognition link the structure and function of the brain.

> The Astonishing Hypothesis is that "You," your joys and your sorrows, your memories and your ambitions, your sense of personal identity and free will, are in fact no more than the behavior of a vast assembly of nerve cells and their associated molecules. As Lewis Carroll's Alice might have phrased it: "You're nothing but a pack of neurons."† This hypothesis is so alien to the ideas of most people alive today that it can truly be called astonishing.
>
> Francis Crick, 1994, *The Astonishing Hypothesis*, p.3

Using neuroimaging methods, it is possible to observe active cortical areas associated with cognitive processes in healthy human volunteers. This capability has stimulated a renewed focus on the physiological bases of cognition. In particular, the implementation of noninvasive, functional imaging techniques such as functional magnetic resonance imaging (fMRI) offers an unprecedented global view of the complexities of the intact working human brain, including local neural circuits (cortical columns), regions, and large-scale systems of interconnected regions. Functional imaging provides a

---

This chapter previously appeared in *Functional MRI: Basic Principles and Clinical Applications,* edited by S. Faro and F. Mohamed. New York: Springer Science+Business Media, LCC 2006.

From: *BOLD fMRI: A Guide to Functional Imaging for Neuroscientists*
Edited by: S.H. Faro and F.B. Mohamed, DOI 10.1007/978-1-4419-1329-6_6
© Springer Science+Business Media, LLC 2010

unique view of the cortical activation patterns associated with specific mental processes such as seeing, hearing, feeling, moving, talking, and thinking. Thus, the potential to realize a neural basis for various aspects of cognition has emerged with the development of neuroimaging.

Conventional definitions of cognition do not directly address the biological components of mental events. For example, *Dorland's Illustrated Medical Dictionary* defines cognition as "operations of the mind by which we become aware of objects of thought or perception; it includes all aspects of perceiving, thinking and remembering."[2] *The American Heritage Dictionary* offers a similar definition for cognition as "the mental process of knowing, including aspects such as awareness, perception, reasoning and judgment, and that which comes to be known, as through perception, reasoning, or intuition, and knowledge."[3] However, in his seminal book, *Cognitive Psychology*, Ulrich Neisser defined cognition as "*all processes* by which the sensory input is transformed, reduced, elaborated, stored, recovered, and used."[4] This definition could be interpreted to encompass biological processes, although none were specifically proposed by Neisser. An essential focus of neuroimaging is to link models of cognition to biological processes.

Medical reports of associations between specific brain injuries and functional deficits provided the initial basis for the assumed linkage between specific brain areas and behavior. As early as 1841, Broca reported language production deficits in patients with specific damage to the left frontal lobe, and in 1874, Wernicke reported deficits in language comprehension and expression in patients following specific damage to the left temporal lobe. Since then, Broca's and Wernicke's Areas have become established as regions of cortex associated with aspects of speech production and comprehension, respectively. Around the same time, Harlow reported profound personality changes following an unfortunate frontal-lobe injury in his now well-known patient, Phineas Gage.[5] Nearly a century later, Penfield pioneered the experimental technique of direct cortical stimulation during neurosurgical procedures. His observations confirmed the functional specializations of the speech-related areas and demonstrated topographical maps associated with sensory and motor functions.[6] Along with the documented associations between lesions and specific functions, Penfield's reports of cortical stimulations that elicited memories, tastes, and other mental events supported the profound link between brain structure and cognitive function widely accepted within the mainstream of clinical neurology and neurosurgery. For example, it had been noted that severing a segment of the optic nerve always resulted in visual field loss (Figure 6.1), and similarly, severing a primary motor projection always resulted in a contralateral plegia.

One of the key principles that links brain function and mental events is the relationship between neural activity and blood flow. In 1881, Angelo Mosso, a physiologist, studied a patient who had survived an injury to the skull. Due to the nature of the injury, it was possible to observe blood-flow–related pulsations to the left frontal lobe that occurred during certain cognitive events. Mosso concluded that blood flow within the brain was coupled to mental events. Roy and Sherrington[7] subsequently proposed a specific mechanism to couple blood flow and neural activity based on direct measurements on dogs. More recently, using $H_2^{15}O$ as a tracer of blood flow in the human brain, Raichle and colleagues[8] confirmed this fundamental relationship between blood flow and local neural activity. This seminal physiology work provided the basis for positron emission tomographic (PET) imaging of active cortical

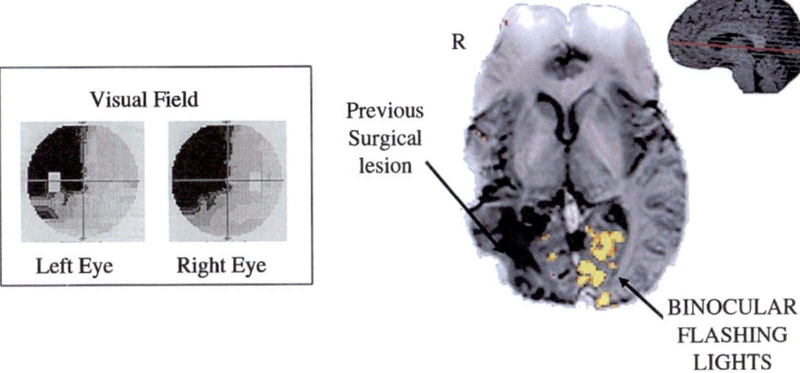

Figure 6.1. Static visual fields indicate a homonymous quadrantic field defect in the left superior quadrant that is associated with damage to the visual projection fibers within the right occipital lobe following resection of a lesion within the right hemisphere occipital region. Functional magnetic resonance imaging activation during binocular viewing of flashing lights (8 Hz) demonstrates unilateral cortical responses (left hemisphere only), reflecting the loss of visual responses in this topographically mapped area of the visual field.

tissue during the execution of a task. The technique was demonstrated by Fox and Raichle[9] with a simple sensory and motor activation paradigm, where hemodynamic variations (as indicated by a radioactive tracer of water molecules) were observed within the pre- and post-central gyri.

Typically, PET activation studies depend upon subtractive comparisons of images acquired during a task and images acquired during a rest or control condition. The logic of this technique is that the difference image represents the neural activity present in the task condition and not in the control; for example, activity associated with viewing a flashing checkerboard minus activity associated with viewing a fixation dot presumably reveals the effect of the flashing checkerboard on specialized neural structures. Unfortunately, the PET camera does not provide a detailed image of brain structure; therefore, computational techniques to register the locations of the gamma ray events to brain anatomy obtained by other higher-resolution techniques such as magnetic resonance imaging (MRI) were developed. These procedures also include algorithms to register the anatomical and PET images of multiple subjects based on a standard human brain atlas. When all subject brains are registered to the same atlas, the difference images of multiple subjects can be averaged to obtain conserved and generalizable results.

These advances in PET techniques enabled the first neuroimaging study of cognitive processes relating to language.[10] The study differntiated cortical patterns of activation associated with four separate word tasks: passively viewing words, listening to words, speaking words, and generating words. These early PET studies firmly established the proof-of-principle that activity associated with cognitive events was observable in the living human brain via hemodynamic variations within locally active neural areas. However, due to risks associated with injections of radioactive tracers, limitations to the number of times a subject can be studied, the relatively coarse resolution, and the relatively few PET facilities available for research, the imaging of cortical activity associated with cognitive processes has advanced most rapidly using a newer, noninvasive, higher-resolution, and more available technique, functional magnetic resonance imaging (fMRI).

Development of Magnetic Resonance Imaging (MRI) to Visualize Living Brain Structure

Since the invention of the microscope in 1664, imaging technology has guided the mainstream of basic research in biology by revealing structures not visible to the naked eye, including the cell, organelles, molecules, and even atoms. Despite its electronic and computational developments, the microscope is not suited for the imaging of living structures occluded beneath surface tissues such as skin, muscle, and bone. This occlusion problem was solved with the development of MRI, where internal structures within the living body can be resolved at submillmeter scales.

The development of MRI incorporated a long chain of discoveries (Figure 6.2), beginning with the discovery of molecular beam magnetic resonance in 1936 by Isidor Rabi at Columbia University. Shortly thereafter, in 1945, Edward Purcell and Felix Bloch independently discovered nuclear magnetic resonance (NMR) in condensed matter, followed by Erwin Hahn's observations of nuclear magnetic relaxation and the discovery of spin echo in 1949. A pinnacle event in the development of MRI was made in 1971 by Raymond Damadian who discovered that biological tissues have different relaxation rates. A year later, the first magnetic resonance image of a tube phantom was produced by Paul Lauterbur using a magnetic gradient to produce spatial resolution of the image. The first MRI of a human body part (a finger) was published in 1976 by Peter Mansfield and colleagues. Mansfield and colleagues also developed a key enhancement of a high-speed imaging sequence, echo planar imaging, which enabled three-dimensional (3D) acquisitions of body organs (such as the brain) within seconds. A year later, Damadian produced the first magnetic resonance image of a human whole body (cross sectional chest) and in 1980 produced the first human whole body commercial MRI scanner.

The Development of fMRI

Recent advances in MRI have extended imaging of brain structures to include the identification of active neural tissue in the cortex. The chain of discoveries that led to the generation of MR images of the working brain include Michael Faraday's discovery in 1845 that dried blood has magnetic properties, and Linus Pauling's discovery in 1936 that the magnetic properties of hemoglobin change with the state of oxygenation.

The BOLD Response

These discoveries lay dormant with respect to functional neuroimaging until after the development of high-speed MRI of brain structure and PET imaging of active neural tissue based on the coupling of blood flow. The fundamental breakthrough discovery of the blood oxygen level-dependent (BOLD) signal in 1990 by Seiji Ogawa and colleagues followed the observation that the MR signal originating from the occipital lobe (the area of the brain specialized for visual processing) in rats had a higher contrast when the room lights were on than when the lights were off. Ogawa reasoned that

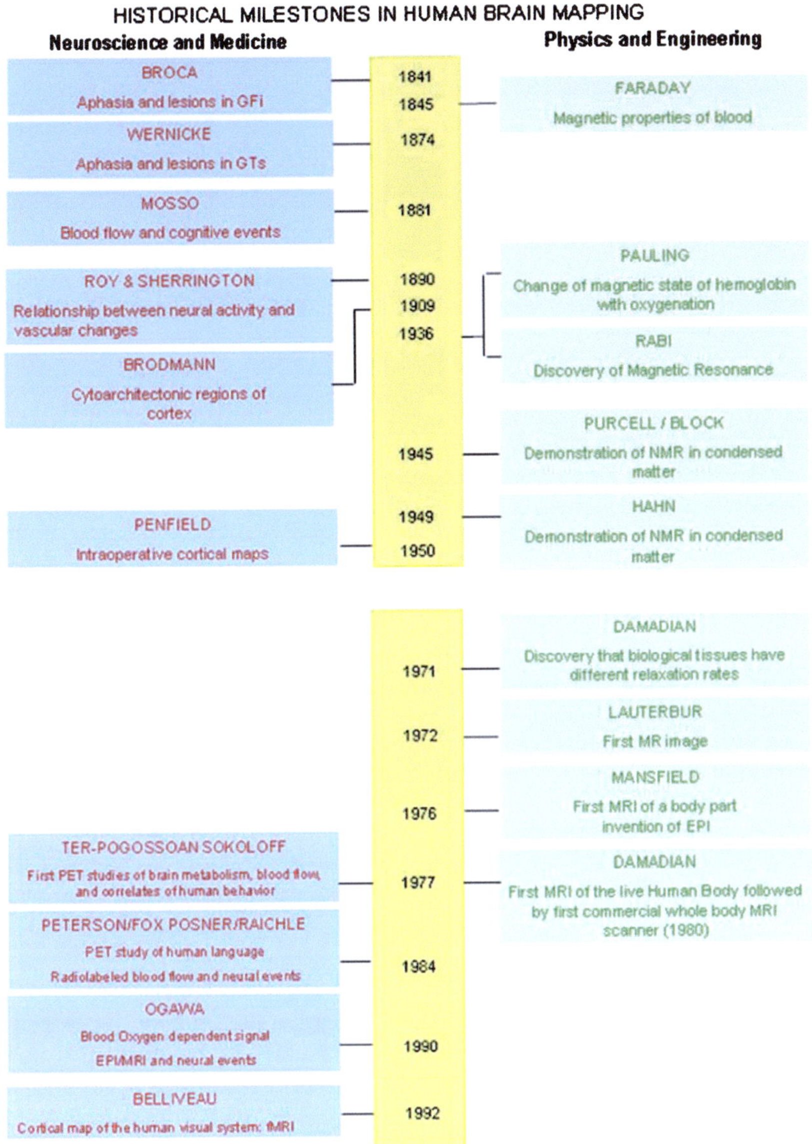

Figure 6.2. Historical milestones in human brain mapping. The timeline marks milestones in neuroscience and medicine in parallel with physics and engineering that lead to the development of functional magnetic resonance imaging (fMRI) and the ability to image active human cortical tissue corresponding to specific cognitive function.

the increased magnetic resonance signal was related to changes in oxygenated hemoglobin resulting from blood flow coupled to neural activity.[11]

Within two years, John Belliveau and colleagues replicated Ogawa's visual stimulation studies in humans using echo planar MRI, demonstrating the potential to reveal not only brain structure, but also brain function using MR. This technique, which exploited the fundamental link between the MR signal, blood flow, and neural events, was referred to as functional magnetic resonance imaging (fMRI) (see review by John Gore[12] for a more

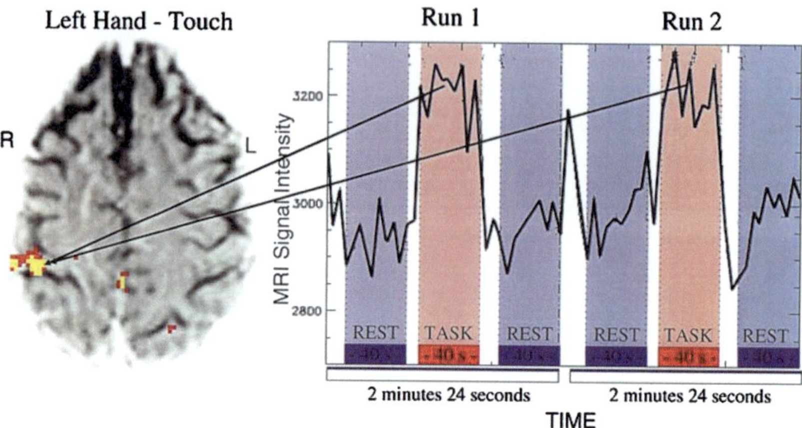

Figure 6.3. Cortical activity associated with tactile stimulation of the left hand. Signals illustrate the BOLD changes in MR susceptibility observed in response to passive tactile stimulation of the left hand of a healthy volunteer. Signals originate from a single voxel (1.5 × 1.5 × 4.5mm) on two separate runs. Each run lasted 2 minutes 24 seconds, during which 36 images were acquired, including 10 images for each of three epochs: initial resting baseline (purple bar), task (left-hand touch) (pink bar), and final resting baseline (purple bar). All voxels in the brain for which the statistical criteria were met (the average amplitude of the signal during the activity epoch was statistically different from the baseline signal) are indicated by either a yellow, or red color superimposed on the T2*-weighted image at the voxel address and signify decreasing levels of statistical confidence. Arrows point to the source voxel, which is centered within a cluster of similar (yellow) voxels and located in the right (R) hemisphere of the brain along the postcentral gyrus. Reprinted with permission from Hirsch J, Ruge MI, Kim KHS, Correa DD, Victor JD, Relkin NR, LaBar DR, Krol G, Bilsky MH, Souweidane MM, DeAngelis LM, Gutin PH. An integrated fMRI procedure for preoperative mapping of cortical areas associated with tactile, motor, language, and visual functions. *Neurosurgery.* 2000;47(3):711–722. Copyright © 2000 Lippincott Williams & Wilkins.

detailed description of these relationships). Figure 6.3 illustrates a BOLD signal (right) originating from the right hemisphere (R) region of postcentral gyrus (indicated by the arrow and yellow cluster) in response to touch of the left hand. The active region is contralateral to the stimulation and well established as an area functionally specialized for tactile sensation.

Hypothesis of Functional Specialization

One of the central assumptions that drives research and clinical applications that link cortical structure and function is that specific brain areas are involved in specific aspects of behavior such as action, perception, cognition, affect, and consciousness. As discussed above, cognitive deficits in patients with brain damage have led to the conclusion that the brain is functionally specialized at a coarse spatial scale (e.g., at the scale of lobes and hemispheres); for example, visual-related cortex includes occipital lobe, inferior temporal lobe, and posterior parietal lobe; auditory-related cortex includes superior temporal lobe; somatosensory-related cortex includes postcentral gyrus; motor-related cortex includes precentral gyrus; and explicit memory-related cortex includes hippocampus and temporal lobe. It is now widely believed that the brain is also functionally specialized at a finer scale.

In the case of the well-studied visual system, over 30 separate and distinct visual cortical areas are organized into well-defined processing pathways. Visual signals from the retina are transmitted to the lateral geniculate nucleus of the thalamus, and then to primary visual cortex where visual information fans out to the extrastriate visual cortical areas. The extrastriate visual areas serve many different aspects of visual perception and visually guided behavior. Among the dimensions suggested for independent visual analysis are: brightness, texture, color, depth, movement, shape, face recognition, and object recognition. While specializations for these functions are active topics for investigation, Figure 6.4 illustrates the well-known specialization of primary visual cortex for primitive stimuli such as on/off full-field stimulation. Similar specializations exist for language, sensory, motor, and auditory systems, and provide the focus for recent developments in cortical function mapping that protect these systems during invasive neurosurgical procedures.

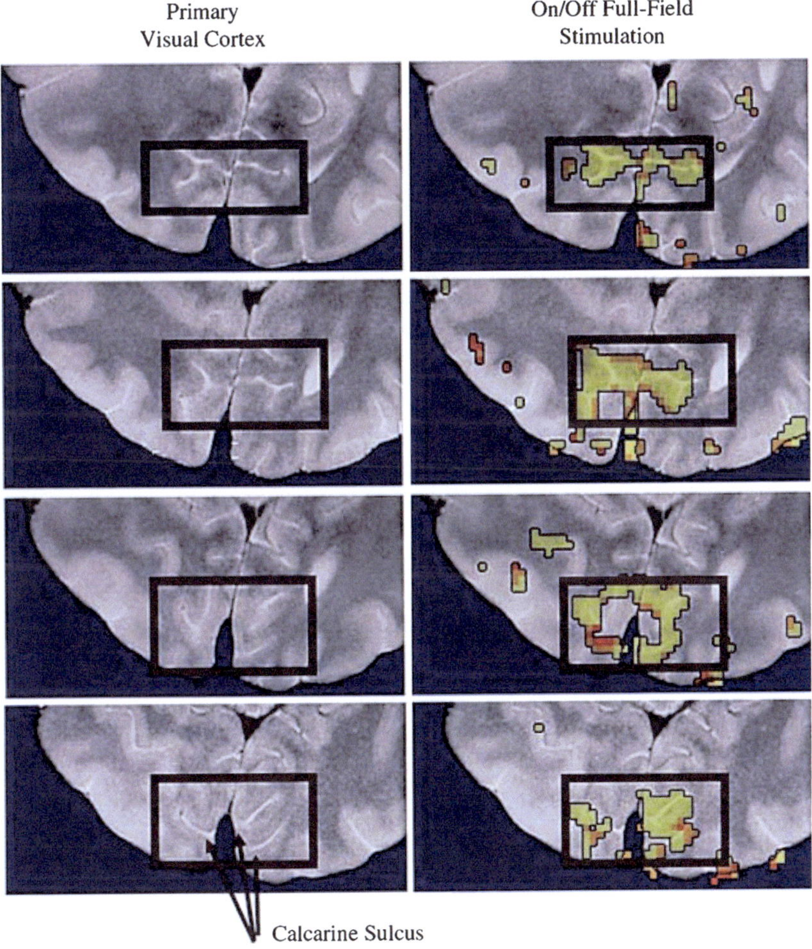

Figure 6.4. Boxed areas surround the anatomical calcarine sulcus in contiguous 3-mm-thick axial slices (left column). The right column illustrates cortical activity (fMRI) observed during viewing of full-field 8Hz on-off stimulation. The proximity of the activity patterns and the calcarine sulcus (primary visual cortex) is consistent with the hypothesis of functional specificity for this simple stimulation.

Identification and Preservation of Cortical Areas Specialized for Essential Tasks

Functional maps for individual subjects aim to identify functional specializations specific to that particular subject. In the case of functional mapping prior to a surgical procedure, the goal is to identify regions of the individual patient's brain that are employed for functions (such as motor movements, tactile sensation, language functions, vision, and audition) that might be at risk because of the location of the surgery. The presence of a space-occupying lesion or long-term seizure-genic conditions can modify or shift functional foci, and normal assumptions do not necessarily apply. In these cases, functional images are acquired at the highest-possible resolution and integrated into the appropriate treatment plan. Ideally, individual effects are studied by comparisons that occur before and after a therapeutic intervention where functional changes would be expected.

The preservation of function during a brain tumor resection is an essential goal of neurosurgery, and various intraoperative and preoperative brain mapping techniques are currently employed for this purpose. These techniques aim to identify cortical areas involved in sensory, motor, and language functions and have become standard practice. They include intraoperative electrophysiology with motor and language mapping, preoperative Wada tests, and visual field examinations. However, the added risk, time, and expense of multiple mapping procedures favors a single, noninvasive, preoperative procedure that could prove effective for mapping these functions. Functional MRI, has emerged as such a technique. Functional MRI maps of sensory and motor functions, either alone or in combination with other neuronavigation techniques,[13–15] have been shown effective in directing brain tumor resection procedures away from cortical regions with residual function.[13,16–22]

Tasks employed for functional mapping of sensory and motor-sensitive regions have generally been developed by separate research groups in the service of neurosurgical planning. As a consequence, many task variants have been employed. For example, motor tasks are sometimes accomplished by single finger–thumb tapping,[19] and in other cases by multiple finger–thumb tapping.[17,23,24] Other approaches include self-paced clenching and spreading of the hand,[22,25–27] or sponge squeezing.[18,20] Tactile stimulation has included palm brushing,[18] compressed air puffs to the hand,[20] and scratching the ventral surface of the hand.[19] Similarly, functional mapping of language areas has also been accomplished by a range of tasks and procedures including object naming and verb generation,[28] production of the names of animals starting with a given letter,[17] word generation in alphabetical order,[29] or auditory noun presentations with a required category response.[30] It is not known, however, how these various tasks compare with respect to sensitivity or targeted regions of interest. Assessment of cortical activity associated with visual stimulation has been accomplished with intermittent binocular photic stimulation,[17,24,31] as well as with various projected pattern stimuli.[32] The length of the activity period and the number of epochs in a run are also non-standard. Additional variation is introduced to the literature by different levels of statistical stringency and multiple data-processing procedures. Although all of these tasks for sensory, motor, language, and visual functions may be individually effective, an integrated and standardized battery of tasks could optimize application for neurosurgical planning.

Within a cohesive task battery, it is desirable to maximize reliability by using multiple tasks to target related functions. One such battery of fMRI tasks targets cortical regions associated with tactile, motor, language, and visual-sensitive cortical areas.[33] The task battery targets functions selective for regions frequently considered most critical for surgical decisions. All functions are repeated using both active (volitional) and passive (receptive) modes to assure that it is applicable to patients with a range of symptoms and performance capabilities. Any subset of these tasks may be selected for specific clinical objectives while retaining the advantages of the standardized procedures with validations based on responses of both healthy volunteers and patients.

A Multifunction Task Battery

The specific tasks selected for this task battery are intended to be nearly universally applicable and employ common stimuli and procedures.[34] The tasks consist of four separate procedures (Figure 6.5) including:

1. Passive tactile stimulation of a hand (either the dominant hand or the hand relevant to the hemisphere of surgical interest) with a mildly abrasive plastic surface that is gently rubbed on the palm and fingers. Simultaneously, the patient views a reversing checkerboard pattern (8Hz). This visual stimulation also aids in head stabilization of the patient.
2. Active hand movement (finger–thumb tapping) using either the same hand, as in the passive tactile stimulation, or both hands during a repeat of the simultaneous visual stimulation (reversing checkerboard).
3. Picture naming by internal (silent) speech in response to visually displayed, black-and-white, line drawings[35] presented at four-second intervals. These drawings are selected from an appropriate range of the Boston Naming test.
4. Listening to recordings of spoken words (names of objects) presented through headphones designed to reduce scanner noise. A visual fixation cross helps prevent head movement.

**fMRI Task Battery for Cortical Mapping of
Sensory, Motor, Language and Vision-Related Areas**

1. **SENSORY** **Touch/hand**	+	**VISION** **Reversing Checkerboard**
2. **MOTOR** **Finger/Thumb tapping**	+	**VISION** **Reversing Checkerboard**
3. **LANGUAGE/active** **Picture Naming**	+	**VISION** **Pictures**
4. **LANGUAGE/passive** **Listening to Words**	+	**AUDITION** **Spoken words**

Figure 6.5. A summary of the functions mapped by the four conditions in the fMRI task battery. Reprinted with permission from Hirsch J, Ruge MI, Kim KHS, Correa DD, Victor JD. Relkin NR, LaBar DR, Krol G, Bilsky MH. Souweidane MM, DeAngelis LM, Gutin PH. An integrated fMRI procedure for preoperative mapping of cortical areas associated with tactile, motor, language, and visual functions. *Neurosurgery.* 2000;47(3):711–722. Copyright © 2000 Lippincott Williams & Wilkins.

The aims of these four conditions include: 1) localization of sensory and motor cortices, and by inference, location of the central sulcus; 2) localization of language-related activity, and by inference, the locations of Broca's and Wernicke's Areas and the dominant hemisphere for speech; and 3) localization of primary and secondary visual areas.

Each of the targeted functions and structures associated with each task is illustrated in Figure 6.6 for a healthy volunteer. The sensory and motor tasks target post- and precentral gyrus (GPoC and GPrC), respectively, and are illustrated in the left panels. These figures also illustrate the expected overlap along the pre- and postcentral gyrus between activity associated with sensory and motor stimulation. The language tasks target putative Broca's and Wernicke's Areas that are found within inferior frontal gurus (GFi) and superior temporal gyrus (GTs), respectively, on the dominant hemisphere for language (middle panels of Figure 6.6). Both areas are redundantly targeted by expressive (active) and receptive (passive) language tasks, and by both visual and auditory modalities. Visual and auditory systems also are revealed by the activity in inferior occipital gyrus (GOi) and the transverse temporal gyrus (GTT), respectively, left and right language panels. Vision-related activity elicited by the reversing black-and-white checkerboard stimulations also targets primary visual cortex found along the calcarine sulcus (CaS), illustrated in the far-right panel of Figure 6.6. Given the high levels of statistical confidence, (p values from ≤ 0.0001 to ≤ 0.0005), it can be assumed that activity not circled also represents true physiological activations that are task-related and distributed outside the targeted regions of interest.

Functions, Tasks and Structures

SENSORY	MOTOR	LANGUAGE		VISION
Touch	Finger/Thumb Tapping	Picture Naming	Listening to Words	Reversing Checkerboard
(Left Hand)	(Left Hand)	(active)	(passive)	(passive)
GPoC	GPrC	GOi	GTT GFi GTs	CaS

Figure 6.6. Selected slices for a healthy brain illustrate targeted (circled) structures labeled according to the Talairach and Tournoux Human Brain Atlas[45] for each of the functions and tasks: sensory, passive touch of the hand (left) using a rough plastic surface targets the post-central gyrus (GPoC); motor, active finger–thumb tapping targets the pre-central gyrus (GPrC); language, picture naming (expressive) and listening to spoken words (receptive) target the inferior frontal gyrus (GFi; Broca's Area) and the superior temporal gyrus (GTs; Wernicke's Area) on the dominant hemisphere; and vision, viewing of the reversing checkerboard and picture naming target the calcarine sulcus (CaS) and the inferior occipital gyrus (GOi). Primary auditory activity expected to be associated with the listening task also is observed bilaterally in the transverse temporal gyrus (GTT), middle panel. Reprinted with permission from Hirsh J, Ruge MI, Kim KHS, Correa DD, Victor JD, Relkin NR, LaBar DR, Krol G, Bilsky MH, Souweidane MM, DeAngelis LM, Gutin PH. An integrated fMRI procedure for preoperative mapping of cortical areas associated with tactile, motor, language, and visual functions. *Neurosurgery.* 2000;47(3):711–722. Copyright © 2000 Lippincott Williams & Wilkins.

Healthy Volunteers and Patients

Development of this test battery was based upon a total of 63 healthy volunteers (24 female and 39 male) who participated in the evaluation of the specific set of tasks targeted to identify brain regions most likely to be surgical regions of interest for 1) primary brain tumor, 2) brain metastasis, 3) seizure disorder, or 4) cerebral vascular malformation. A total of 125 patients also participated. These patients were surgical candidates and presented with surgical regions of interest that included sensorimotor ($n = 63$), language ($n = 56$), or visual ($n = 6$) functions.

Sensitivity of Task Battery: Healthy Volunteers

Each task was associated with the targeted region of interest, and the percentage of cases showing activity in those regions (sensitivity) was determined (Table 6.1A). This task battery provides two opportunities to observe the targeted region; for example, whereas the superior temporal gyrus (GTs) was activated in only 73% of cases during picture naming, it was activated in 100% of healthy volunteers during listening to spoken words (Table 6.1, column 5). Overall, the sensitivity of the entire battery to identify language-related cortex in the superior temporal gyrus is 100% for the population of healthy volunteers, as indicated on the bottom row, Composite Sensitivity. Specifically, the composite sensitivity is the result of a logical operating room (OR) decision rule based on two tasks that target a specific region. Central sulcus and visual cortex were identified in 100% of cases and Broca's Area in 93%.

Sensitivity of Task Battery: Surgical Population

Following task-sensitivity determinations for healthy volunteers, similar determinations were made for surgical candidates with pathology in the specified cortical regions of interest. This enabled assessment of the fMRI task within the affected pathological cohort. These subgroups served as the basis for evaluation of the respective tasks, although all patients completed all tasks in the battery, regardless of the region of surgical interest. Table 6.1B reports the task sensitivity within each surgical group, thus indicating the sensitivity in the presence of pathology. The tactile stimulation revealed activity in the postcentral gyrus in 94% of patients with lesions in or close to the motor strip, whereas the finger–thumb-tapping task predominantly demonstrated function in the area of the precentral gyrus in 89%. Of the two patients for whom the central sulcus was not identified, one was characterized by excessive (not correctable) head movement and marginal compliance. Neurological deficits were the most likely contributing factor in the second case. Overall, the location of central sulcus, as indicated by either its posterior or anterior margins, was obtained in 97% of the cases with pathology in this region and is indicated as the composite sensitivity (bottom row). This boost in sensitivity is achieved by exploiting the two approaches to locate central sulcus and the employment of a logical OR combination decision rule between the two tasks.

Table 6.1. Evaluation of Task Sensitivity

Task	Structure	A. Healthy Subjects Targeted regions of interest				B. Surgical Patients Surgical regions of interest			
		Central Sulcus ($n = 30$)	Broca's Area ($n = 45$)	Wernicke's Area ($n = 45$)	Visual Cortex ($n = 15$)	Central Sulcus ($n = 63$)	Broca's Area ($n = 22$)	Wernicke's Area ($n = 34$)	Visual Cortex ($n = 6$)
Touch	GPoC	100%				94%			
Finger-Thumb Tapping	GPrC	100%				89%			
Picture	GFi		90%				72%		
Naming	GTs			73%				65%	
Listening to	GFi		93%				54%		
Spoken Words	GTs			100%				88%	
Checkerboard	CaS				100%				100%
Pictures	GOi				100%				100%
Composite Sensitivity (Logical OR)		100%	93%	100%	100%	97%	77%	91%	100%

Reprinted with permission from Hirsch J, Ruge MI, Kim KHS, Correa DD, Victor JD, Relkin NR, LaBar DR, Krol G, Bilsky MH, Souweidane MM, DeAngelis LM, Gutin PH. An integrated fMRI procedure for preoperative mapping of cortical areas associated with tactile, motor, language, and visual functions. *Neurosurgery.* 2000;47(3):711–722. Copyright © 2000 Lippincott Williams & Wilkins.

With the combined performances of the picture-naming task, as well as the passive listening task, the fMRI signal was observed in Wernicke's Area in 31 of 34 (91%) patients with pathology in superior temporal gyrus and Broca's Area in 17 of the 22 patients (77%) with pathology in inferior frontal gyrus. Explanations for the three unsuccessful Wernicke's Area patients included movement artifact ($n = 1$) and probable lack of compliance ($n = 2$). Explanations for the five unsuccessful Broca's Area patients included neurological deficits ($n = 3$), probable marginal compliance ($n = 1$), and head-movement artifact that was not correctable ($n = 1$), although a false–negative finding cannot be ruled out. The fMRI signal was observed in the visual cortex (calcarine sulcus and inferior occipital gyrus) in all six patients with lesions in these cortical areas.

Comparison of Task Sensitivity for Patients and Healthy Volunteers

Although the sensory and motor probes of GPoC and GPrC were each 100% effective in healthy volunteers, they were individually 94% and 89% effective in patients with tumors in those regions. These observations include patients with severe symptoms such as hemiparesis and loss of sensory function. However, by combining the two tasks with the Either/Or decision rule, the central sulcus was identified in 97% of cases. By combining the hit rates of the picture-naming and the listening to spoken words tasks for the healthy volunteers, the targeted Broca's Area (GFi) and Wernicke's Area (GTs) were activated in 93% and 100% of cases, respectively. Correspondingly, for the surgical cases, these areas were activated in 77% and 91% of the cases, respectively. The reduction in patient sensitivity for the language areas presumably reflects tumor-related receptive and expressive aphasias, as well as related cognitive losses. The visual functions within CaS and GOi were 100% effective in both healthy subjects and also for surgical patients where the unaffected hemisphere provided the comparison. Accuracy of the fMRI observations also can be assessed in all surgical patients for whom multiple procedures were included in the treatment plan by comparison of the fMRI maps with conventional techniques such as intraoperative mapping, WADA and visual fields testing methods. This method of comparison serves to establish the concordance of the fMRI technique with other accepted techniques.

Accuracy of Task Battery: Comparison with Intraoperative Electrophysiology

Both fMRI preoperative maps and intraoperative electrophysiology were performed in 16 cases. Intraoperative recording of somatosensory evoked potentials (SSEPs) were performed to localize the central sulcus,[36] and successful recordings were obtained in 15 cases. Direct cortical stimulation was performed in 11 of these cases with successful stimulations in nine. The areas of electrophysiological response were referenced to axial images with the use of an intraoperative frameless-based stereotactic navigation device and compared to the preoperative fMRI images. Due to the differences in the orientations of the acquired slices, however, precise measurements of the localizations of the two techniques were not possible. In each case, the surgeon judged the correspondence as consistent. (See case example below).

The fMRI maps revealed precentral gyrus activity in 16 of 16 (100%) cases and postcentral gyrus in 13 of 16 (81%) cases. However, the combined maps revealed the location of the central sulcus in all cases. When both methods (fMRI and electrophysiology) reported the central sulcus, the locations concurred in 100% of the cases for the SSEPs (15 of 15), and 100% for the direct cortical stimulation (9 of 9), as determined within the spatial accuracy of both methods, and in accord with previous findings of other investigators.[20,37,38]

Comparison of fMRI, Wada, and Intraoperative Language Mapping

Hemispheric language dominance as predicted by the fMRI language-related maps was compared to preoperative Wada procedures[39] in 13 cases. The dominant hemisphere for language as determined by Wada testing was consistent with fMRI results in all 13 cases (double-blind study), and is consistent with findings of previous investigations.[30] In a subsequent cohort of five patients, this integrated battery of tasks was applied prior to intraoperative language mapping, with consistent findings between the two methods.[40]

Comparison of fMRI and Visual Fields

Homonymous visual field defects were compared with fMRI response patterns in primary visual cortex in six cases (illustrated in Figure 6.2). Visual fields determined by formal static perimetry indicated hemianopic or quadrantanoptic field deficits consistent with known disruptions of visual projection pathways and were consistent with the fMRI cortical maps when compared with activity within the unaffected hemisphere. That is, gross absences of hemispheric symmetry along the calcarine sulcus in regions expected to correspond to the visual field were taken as demonstrations of field and fMRI consistency.

Case Example 1: Motor and Language Mapping

In this case, a 43-year-old, right-handed man presented with mild headaches and brief episodes of receptive language disturbance, as well as occasional word-finding difficulties. Preoperative neuropsychological evaluation revealed no language deficits. Magnetic resonance imaging revealed a rounded, partially hemorrhagic lesion, 4.5 centimeters in diameter located in the left posterior temporal lobe. To optimize a therapeutic plan, functional maps were obtained using the multifunction task battery; results are summarized in Figure 6.7. The central sulcus was identified clearly by the sensory and motor tasks (top rows). The language tasks revealed language-related activity on the left hemisphere adjacent to both the posterior margins and the anterior margins of the mass (GTs and GFi; middle rows). The visual stimulation was reliably associated with signals within and along the primary visual areas (CaS). Due to the proximity of the language-related activity to the tumor, an awake craniotomy with electrophysiological mapping of motor and language functions was performed.

Summary of fMRI Task Battery		(Illustrative Case)	
FUNCTION	TASK	AREA	fMRI
Motor	Finger-Thumb Tapping	GPrC	
Sensory	Touch	GPoC	
Broca's Area	Picture Naming	GFi	
Wernicke's Area	Listening to Spoken Words	GTs	
Visual Cortex	Reversing Checkerboard	CaS	

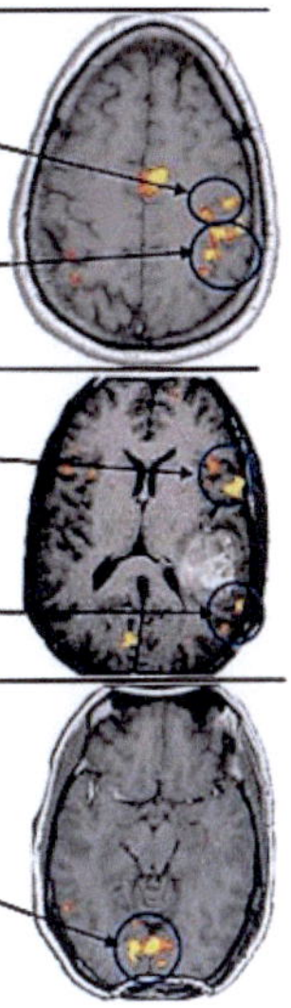

Figure 6.7. Selected slices (right) illustrate cortical responses associated with each of the tasks and the targeted regions of interest for case example 1. Sensory and motor tasks elicited activity within pre- and post-central gyri and predicted the location of the central sulcus on multiple contiguous slices. The slice illustrated in the right top row shows a relatively inferior representation. The two language tasks—picture naming and listening to spoken words—elicited activity in the left hemisphere within the inferior frontal gyrus (GFi) and the superior temporal gyrus (GTs; arrows). In this case, the specific locations of the activity within the GFi and GTs were replicated on both tasks and the overlapping regions were taken as the best predictor of Broca's and Wernicke's Areas, respectively. Finally, the reversing checkerboard (bottom row) indicated primary visual cortex, as illustrated by the activity labeled calcarine sulcus (CaS). Similar to the language-related regions, these regions were replicated across the multiple visual tasks and served to increase confidence in these results. Reprinted with permission from Hirsch J, Ruge MI, Kim KHS, Correa DD, Victor JD, Relkin NR, LaBar DR, Krol G, Bilsky MH, Souweidane MM, DeAngelis LM, Gutin PH. An integrated fMRI procedure for preoperative mapping of cortical areas associated with tactile, motor, language, and visual functions. *Neurosurgery.* 2000;47(3):711–722. Copyright © 2000 Lippincott Williams & Wilkins.

Integrative Mapping of Sensory and Motor Functions

Recording of SSEPs indicated the location of the central sulcus (Figure 6.8, left columns), which was confirmed by direct cortical stimulation of precentral gyrus (middle columns). Comparison with the location of central sulcus by fMRI (right column) indicates good agreement with both techniques, as illustrated by the arrows.

Interoperative Mapping of Language Functions

Direct cortical stimulation of the left inferior frontal gyrus with the Ojemann Bipolar stimulator disrupted the patient's ability to count, and a similar stimulation of the superior temporal gyrus produced language disturbances, including literal paraphasic errors and word-finding difficulties, respectively (Figure 6.9). Sites of observable responses were tagged with numbers, photographically documented, and cross referenced to the fMRI, as illustrated by arrows.

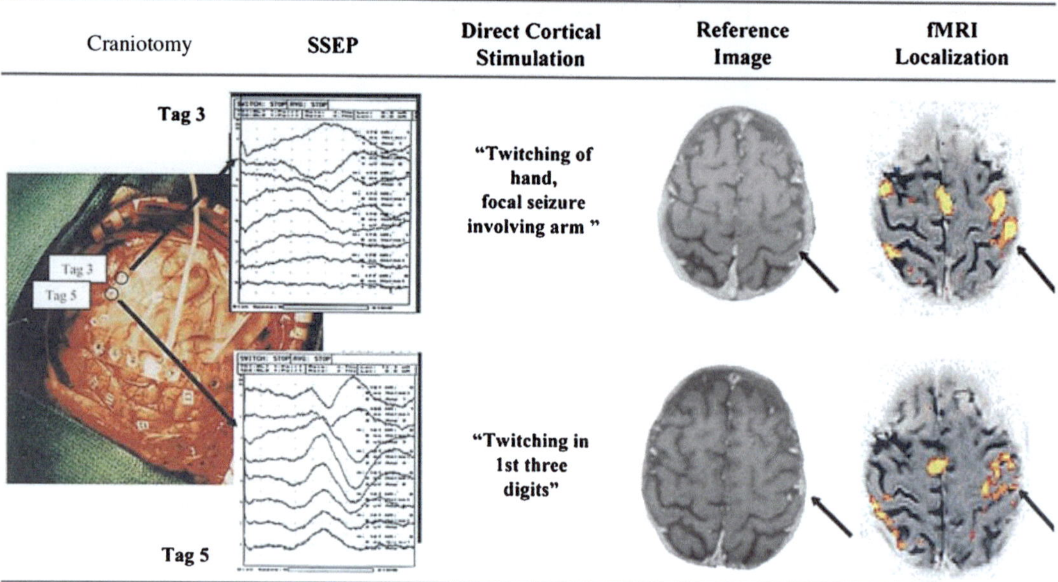

Sensory Motor Mapping

Figure 6.8. Needle-recording electrodes were placed at Erb's Point and stimulating electrodes were placed over the left or right median nerve at the wrist. Following craniotomy and exposure of cortex, subdural strip electrodes were placed in the operative field. The median nerve was stimulated to elicit epicortical responses measured with the electrodes. A consistent phase reversal between electrode sites (tags 3 and 5, column 2) was taken as the physiological identification of sensorimotor cortex, and therefore, the central sulcus (indicated by arrows on the reference images in column 4). These recordings of somatosensory-evoked potentials (SSEP) were made with an 8-Channel Viking IV7 and standard filter settings (30Hz to 3kHz). Direct cortical stimulation of the exposed cortex directed by the SSEP results was performed using the Ojemann bipolar stimulator (one second trains of one millisecond pulses at 60Hz) varied from two milliamperes (mA) to 18mA, peak to peak, resulting in hand twitching and a focal seizure of the right arm (top row) and twitching of the first three digits of the hand (bottom row). Using a frameless-based intraoperative navigation system (BrainLAB GmbH, Munich, Germany), the tagged locations were referenced to anatomical axial MR images localized using a viewing wand and subsequently compared with areas of activation on corresponding fMRI images, as illustrated by comparison of the images in columns 4 and 5 (arrows). The T2* images (right column) and the conventional T1 images (reference image) were not acquired at exactly corresponding plane orientations, accounting for the variation in the two structural images and limiting the precision with which the electrophysiological and fMRI locations can be compared. Reprinted with permission from Hirsch J, Ruge MI, Kim KHS, Correa DD, Victor JD, Relkin NR, LaBar DR, Krol G, Bilsky MH, Souweidane MM, DeAngelis LM, Gutin PH. An integrated fMRI procedure for preoperative mapping of cortical areas associated with tactile, motor, language, and visual functions. *Neurosurgery*. 2000;47(3):711–722. Copyright © 2000 Lippincott Williams & Wilkins.

Postsurgical Status

A total resection was achieved that spared these functional regions. The pathology was consistent with an ependymoma. Immediately postsurgery, no impairments in language function were detected. However, the postoperative recovery of the patient was complicated by a temporary mixed aphasia and seizures. Subsequently, within 10 days, the patient's condition was substantially improved, and no further adjuvant treatment was planned. A six-month postsurgical fMRI scan was consistent with previous findings, and neuropsychological evaluation revealed residual, mild word-finding difficulties and occasional literal paraphasic errors.

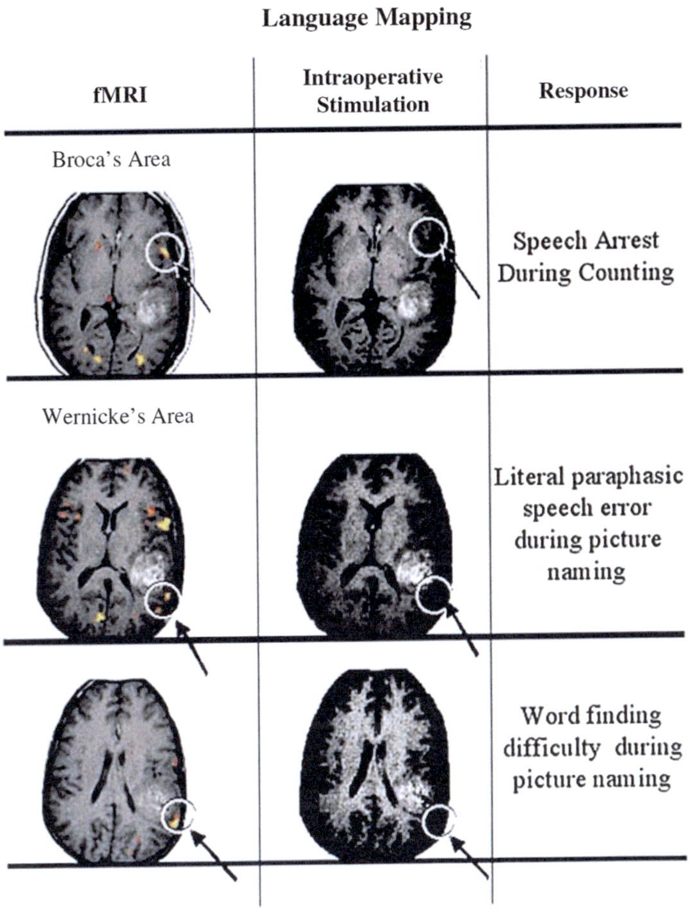

Figure 6.9. After craniotomy and recording of SSEPs, the patient was awakened and asked to count forward and backward while the cortex in putative Broca's Area was stimulated. Subsequently, the picture-naming paradigm used in the fMRI battery of tasks was administered and stimulation at the site where fMRI maps indicated the location of Broca's Area resulted in speech disruption (top row). Stimulation was systematically repeated and extended to temporal lobe cortex, and sites of activation revealed by the fMRI maps were specifically targeted as indicated by the circles in the middle and bottom column. These stimulations resulted in paraphasic speech errors and word-finding difficulties as indicated, consistent with disruption of Wernicke's Area-related functions that occurred in the two separate locations as indicated. The corresponding preoperative fMRI maps shown on the left column confirm the correspondence of cortical areas (circles and arrows). Reprinted with permission from Hirsch J, Ruge MI, Kim KHS, Correa DD, Victor JD, Relkin NR, LaBar DR, Krol G, Bilsky MH, Souweidane MM, DeAngelis LM, Gutin PH. An integrated fMRI procedure for preoperative mapping of cortical areas associated with tactile, motor, language, and visual functions. *Neurosurgery*. 2000;47(3):711–722. Copyright © 2000 Lippincott Williams & Wilkins.

Case Example 2: Language Mapping—Late Bilingual Patient

In this case, the patient was a native of Italy who emigrated to the United States as a young adult and then learned English. When she was 44 years old, she began to experience episodes of word-finding difficulty in both

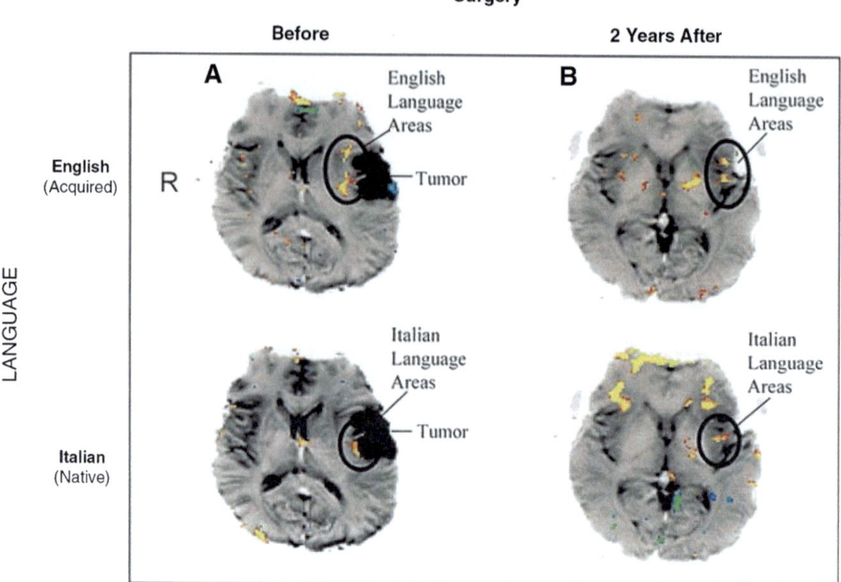

Figure 6.10. Language mapping of a late bilingual patient. Object naming was performed in the native language (Italian), and also in the acquired language (English). Typical of Late Bilingual individuals, the languages occupied distinct regions of Broca's Area (A). These distinct regions were preserved following surgery and are consistent with her clinical outcome of no deficits in either language (B).

Italian and English, as well as slowed speech production. An MRI obtained during a medical evaluation revealed a large tumor in the left inferior posterior frontal region of her brain expected to be associated with speech production (Figure 6.10A). In order to determine the location of her language areas relative to her tumor, a functional MRI was acquired using the task battery described above for each language, which revealed: 1) separate locations for her native (Italian) and second language (English), and 2) that both languages were displaced from the expected locations by the tumor. These displacements were confirmed during surgery and the tumor was resected without damage to either language function. Approximately two years later, she remains tumor free, with excellent English and Italian language function. A follow-up fMRI scan indicated the language areas associated with each language have shifted back to the expected locations within the brain (Figure 6.10B). The separation of the locations active during the native language and the second language within Broca's Area is consistent with previous findings of separation between L1- and L2-sensitive areas, when L2 was acquired during adulthood.[41]

Case Example 3: Language Mapping—Early Bilingual Patient

A 23-year-old right-handed bilingual woman who works as a waitress in her father's Italian restaurant was seen on an emergency basis following the sudden onset of supplementary motor seizures. An MRI revealed the presence of a left posterior frontal cystic lesion suggestive of cystic astrocytoma.

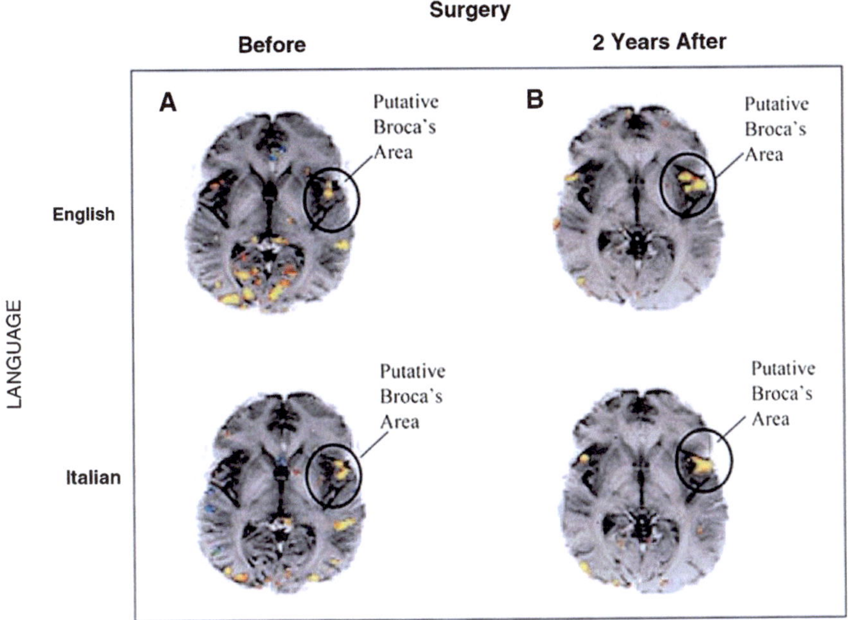

Figure 6.11. Language mapping of an early bilingual patient. Object naming as for the Case 2 patient (Figure 6.10) was performed in both languages, Italian and English. Typical of early bilingual individuals, the activity clusters associated with both languages were largely overlapping within Broca's Area (A). This single language area was preserved following resection (B), consistent with the absence of post-surgical morbidity.

Although the patient was born and educated in the United States, she was raised in a household that spoke Italian and became bilingual during her early language development. Functional MRI of her language areas for both languages revealed over-lapping clusters in putative Broca's Area (left inferior frontal gyrus) as illustrated in Figure 6.11A, which was not changed following surgery (Figure 6.11B), consistent with the absence of postsurgical morbidity.

Cases 2 and 3 illustrate earlier findings that document different cortical organization with respect to early and late acquisition of a second language. Kim and colleagues[41] showed that the average centroid separation in putative Broca's Area during L1 and L2 production in late bilingual subjects was approximately seven millimeters, whereas in early bilingual subjects, the language activations were indistinguishable (Figure 6.12).

Case Example 4: Motor Mapping

An 11-year-old female with a completely unremarkable medical history presented following the occurrence of a grand mal seizure. Imaging revealed a large mass along the lateral margin of right central sulcus (Figure 6.13A. Due to the risk to sensory and motor functions, a surgical resection was recommended, and recommended treatment consisted of seizure management.

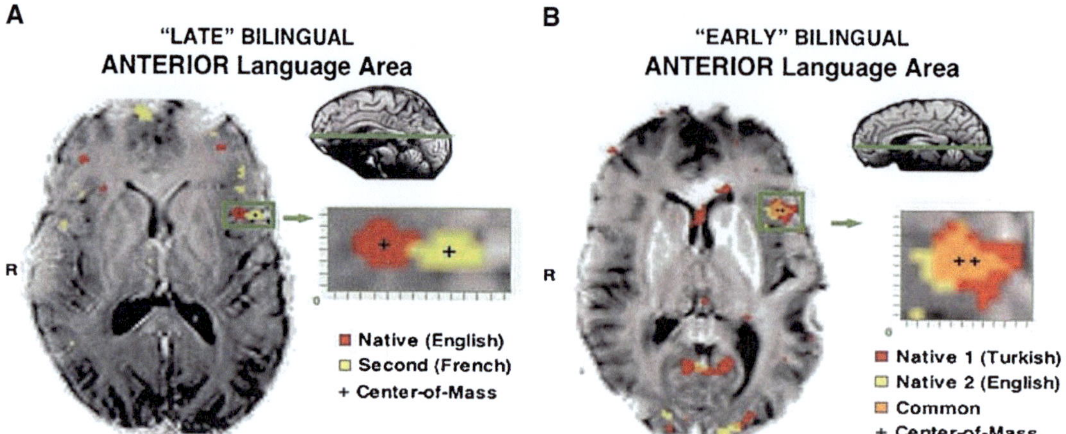

Figure 6.12. Examples of main findings based on two samples of healthy volunteers who were either late (A) or early (B) bilinguals. Cluster centroids and variances (spreads) were determined for activity associated with each language. A significant separation between centroids of activity was found for late bilingual subjects and not for the early bilingual subjects in Broca's Area. No differences were observed within Werniche's Area. Reprinted with permission from Kim KHS, Relkin NR, Lee K-M, Hirsch J. Distinct cortical areas associated with native and second languages. *Nature.* 1997;388:171–174.

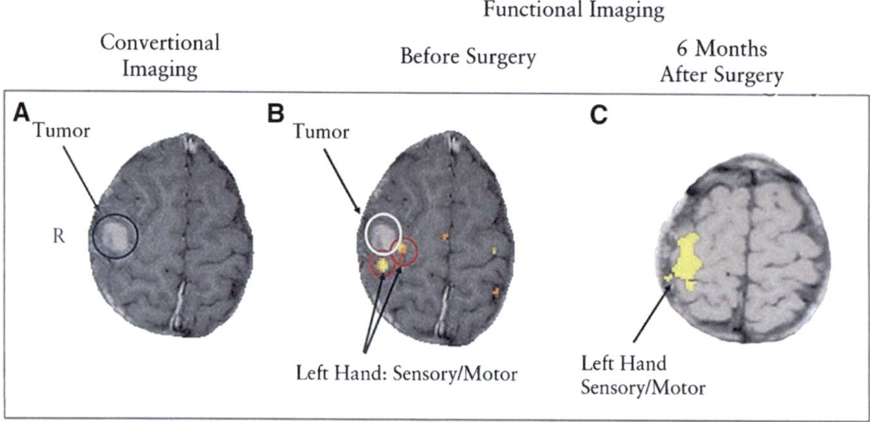

Figure 6.13. (A) Conventional T1 image reveals right hemisphere mass located on the margins of the central sulcus. (B) Functional map of tactile and finger–thumb tapping suggests displacement of eloquent cortex. (C) Six months after surgery, the patient is disease-free, without deficits consistent with the sensory and motor activity revealed by fMRI.

Seeking a second opinion, parents sought a medical center with fMRI mapping capability; the functional map revealed that the tumor had displaced eloquent sensory and motor sensitive cortex medially and posteriorly from the expected positions (Figure 6.13B). Based on this information, an anterior surgical route resulted in a complete and total resection of a ganglioglioma without functional deficit. Six months postsurgery she returned for a follow-up map that revealed the expected functional pattern (Figure 6.13C). She had returned to her normal activities, including soccer, dance, and rock climbing.

A novel feature of this battery of integrated fMRI tasks is the redundancy in the measurements; for example, language-sensitive regions are mapped by both active (expressive) and passive (receptive) tasks, as are the regions sensitive to motor (active tapping) and sensory (passive touching) tasks. Visual areas also are assessed by passive viewing of the reversing checkerboard stimulus (no response required) and active viewing of pictures during a naming task in which a response was required. Advantages to employing more than one task associated with a particular function to isolate eloquent cortical areas include improved confidence when replications are observed, and improved sensitivity when the activity is observed during either an active or a passive performance. This feature translates into a greater likelihood of a successful map for patients with neurologic deficits. Together, the task sensitivity and accuracy observed for these fMRI maps suggests that this multifunction task battery yields a reliable estimate of the locations of critical functions potentially at risk during brain surgery, and thus extends the potential of a single preoperative fMRI brain mapping procedure to facilitate optimal outcomes for neurosurgery.

Based on our experience with this fMRI task battery, the images serve both pre- and intraoperative objectives. On the preoperative side, the fMRI maps have contributed to our estimates of the risk–benefit ratio and to the decision whether or not to offer surgery to the patient, although these decisions are based on the entire medical situation taken together, and not on any single factor. Communication between the surgeon and the patient is also facilitated by images that summarize the relevant structure and function issues. On the intraoperative side, as illustrated above, the fMRI results have also served to direct the intraoperative electrophysiology, and thereby have contributed to the efficiency of the intraoperative procedures. However, it has been observed that the information offered by the preoperative fMRI map is often more distributed than that of the intraoperative map, and the question of which active regions are essential to the function is not directly addressed by fMRI.[42] A false–positive interpretation is therefore possible based on these associated patterns of activity, whereas a false–negative finding is also possible due to sensitivity, compliance, and imaging artifacts. The likelihood of both types of errors is reduced with repetitions and checks for internal consistency, as suggested by this integrated task battery. However, advances to resolve these issues may depend upon additional techniques, such as transcranial magnetic stimulation (TMS) to confirm the essential nature of an area identified by fMRI.

Many future enhancements of this initial task battery are possible using methods that determine task sensitivity and clinical validity, as well as improve confidence by reducing the risk of either false–positive or false–negative findings. The battery could be extended to include memory functions, high-level cognitive tasks, and perhaps even emotion and affect, and continued development could improve the tasks to target the sensory/motor and language areas. Techniques employed for the development of this integrated battery of functions could serve as a basis to develop other similar probes, and thus extend the potential role of fMRI in neurosurgical planning to encompass more precision and diversity in structure and function relationships.

Determination of the Anatomy and Topography of Cortical Areas Specialized for Cognitive Tasks

In contrast to language, sensory/motor, and visual systems, our current understanding of the mechanisms of higher functions is not so closely linked to a specified neurophysiological substrate. This is due, in part, to the fact that many aspects of cognition cannot be studied in animals; therefore, the burden of our understanding falls historically on research in human subjects. The emergence of neuroimaging provides a new opportunity to test hypotheses and map the underlying mechanisms of cognition in healthy individuals without reliance on lesions or disease processes. The neural bases of various aspects of cognition are now observable using imaging techniques. Determinations of the anatomy and topography of cortical areas specialized for cognitive tasks are possible and can contribute to models that integrate multiple functionally specialized areas to perform cognitive tasks. These objectives are discussed below in the context of specific functions, including attention, working memory, executive processes, and consciousness, with an emphasis on the unifying notion that the neurobiological pathways are multiregional with complex covariations.

> While there has been general agreement that operations performed by the sensory and motor systems are localized, there has been much more dispute about higher-level cognitive processes. It is still undetermined whether higher-level processes have defined locations, and if so, where these locations would be.
>
> Posner and Raichle, *Images of Mind*, 1994, p.16

As discussed above, the functional neuroanatomy of cognitive processes is revealed by comparing the BOLD response elicited by various experimental and control tasks and is typically characterized by a voxel-by-voxel statistical comparison of the signal amplitude during the activity epoch, with the average signal amplitude during a baseline resting or control epoch. The basic assumption is that neuronal activity is increased in a functionally specialized area during the execution of a task that employs that specialization. Locations of active areas, cluster sizes, and dynamic properties of the signal can be compared across cognitive conditions. Tasks are designed to either include or exclude the cognitive component of interest and the signals elicited from these tasks are compared.

Conservation of Effects versus Individual Differences: Generalizing the Results

Investigations of the neural basis for cognitive processes are aimed toward findings generalizable to the population at large. Neuroimaging studies on single subjects can be assumed to include effects that are conserved across all subjects (generalizable), as well as effects that are specific to that individual subject. Results that are present in all or most cases given a sufficiently large sample size can be assumed to reflect a fundamental specialization characteristic of the population, whereas intermittently present results can be assumed to represent other less-conserved (individual) processes. A theoretical basis for inferences to a population based on functional imaging data is currently under development. However, preliminary estimates of a sufficient sample size based on expected levels of variation exceed six subjects.[43] This proposed minimum is consistent with the general practice to employ six to ten subjects per condition in fMRI studies. However, based on other models using a two-tailed test of significance at a criterion level of $p \leq 0.05$ and a power of 80%, Desmond and Glover[44] suggested a sample size of 11 to 12, and most recent analyses of covariation and connectivity may require sample sizes up to 20 subjects.

Inferences to a population based on imaging data generally require registration of individual brains and a standard stereotactic coordinate system. Although registration procedures are an area of active development, the conventional method (originally developed for PET studies) employs the *Co-Planar Stereotaxic Atlas of the Human Brain*.[45] Acquired brain images are registered to that atlas by reference to the anterior–posterior commissure line and active areas are labeled accordingly and assigned an address in x, y, z stereotactic coordinates. One popular tool for accomplishing this objective is available in Statistical Parametric Mapping (SPM),[46] a software package developed for processing neuroimaging data. Other representations of brain structure and functions include flat maps and inflated brains.

Method of Cognitive Subtraction

The cognitive subtraction paradigm requires two tasks: an experimental task that engages the cognitive component of interest, and a baseline or control task that engages all of the processes included in the cognitive task except for the cognitive component of interest. The neural correlates of the cognitive task of interest are presumed to be revealed by a subtraction of the baseline activity from the activity observed during the experimental task. Examples of the cognitive subtraction design are found in the early PET studies, where, for example, the effect of viewing a fixation dot was subtracted from the effect of viewing a flashing checkerboard to reveal the neural effect of the checkerboard alone. Although the subtractive approach was employed successfully in those early studies, it is limited by the difficulty of selecting tasks that differ only with respect to the cognition of interest. If differences between the experimental task and the comparison baseline task are due to a combinatorial effect not present with either task alone, then the conclusion could be misguided. These assumptions often are referred to as the assumptions of linear additivity or pure insertion, and depend upon the partitioning of complex cognitive tasks into independent subcomponent processes.

Method of Cognitive Conjunction

In contrast to the identification of differences between the elicited activity of two cognitive tasks by subtraction, a conjunction analysis reveals the activity common to multiple tasks. For example, in an investigation to identify the neural substrate specialized for object naming, the same task can be performed using multiple sensory systems—that is, objects that are seen, heard, and felt are named during an imaging study. The conjunction of neural activity present in all three naming tasks is assumed to represent the neural activity associated with naming alone, and the processes associated with the

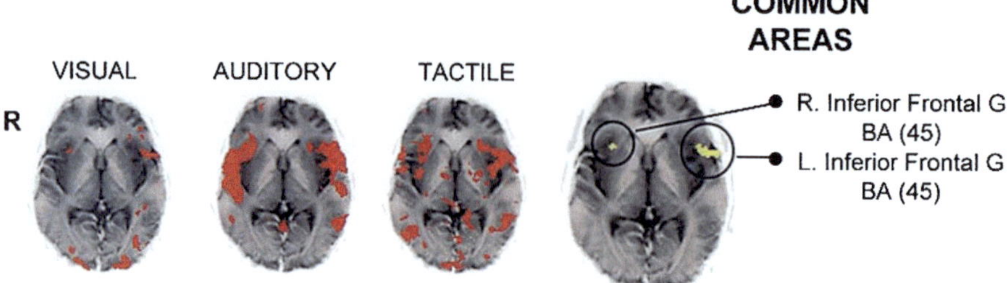

Figure 6.14. Conjunction of BOLD responses during object naming across three sensory modalities. Voxels active during visual stimulation (left), auditory stimulation (middle), and tactile stimulation (right) are indicated in orange for one slice of brain. The conjunction image (yellow) illustrates the supramodal activity common to all three modalities of stimulation following a Boolean AND operation. This activity occurs in left and right inferior frontal gyrus (BA 45) and is taken to represent the aspects of object naming not primarily associated with a specific sensory modality for this single subject. Reprinted from Hirsch J, Rodriguez-Moreno D, Kim KHS. Interconnected large-scale systems for three fundamental cognitive tasks revealed by functional MRI *J Cogn Neurosci.* 2001;13(3):1–16. Reprinted with permission from MIT Press Journals.

sensory-related activity are assumed to be excluded by virtue of the fact that such activity is not common to all tasks (as illustrated in Figure 6.14).

Some of the same assumptions for the subtractive approach described above apply. First, it is assumed that the cognitive processes engaged by each task are performed similarly across the sensory modalities. However, there is considerable evidence for intermingling of modality-specific and domain-general mechanisms in some tasks. For example, mental imagery tasks may draw upon modality-specific subsystems, which would not be observed by this method. Thus, the conjunctive method applied to cross-modal studies identifies a subset of domain-general processes, but may fail to recognize all components critical to task performance.

On the other hand, the conjunctive approach, applied to within-modal studies, can serve to enhance confidence in a result by isolating activity that is repeated on multiple runs of the same task. This strategy is based on the assumption that signals originating from noise sources are distinguished from signals originating from real events by the probability of a repeat occurrence at the same location. Voxels that are reliably activated on multiple separate occasions result in a low false–positive rate that can be empirically determined based on images acquired either during resting states or on images acquired on a spherical container of copper sulfate solution that simulates brain (phantom). For this reason, conjunctions often are employed in clinical and neurosurgical applications to enhance confidence in a result by isolating the activity that is elicited on at least two runs of the same task.[34,40,41] However, because repeated stimuli do not usually elicit as robust a response as novel stimuli, all repetitions of a task are optimally performed using equal but different stimuli. Thus, in the case of an object-naming task, all objects would be novel but equated for variables such as familiarity and difficulty, etc., during the multiple runs in order to be optimized for the within-modal conjunction approach.

Integration of Functionally Specialized Areas Associated with Cognitive Tasks: The Network Approach

Although functional differentiation of single brain areas is a well-established principle of cortical organization, recent approaches to human cognition have focused on the integration of groups of specialized areas into long-range units that may collectively serve as the comprehensive neural substrate for specific cognitive tasks. An early empirical foundation for this emerging view is found in the work of Mishkin and Ungerleider,[47] who described ventral and dorsal pathway segmentation during visual tasks that required either object identification or object localization, respectively. More recently, direct interactions between brain regions that participate in specific functions have been proposed as evidence for this systems model; for example, covariations between BOLD responses in separate cortical areas during complex attention tasks have been examined using a statistical approach called structural equation modeling, which can determine whether the covariances between areas are due to direct or indirect interactions.[48] This analysis technique identifies the groups of areas associated with a task, and also characterizes changes in regional activity and interactions between regions over time. Other approaches to identify function-specific long-range systems associated with language and attention processes are illustrated below.

> A central feature in the organization of the large-scale network is the absence of one-to-one correspondences among anatomical sites, neural computations and complex behaviors. According to this organization, an individual cognitive or behavioral domain is subserved by several interconnected macroscopic sites, each of which subserves multiple computations, leading to a distributed and interactive but also coarse and degenerate (one-to-many and many-to-one) mapping of anatomical substrate onto neural computation and computation onto behavior.
>
> M.—Marsel Mesulam, 1998[49]

Functional Neuroanatomy of Language Processes: A Large-Scale Network

Models of the neural correlates for elementary language processes often include left hemisphere regions involved in a variety of language functions, including Broca's and Wernicke's Areas, and are generally consistent with a network model. To demonstrate this network, an object naming task using auditory, visual, and tactile stimuli can be employed. A cross-modality conjunction technique (above) isolates effects not dependent upon sensory processes. Results are consistent with the view that the task of naming objects elicits activity from a set of areas within a neurocognitive system specialized for language-related functions (Figure 6.15). The colored circles on the glass brain represent average locations of activity centroids on the standard atlas brain (x, y, z coordinates) as indicated on the table. There are five regions in this neurocognitive system (all located within the left hemisphere), including putative Broca's Area (inferior frontal gyrus, BA 44 and 45), putative Wernicke's Area (superior temporal

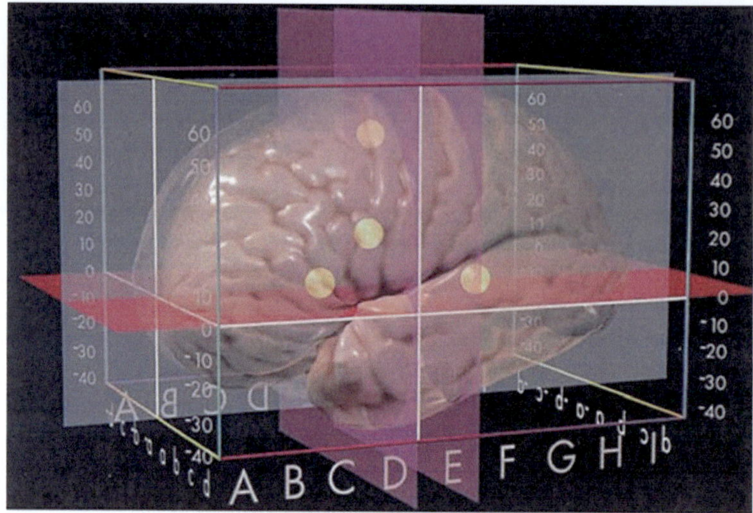

Anatomical Region	Area	Center of mass		
		x	y	z
Medial Frontal Gyrus (GFd)	6	9	−6	53
Superior Temporal Gyrus (GTs)	22	57	−26	9
Inferior Frontal Gyrus (Gfi)	44	49	10	25
Inferior Frontal Gyrus (Gfi)	45	40	25	8

Figure 6.15. A fixed large-scale network for object naming. The network of areas that subserve object naming as determined by conjunction across three sensory modalities consists of medial frontal gyrus (GFd, BA 6), superior temporal gyrus (GTs, BA 22; putative Wernicke's Area), and inferior frontal gyrus (Gfi, BA 44,45; putative Broca's Area) in the left hemisphere. These areas are portrayed as colored circles in a three-dimensional glass brain based upon the Talairach and Tournoux Human Brain Atlas[45] and stereotactic coordinate system. The table appearing below contains the average group coordinates (x, y, z) of the included regions. Reprinted from Hirsch J, Rodriguez-Moreno D, Kim KHS. Interconnected large-scale systems for three fundamental cognitive tasks revealed by functional MRI. *J Cogn Neurosci.* 2001;13(3):1–16. Reprinted with permission from MIT Press Journals.

gyrus, BA 22), and medial frontal gyrus (BA 6). Thus, these results are consistent with the view that the functional specialization for this elementary language task involves a system of language-related areas rather than a single area.

Functional Neuroanatomy of Attention Processes: A Large-Scale Network

Like language, the ability to direct attention is involved in a range of cognitive tasks. Functional imaging studies by Mesulam[49] and others suggest that spatial attention is mediated by a large scale distributed network of interconnected cortical areas within the posterior parietal cortex, the region of frontal eye fields, and the cingulate cortex. Kim and colleagues[50] used a conjunction analysis to compare activity associated with two different types of visuospatial attention shifts: one based on spatial priming and the other based on cues that directed spatial expectancy to test the hypothesis of a fixed area network for both tasks. The activation foci observed for the two tasks were nearly overlapping, indicating that both were subserved by a common network of cortical and subcortical areas. The main findings of this study were consistent with a model of spatial attention that is associated with a fixed large-scale distributed network specialized to co-ordinate multiple aspects of attention. Alternative hypotheses that predict that task variations are associated with an increase in the number of involved areas can be rejected. However, an observed right-ward bias for the spatial priming task suggested that activation within the system showed variations specific to the attributes of the attentional task (Figure 6.16).

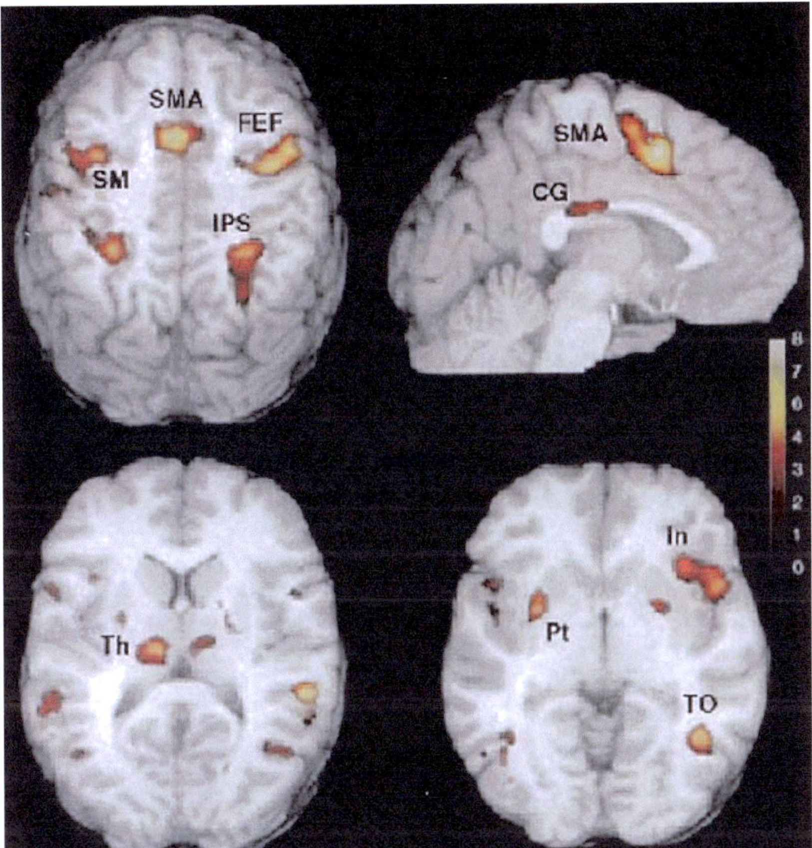

Figure 6.16. A fixed large-scale network for spatial attention. The network of areas that subserve visuospatial attention shifts consists of supplementary motor area— anterior cingulate cortex (SMA, BA 6), frontal eye fields (FEF, BA 6), and the banks of the intraparietal sulcus (IPS, BA 7,40). This network was determined by a conjunction analysis of activation related to visuospatial attention tasks based on two different types of information, spatial priming and spatial expectancy. Although the same areas are involved in both tasks, a right-ward bias in the intraparietal sulcus (IPS) was observed for the spatial priming task and suggests that, within this network, task-related variations are present. Reprinted from *NeuroImage* Vol. 9. Kim Y-H, Gitelman Dr, Nobre AG, Parrish TB, LaBar KS, Mesulam M-M. The large-scale neural network for spatial attention displays multifunctional overlap but differential asymmetry, 269–277. Copyright © 1999, with permission from Elsevier. (Neurologic coordinates).

Tests of Cognitive Theory Based on Mapping of Neural Correlates

Advances in our understanding of the biological components of cognition are dependent upon the development of functional tasks that reveal specific cognitive processes; therefore, tasks are selected to target some aspect of cognition that can be varied so that the specific processing requirements are increased or decreased. Current neuroimaging investigations of language, attention, memory, executive processes, and even consciousness generate hypotheses based on theoretical frameworks and behavioral models and develop stimulation paradigms that cause the subject to engage the targeted functions. This section presents a selection of models, hypotheses, cognitive functions, and tasks that have been investigated by neuroimaging techniques. Although more in-depth coverage of many of these topics is presented elsewhere, the objective here is to illustrate the advantages of neuroimaging for understanding the biological components of various cognitive processes rather than to provide a comprehensive survey of each of these cognitive processes.

Functional Neuroanatomy of Working Memory: A Fixed- or Variable-Area Network

Mechanisms for cognitive functions such as reasoning, problem solving, and language are critically dependent upon working memory processes that briefly maintain a limited amount of information in a mental scratch pad for ongoing processing. To test the hypothesis that a working memory system is subserved by a fixed number of brain areas, Smith and Jonides[51] employed a memory task (*N*-Back) that varied cognitive load. The logic of the experiment follows: If the hypothesis of a fixed number of regions was supported, then increasing the difficulty of the task, and thereby the cognitive load, would increase the amount of activity in each of the component areas. However, if the hypothesis of a variable area network was supported, then increasing the difficulty of the task would activate additional areas.

The *N* Back Task and a Test of a Cognitive Theory

The *N*-Back task, illustrated in Figure 6.17, was developed as a cognitive tool to vary memory task difficulty (load). The subject views a series of letters separated by fixation points. In the 0-Back condition, the subject responds whenever one of the presented letters matches a standard presented at the beginning of the run. In the 1-Back condition, the subject responds when there is a match to the preceding letter. In the 2-Back condition, the subject responds when there is a match to the letter 2-Back in the series, and similarly for the 3-Back condition.

Results of this study showed a clear increase in the volume of activity, with the increase in difficulty (load) of the task (Figure 6.18). However, the specific regions involved did not vary with increases in load supporting the fixed-number-of-areas hypothesis for a working memory system.

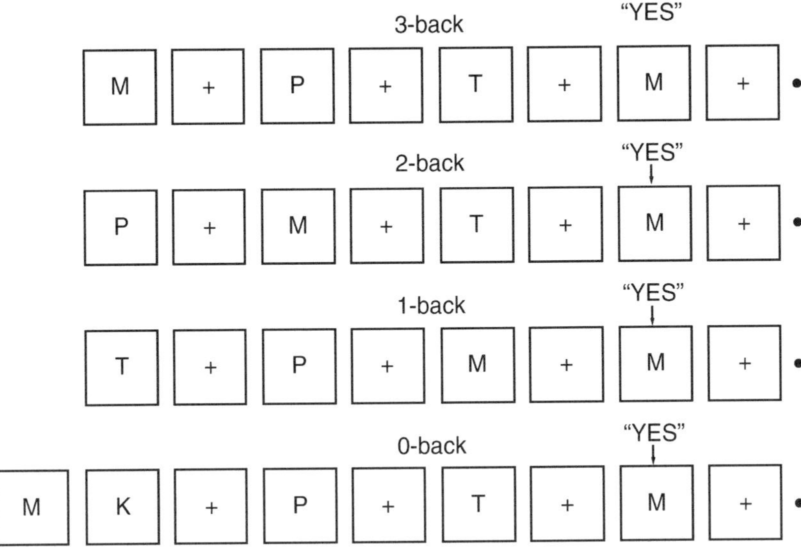

Figure 6.17. Variation in working memory load based on the *N*-Back task. The *N*-Back task engages working memory by requiring the subject to remember a previous event and respond if a present stimulus (target) is identical to that previously presented stimulus. Task load can be increased by increasing the distance between the target and its match, e.g., 0-, 1-, 2-, 3-Back. Reprinted from *Cognitive Psychology*, Vol. 33, Smith EE, Jonides J. Working memory: A view from neuroimaging, 5–42. Copyright © 1997, with permission from Elsevier.

Functional Neuroanatomy of Selective Attention: A Neurological Model of Cognitive Interference

The ability to filter task-related stimuli to guide responses is referred to as selective attention. An experimental task that requires the subject to attend to certain stimulus characteristics while ignoring others that elicit a competing response engages a system of selective attention. The Stroop task is a classical cognitive task first developed for use in behavioral studies of cognitive interference and is an ideal task for functional imaging studies that seek to identify the neural substrate associated with selective attention mechanisms.

The Stroop Task

In the classical Stroop task, a subject views a series of words in different colored inks. Each word is the name of a color. The subject is instructed to produce the color of the ink. In the incongruent case, the word and the ink color of the written word are different, resulting in longer reaction times than in the congruent case where the word and ink color match. For example, if the ink color was blue but the word was red (incongruent), the reaction time to report "blue" (the ink color) would be longer than when the word and the ink color were both blue (congruent) (Figure 6.19).

Cognitive models that account for results obtained by the Stroop task propose that subjects must inhibit the automatic reading response and

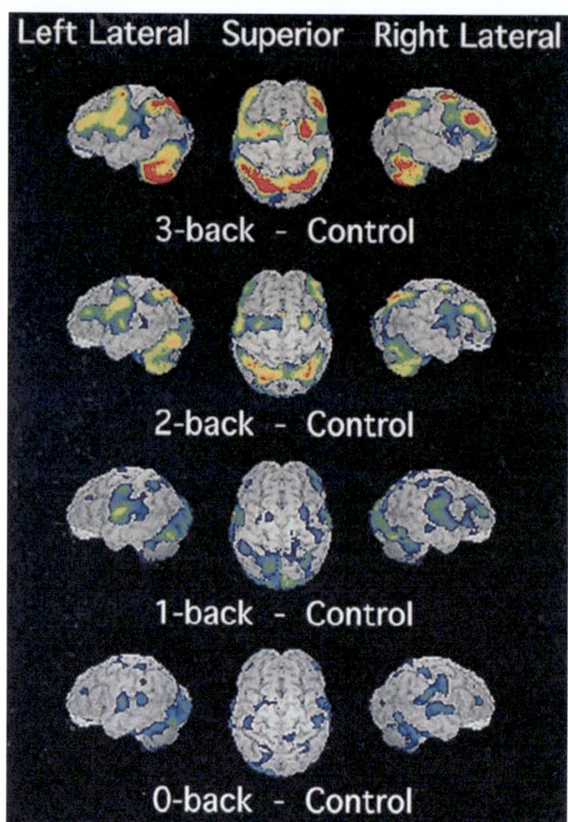

Figure 6.18. Cortical responses during the *N*-Back task. Left and right lateral, as well as a superior, views of the average PET images are shown. All images are difference images that reflect the subtraction of a control condition in which subjects responded to every stimulus. The different colors reflect the significance of the activation, with red areas being most significant. Robust responses for the 3-Back condition relative to 0-, 1-, and 2-Back conditions are taken as evidence of increased neural activity associated with increased memory load. Reprinted from *Cognitive Psychology*, Vol. 33, Smith EE, Jonides J. Working memory: A view from neuroimaging, 5–42. Copyright © 1997, with permission from Elsevier.

selectively attend to the color of the letters in order to successfully perform the color-naming task. A neuroimaging study designed to probe the neural basis for this type of cognitive interference, that is, the mechanisms of selective attention,[52] compared BOLD responses to congruent and incongruent conditions in an event-related neuroimaging study (see following section on event-related paradigms). The results are shown in Figure 6.20 for incongruent (A) and congruent conditions (B), respectively. The incongruent condition is associated with robust distributed responses as compared to the congruent condition, suggesting that a distributed large-scale neural network is employed during selective attention. The results also suggest a possible correspondence between the selective attention mechanisms engaged in this study and visuospatial attention mechanisms.

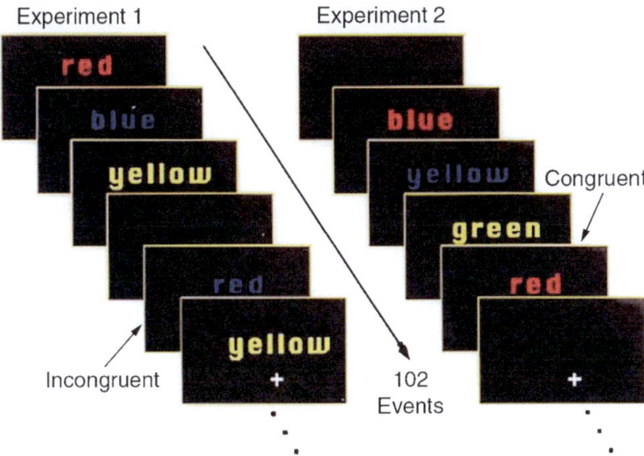

Figure 6.19. The classical Stroop color word interference task. In congruent cases, the color of the ink matches the color of the word. In incongruent cases, the color of the ink is different from the color of the word. The words are presented sequentially to subjects who respond by indicating the color of the ink for each word. Reprinted from Leung H-C, Skudlarski P, Gatenby JC, Peterson BS, Gore JC. An event-related functional MRI study of the Stroop color word interference task. *Cereb Cortex*. 2000;10:552–560. Reprinted by permission of Oxford University Press.

Functional Neuroanatomy of Executive Processes: Separate or Combined Systems

Current models of cognition often include undefined mechanisms (frequently referred to as a black box) to account for executive processes such as the allocation of attentional resources among competing tasks. Functional neuroimaging techniques and experimental paradigms, such as the dual performance task and the Go No-Go task, have been developed to observe the neural correlates of these executive functions and attempt to define the black box in neurophysiological terms.

D'Esposito and colleagues[53] introduced an fMRI task paradigm that required subjects to perform two tasks simultaneously, referred to as a dual performance task (see diagram on page 172). Comparison of the BOLD responses elicited during each task alone and both tasks together enabled tests of hypotheses about the neural system involved in the execution of competing tasks. Specifically, the hypothesis of a modular executive system predicts the recruitment of additional regions during the dual task condition, whereas the fixed-areas hypothesis predicts an increase in volume of the areas activated by a single task.

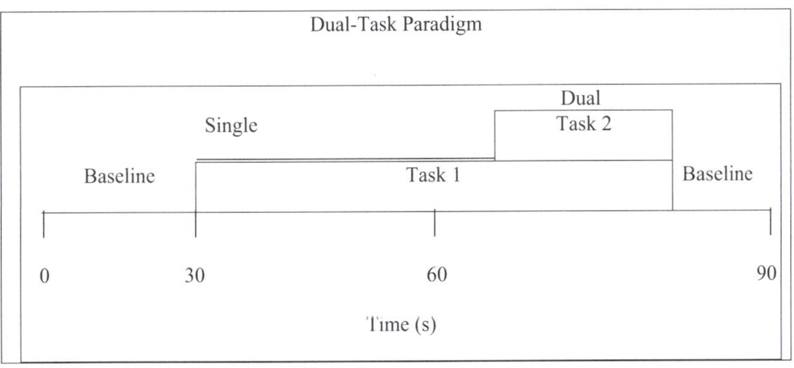

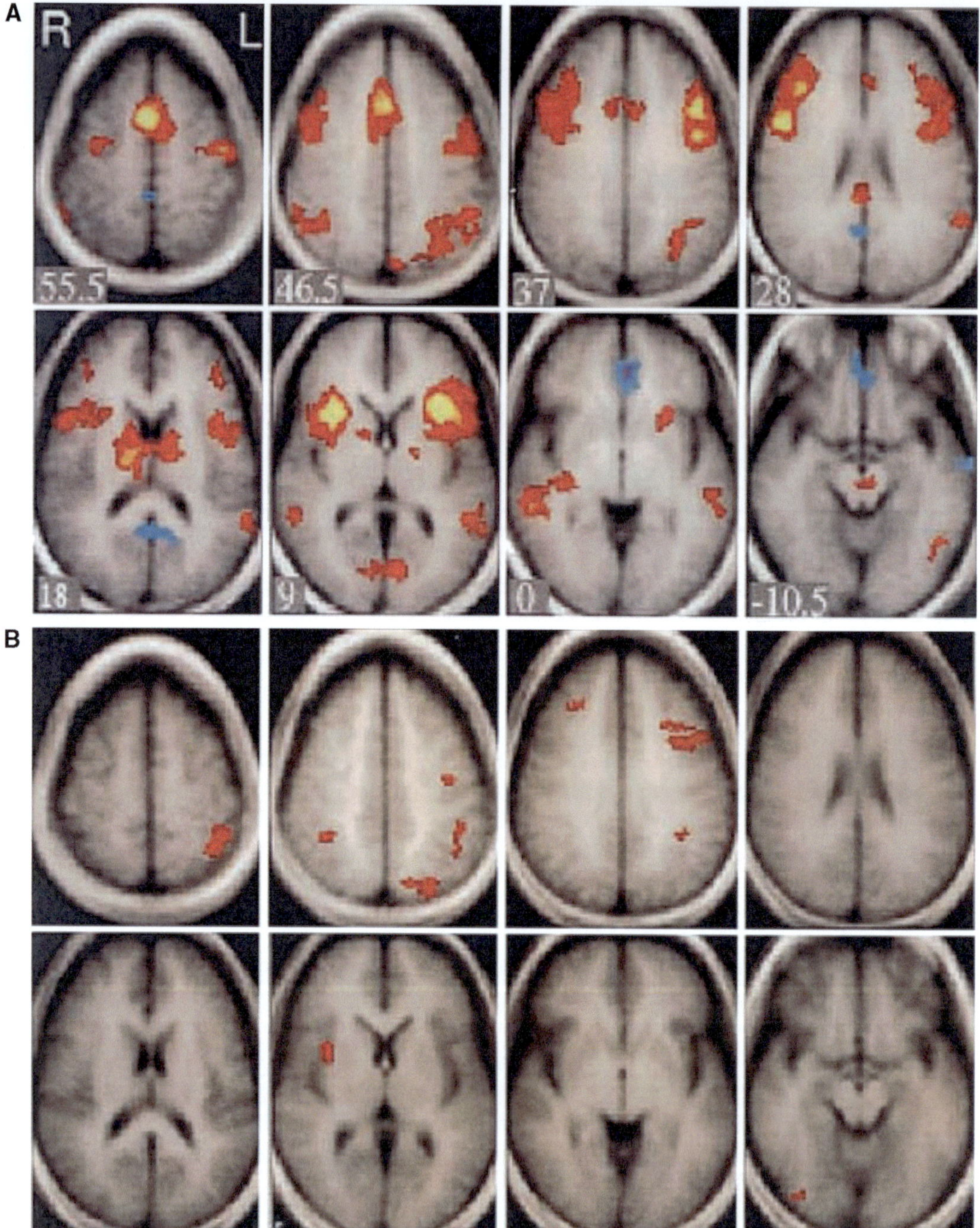

Figure 6.20. Activation related to the classical Stroop task versus the inverse Stroop task. Images represent composite maps of 13 subjects performing the Stroop task. In Experiment 1, the classical Stroop task was employed, that is, incongruent words appear infrequently whereas congruent words appear frequently (A). In Experiment 2 (B), an inverse Stroop task was employed, that is, congruent words are infrequent events and incongruent words appear frequently. The robust response for the incongruent condition (A) relative to the congruent condition (B) is taken as evidence of a neural basis for response inhibition. Reprinted from Leung H-C, Skudlarski P, Gatenby JC, Peterson BS, Gore JC. An event-related functional MRI study of the Stroop color word interference task. *Cereb Cortex* 2000;10:552–560. Reprinted by permission of Oxford University Press.

Adcock and colleagues[54] employed this paradigm with paired combinations of spatial rotation tasks (visual), semantic categorization tasks (auditory), and facial identification tasks (visual). Results indicated that the activated areas varied with the sensory modality of component tasks as expected based on these domain-specific functional specializations. However, all of the areas activated during the dual task performance were also activated during the component tasks; that is, there was no evidence for a separate executive system. Increases in activity within a given area during the dual task are related to the additional load of the second task. These results can be interpreted as generally consistent with the hypothesis that these executive processes may be implemented by interactions between anatomically and functionally distinct systems engaged in the performances of component tasks rather than by a specific area or areas dedicated to a modular and separable executive system.

The Go-No Go Task

Another classical executive function is the ability to inhibit a prepotent or habitual response that has been studied psychophysically using a Go No-Go task paradigm. Neuroimaging investigations of the neural correlates of response inhibition have employed a version of the task to investigate the neural correlates of response inhibition in children and adults.[55] The hypothesis was that the ability to successfully inhibit a response varies with maturity. This variation could be neurally represented as either the recruitment of different areas in children versus adults or variations in the volumes within a fixed set of areas. During the Go-No Go task, the subject views a series of letters presented sequentially and presses a button on each successive presentation except when the letter is an X. On the X trials, the subject must inhibit the response.

The BOLD responses for children (ages 7–12) and adults were compared within five selected areas of the prefrontal cortex using an event-related paradigm and an analysis of variance (ANOVA) where subject age and the task conditions (Go vs. No-Go) were taken as factors. The areas demonstrating significant activity related to the No-Go task include anterior cingulate and four frontal gyri, including inferior, middle, orbital, and superior. The areas involved in the response inhibition function did not vary between adults and children. However, during No-Go trials, the amount of activity was higher in children, particularly in the dorsal and lateral prefrontal sites.

This observation is consistent with the hypothesis of a distributed system for response inhibition and further suggests that the elements within that system are modified with development. In both children and adults, the percent change in the amplitude of the BOLD signal responses in the anterior cingulate and the orbital frontal gyri was correlated with the number of false alarms, which also suggests putative within-system processes associated with the emergent response inhibition behavior.

Integration of Temporal and Spatial Information to Map Executive Processes

A common theme in the aforementioned neuroimaging studies of cognitive functions is the identification of the underlying cortical networks associated with each function and the question of fixed versus variable areas for related functions. In the case of the language, attention, memory, and cognitive control systems illustrated above, the results suggest that a fixed number of areas (rather than the recruitment of new areas) are modulated with increased load. This is an active area of research, and new evidence from studies using techniques such as electrophysiological recordings and event-related fMRI to probe within-system effects may be required to elucidate the modulation of processes both within and across these systems.

Integration of ERP and fMRI

New investigations that focus on within-system processes and the modulation of a specialized system consisting of a fixed set of distributed areas require probes of the computations performed within neural systems. A new class of multi-technique experiments are currently being developed that elucidate the spatial localization of active regions (fMRI), as well as the temporal co-variations between these cortical or subcortical regions, as reflected in event-related potentials. These techniques may be employed either simultaneously or sequentially and require an adaptation of the blocked fMR experiments (event-related fMRI) and a task specialized for both fMRI and electrophysiological approaches.

Event-Related fMRI

As in conventional event-related electrophysiology, individual trials (events) are presented separately (rather than in a continuous block), and the signal is selectively averaged across like trials. This acquisition scheme is illustrated in Figure 6.21, where both block and event-related schemes are shown.[56]

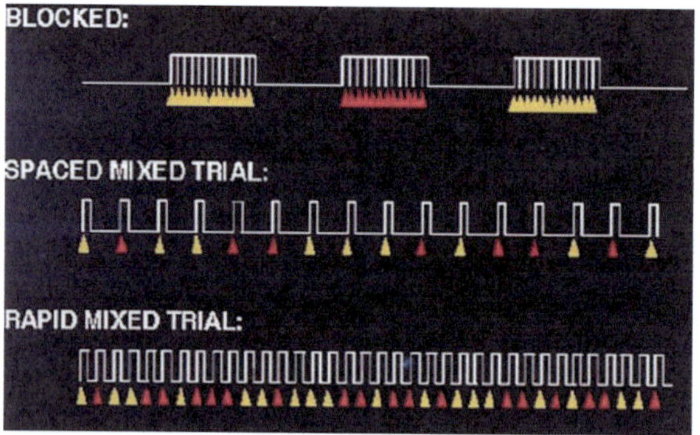

Figure 6.21. Blocked-versus event-related fMRI paradigms. Schematic diagrams illustrate the difference between two forms of imaging paradigms: blocked trials and event-related trials. Each schematic shows two trial types indicated by either yellow or red arrows. In blocked trial paradigms (labeled Blocked), the trial types are clustered together in succession so that the same trial type or condition occurs for an extended period of time. Event-related trials, by contrast, intermix different trial types either by spacing them widely apart to allow the hemodynamic response from one trial to decay before the next trial occurs (labeled Spaced Mixed Trial), or by presenting them rapidly (labeled Rapid Mixed Trial). Reprinted from Dale AM, Buckner RL. Selective averaging of rapidly presented individual trials using fMRI. *Hum Brain Mapp.* 1997;5:329–340. Copyright © 1997 Wiley. Reprinted with permission of Wiley-Liss, Inc., a subsidiary of John Wiley & Sons, Inc.

Event-related fMRI offers an additional class of task designs that expand and elaborate investigations of cognitive processes. Given that the BOLD response tracks neuronal activity with hemodynamic delays on the order of about two to four seconds, it is possible to reliably identify the activity associated with each successive trial.

There are several advantages to event-related fMRI:

1) By detecting signals that are linked to individual trial events rather than to blocks, the observations can parallel other behavioral and evoked response potential studies that are also linked to individual events. Thus, the added value of precise temporal data from other integrated methods in combination with the high-resolution data of fMRI extends the range of questions that can be addressed.
2) An event-related approach is particularly useful when subject response is a factor, as in the case where it is necessary to separate trials in which there was a correct response from trials in which the response was not correct or trials where the stimulus was novel from trials where the stimulus was repeated or to isolate the acquisitions associated with bistable perspectives of ambiguous figures as reported by the subject during the experiment. Thus, the event-related approach allows trials to be categorized post hoc on the basis of the subject's behavior.
3) Some events cannot be presented in a blocked design, as in cases involving a surprise element or the occurrence of an oddball stimulus that is distinguished from the expected context. In those cases, an event-related approach is required.

The Oddball Task

Cortical mechanisms specialized for novelty oddball detection compare incoming information with relevant memories to register a novel event. Opitz and colleagues[57] reported the spatial and temporal properties of cortical mechanisms involved in the detection of novel tones by combining evoked response potential and fMRI measures. The evoked response potential methods lack precision with respect to the spatial source of the signal as detected by scalp electrodes because these sources must be inferred from two-dimensional scalp topography and using dipole fitting algorithms. Temporal resolution of signals, however, is within milliseconds. By combining evoked response potential and fMRI, both temporal and spatial properties of the cortical responses corresponding to novelty can be investigated. Although registration of these separate data domains remains a challenge, results of the Opitz study relate specific evoked response potential responses to bilateral superior temporal gyrus and right pre-frontal cortex, suggesting coordinated activity between areas previously associated with novelty using event-related fMRI techniques.

A similar evoked response potential and fMRI experiment by Kruggel and colleagues[58] employed a visual oddball task using illusory contours that deviated from the prevailing visual stimuli (no illusory contours). Results replicated previous fMRI findings, indicating the activation of extrastriate visual cortex in the appreciation of the illusory contours (perceived between the corner elements of Kanizsa squares) and the lack of this activation during viewing of stimuli in which the corner elements were rotated out of alignment. Additionally, the evoked response potential results confirmed a sequential activation of striate to extra striate visual cortex consistent with hierarchal models of visual processing. Thus, integration of approaches that optimize both spatial and temporal information relating to neural mechanisms and both perceptual and cognitive processes offers new directions and precision to probe the neural basis of mental events.

The Functional Neuroanatomy of Very High Level Cognitive Processes

Guided by the Astonishing Hypothesis of Francis Crick,[1] it is assumed that the biological components of even very high-level cognitive processes, such as consciousness, are observable. Although still in a nascent stage, the study of consciousness with neuroimaging techniques is a rapidly developing area of research. As in the neuroimaging of related cognitive processes, including language, attention, working memory, and executive control, an investigation of consciousness is largely dependent upon the development of appropriate paradigms and evaluation of relevant theory.

Dehaene and Naccache[59] have developed one theoretical framework for the investigation of consciousness that consists of a global neuronal work space. This framework postulates that, "at any given time, many modular cerebral networks are active in parallel and process information in an unconscious manner." As information becomes conscious, however, the neural population that represents the information is mobilized by top-down attentional amplification into a state of coherent activity that involves many neurons distributed throughout the brain. The long-distance connectivity of these workspace neurons can, when they are active for a minimal duration, make the information available to a variety of processes, including perceptual categorization, long-term memorization, evaluation, and intentional action. According to this theoretical framework, the global availability of information throughout the workspace is what is subjectively experienced as a conscious state.

The fact that consciousness is a private, first-person phenomenon makes it more difficult to study than other cognitive phenomena that, although being equally private, also have characteristic behavioural signatures. Nonetheless, by combining cognitive and neurobiological methods, it is possible to approach consciousness, to describe its cognitive nature, its behavioral correlates, its possible evolutionary origin and functional role; last but not least, it is possible to investigate its neuroanatomical and neurophysiological underpinnings.

Antonio R. Damasio, 1998[60]

A major obstacle to applying neuroimaging techniques to the investigation of consciousness is the inability to establish a task that varies the state of consciousness; that is, consciousness is not started and stopped in synchrony with a particular task, as is assumed in many cognitive tasks. The global workspace hypothesis suggests a distributed neural system or workspace with long-distance connectivity that interconnects multiple specialized brain areas in a coordinated, although variable, manner.[61] This framework challenges current neuroimaging paradigms based on conventional experimental paradigms and views of functional specialization.

One approach to circumvent this obstacle is based on the specific hypothesis that conscious humans are engaged continuously during resting states in "adaptive cognitive processes that involve semantic knowledge retrieval, representation in awareness and directed manipulation of represented knowledge for organization, problem solving and planning." Thus, comparison of resting activation and task activations during a neuroimaging study might reveal neural processes associated with consciousness. Binder and colleagues[62] used fMRI to measure brain activity during rest and during several contrasting activation paradigms, including a perceptual task (tone-monitoring) designed to interfere with ongoing thought processes and a semantic retrieval task (noun categorization) designed to engage on-going thought processes similar to those hypothesized to occur during rest. Higher signal values were observed during the resting state than during the tone-monitoring task in a network of left hemisphere cortical regions. These areas were equally active during the semantic task.

This finding is consistent with the hypothesis that perceptual tasks interrupt specific ongoing processes during rest that are associated with many of the same brain areas engaged during semantic retrieval. Thus, neuroimaging observations suggest that on-going processing during a conscious resting state involves an underlying neural substrate similar to that employed in cognitive tasks such as semantic processing.

Another paradigm that employs masked (too brief for cognitive awareness) presentations of emotional facial expressions has been found to modulate BOLD and PET-related hemodynamic responses originating in the amygdala.[63,64] In these studies, the amygdala was involved in 1) nonconscious responses that reflected the emotional valence of stimuli, and 2) was spatially differentiated depending upon level of awareness. Both findings confirm a neural substrate that is active and responsive without awareness.

The resting-state and masking paradigms, as well as other ongoing neuroimaging investigations of related aspects of consciousness, including perceptual awareness, awareness during varying levels of anesthesia, and awareness in patients in vegetative and minimally conscious states, can be expected to contribute to an emerging understanding of the neural basis of consciousness and the neural basis for related events that occur without awareness. Imaging paradigms that are established to investigate the neural underpinnings of cognition also provide foundations for emerging investigations of the neural underpinnings of consciousness and bring neural science closer to the goal of understanding the biological underpinnings of the mind.

The BOLD Signal

Physiology	**Physics**
Neural activation is associated with an increase in blood flow O_2 extraction is relatively unchanged	**Deoxy HGB is paramagnetic** and distorts the local magnetic field, causing signal loss
Result Reduction in the proportion of deoxy HGB in the local vasculature	**Result** Less distortion of the magnetic field results in local signal increase

---

Acknowledgments: This chapter was written in collaboration with Sarah Callahan, a psycholinguistic student in my laboratory, who not only researched and provided essential original sources, but also was a partner in the development of the ideas and conceptual organization. Without her critical contributions, this chapter would not have emerged in print.

References

1. Crick F. *The Astonishing Hypothesis: The Scientific Search for the Soul.* New York: Charles Scribner's Sons; 1994.
2. *Dorland's Illustrated Medical Dictionary.* 27th ed. Philadelphia, PA: W.B. Saunders Co. (Harcourt Brace Jovanovich Inc.); 1988.
3. *The American Heritage Dictionary of the English Language.* 4th ed. Boston, MA: Houghton Mifflin Co.; 2000.
4. Neisser U. *Cognitive Psychology.* New York; Appleton: 1967.
5. Damasio H, Grabowski T, Frank R, Galaburda AM, Damasio AR. The return of Phineas Gage: Clues about the brain from the skull of a famous patient. *Science.* 1994;264:1102–1105.
6. Penfield W. *The Mystery of the Mind.* Princeton, NJ; Princeton University Press: 1975.
7. Sherrington R. *J Physiol.* 1890;11:85.
8. Raichle ME, Martin WRW, Herscovitch P, Mintun MA, Markham J. Brain blood flow measured with intravenous H2150. II. Implementation and validation. *J Nucl Med.* 1983;24:790–798.
9. Fox PT, Raichle ME. Stimulus rate dependence of regional cerebral blood flow in human striate cortex demonstrated by positron emission tomography. *J Neurophysiol.* 1984;51:1109–1120.
10. Peterson SE, Fox PT, Posner MI, Mintun M, Raichle ME. Postiron emission tomographic studies of the processing of single words. *J Cogn Neurosci.* 1989;1(2): 153–170.
11. Ogawa S, Lee T-M, Nayak AS, Glynn P. Oxygenation-sensitive contrast in magnetic resonance image of rodent brain at high magnetic fields. *Magn Reson Med.* 1990;14:68–78.

12. Gore JC, Principles and practice of functional MRI of the human brain. *J Clin Invest.* 2003;112:4–9.

13. George JS, Aine CJ, Mosher JC, Schmidt MD, Ranken DM, Schlitt HA Wood CC, Lewine JD, Sanders JA, Belliveau JW. Mapping function in the human brain with magneto encephalography, anatomical magnetic resonance imaging, and functional magnetic resonance imaging. *J Clin Neurophysiol.* 1995;12:406–429.

14. Nimsky C, Ganslandt O, Kober H, Moller M, Ulmer S, Tomandl B, Fahlbusch R. Integration of functional magnetic resonance imaging supported by magnetoencephalography in functional neuronavigation. *Neurosurgery.* 1999;44(6):1249–1255.

15. Stapleton SR, Kiriakopoulos E, Mikulis D, Drake LM, Hoffman HJ, Humphreys R, Hwang P, Otsubo H, Holowka S, Logan W, Rutka JT. Combined utility of functional MRI, cortical mapping, and frameless stereotaxy in the resection of lesions in eloquent areas of brain in children. *Pediatr Neurosurg.* 1997;26:68–82.

16. Atlas SW, Howard RS, Maldjian J, Alsop D, Detre JA, Listerud J, D'Esposito M, Judy KD, Zager E, Stecker M. Functional magnetic resonance imaging of regional brain activity in patients with intracerebral gliomas: findings and implications for clinical management. *Neurosurgery.* 1996;38(2):329–338.

17. Latchaw RE, Xiaoping HU, Ugurbil K, Hall WA, Madison MT, Heros RC. Functional magnetic resonance imaging as a management tool for cerebral arteriovenous malformations. *Neurosurgery.* 1995;37(4):619–625.

18. Lee CC, Jack CR Jr, Riederer SJ. Mapping of the central sulcus with functional MR: Active versus passive activation tasks. *Neuroradiology.* 1998;19:847–852.

19. Mueller WM, Yetkin FZ, Hammeke TA, Morris GL III, Swanson SJ, Reichert K, Cox, Haughton VM. Functional magnetic resonance imaging mapping of the motor cortex in patients with cerebral tumors. *Neurosurgery.* 1996;39(3):515–521.

20. Puce A, Constable T, Luby ML, Eng M, McCarthy G, Nobre AC, Spencer DD, Gore JC, Allison T. Functional magnetic resonance imaging of sensory and motor cortex: comparison with electrophysiological localization. *J Neurosurg.* 1995;83:262–270.

21. Schulder M, Maldijian JA, Liu WC, Holodny AI, Kalnin AT, Mun IK, Carmel PW. Functional image-guided surgery of intracranial tumors located in or near the sensorimotor cortex. *Neurosurgery.* 1998;89:412–418.

22. Yousry TA, Schmid UD, Jassoy AG, Schmidt D, Eisener WE, Reulen HJ, Reiser MF, Lissner J. Topography of the cortical motor hand area: prospective study with functional MR imaging and direct motor mapping at surgery. *Radiology.* 1995;195:23–29.

23. Debus J, Essig M, Schad LR, Wenz F, Baudendistel K, Knopp MV, Engenhart R, Lorenz WJ. Functional magnetic imaging in a stereotactic setup. *Magn Reson Imaging.* 1996;14(9):1007–1012.

24. Fried I, Nenov VI, Ojemann SG, Woods RP. Functional MR and PET imaging of rolandic and visual cortices for neurosurgical planning. *J Neurosurg.* 1995;83:854–861.

25. Chapman PH, Buchbinder BR, Cosgrove GR, Jiang HJ. Functional magnetic resonance imaging for cortical mapping in pediatric neurosurgery. *Pediatr Neurosurg.* 1995;23:122–126.

26. Fandino J, Kollias S, Wieser G, Valavanis A, Yonekawa Y. Intraoperative validation of functional magnetic resonance imaging and cortical reorganization patters in patients with brain tumors involving the primary motor cortex. *J Neurosurg.* 1999;91:238–250.

27. Pujol J, Conesa G, Deus J, Lopez-Obarrio L, Isamat F, Capdevila A. Clinical application of functional magnetic resonance imaging in presurgical identification of the central sulcus. *J Neurosurg.* 1998;88:863–869.

28. Herholz K, Reulen H, von Stockhausen H, Thiel A, Ilmberger J, Kessler J, Eisner W, Yousry TA, Heiss W. Preoperative activation and intraoperative stimula-

tion of language-related areas in patients with glioma. *Neurosurgery*. 1997;41(6): 1253–1262.

29. Hinke RM, Hu X, Stillman AE, Kim SG, Merkle H, Salmi R, Ugurbil K. Functional magnetic resonance imaging of Broca's area during internal speech. *NeuroReport*. 1993;4:675–678.

30. Binder JR, Frost JA, Hammeke TA, Bellgowan PSF, Rao SM, Cox RW. Conceptual processing during the conscious resting state: A functional MRI study. *J Cogn Neurosci*. 1999;11(1):80–93.

31. Kollias SS, Landau K, Khan N, Golay X, Bernays R, Yonekawa Y, Valavanis A. Functional evaluation using magnetic resonance imaging of the visual cortex in patients with retrochiasmatic lesions. *Neurosurgery*. 1998;89:780–790.

32. Tootell RB, Reppas JB, Kwong KK, Malach R, Born RT, Brady TJ, Rosen BR, Belliveau JW. Functional analysis of human MT and related visual cortical areas using magnetic resonance imaging. *J Neurosci*. 1995;15:3215–3230.

33. Hirsch J, Rodriguez-Moreno D, Kim KHS. Interconnected large-scale systems for three fundamental cognitive tasks revealed by functional MRI. *J Cogn Neurosci*. 2001;13(3):1–16.

34. Hirsch J, Ruge MI, Kim KHS, Correa DD, Victor JD, Relkin NR, Labar DR, Krol G, Bilsky MH, Souweidane MM, DeAngelis LM, Gutin PH. An integrated fMRI procedure for preoperative mapping of cortical areas associated with tactile, motor, language, and visual functions. *Neurosurgery*. 2000;47(3):711–722.

35. Kaplan EF, Goodglass H, Weintraub S. The Boston naming test. 2nd ed. Philadelphia, PA: Lea & Febiger: 1983.

36. Dinner DS, Luders H, Lesser RP, Morris HH. Cortical generators of somatosensory evoked potentials to median nerve stimulation. *Neurology*. 1987;37:1141–1145.

37. Cedzich C, Taniguchi M, Schafer S, Schramm J. Somatosensory evoked potential phase reversal and direct motor cortex stimulation during surgery in and around the central region. *Neurosurgery*. 1996;38:962–970.

38. Puce A. Comparative assessment of sensorimotor function using functional magnetic resonance imaging and electrophysiological methods. *J Clin Neurophysiol*. 1995;12:450–459.

39. Wada J, Rasmussen T. Intracarotid injection of sodium amytal for the lateralization of cerebral speech dominance. *J Neurosurg*. 1960;17:266–282.

40. Ruge MI, Victor JD, Hosain S, Correa DD, Relkin NR, Tabar V, Brennan C, Gutin PH, Hirsch J. Concordance between functional magnetic resonance imaging and intraoperative language mapping. *J Stereotact Funct Neurosurg*. 1999;72:95–102.

41. Kim KHS, Relkin NR, Lee K-M, Hirsch J. Distinct cortical areas associated with native and second languages. *Nature*. 1997;388:171–174.

42. Ojemann G, Ojemann J, Lettich E, Berger M. Cortical language localization in left, dominant hemisphere. *J Neurosurg*. 1989;71:316–326.

43. Friston KJ, Holmes AP, Price CJ, Büchel C, Worsley KJ. Multisubject fMRI studies and conjunction analysis. *Neuroimage*. 1999;10:385–396.

44. Desmond JE, Glover GH. Estimating sample size in functional MRI (fMRI) neuroimaging studies: statistical power analyses. *J Neurosci Methods*. 2002;118: 115–128.

45. Talairach J, Tournoux P. *Co-Planar Stereotaxic Atlas of the Human Brain*. New York; Thieme: 1988.

46. Friston KJ, et al. *Human Brain Mapping*. 1995;2:189.

47. Mishkin M, Ungerleider LG. Contribution of striate inputs to the visuospatial functions of parieto-preoccipital cortex in monkeys. *Behav Brain Res*. 1982;6(1): 57–77.

48. Buchel C, Friston KJ. Modulation of connectivity in visual pathways by attention: Cortical interactions evaluated with structural equation modelling and fMRI. *Cerebral Cortex*. 1997;7(8):768–778.

49. Mesulam M-M. From sensation to cognition. *Brain*. 1998;121:1013–1052.

50. Kim Y-H, Gitelman DR, Nobre AC, Parrish TB, LaBar KS, Mesulam M-M. The large-scale neural network for spatial attention displays multifunctional overlap but differential asymmetry. *NeuroImage.* 1999;9:269–277.
51. Smith EE, Jonides J. Working memory: A view from neuroimaging. *Cogn Psychol.* 1997;33:5–42.
52. Leung H-C, Skudlarski P, Gatenby JC, Peterson BS, Gore JC. An event-related functional MRI study of the Stroop color word interference task. *Cereb Cortex.* 2000;10:552–560.
53. D'Esposito M, Detre JA, Alsop DC, Shin RK, Atlas S, Grossman M. The neural basis of the central executive system of working memory. *Nature.* 1995;378: 279–281.
54. Adcock RA, Constable RT, Gore JC, Goldman-Rakic PS. Functional neuroanatomy of executive processes involved in dual-task performance. *Proc Natl Acad Sci USA.* 2000;97(7):3567–3572.
55. Casey BJ, Trainor RJ, Orendi JL, Schubert AB, Nystrom LE, Giedd JN, Castellanos FX, Haxby JV, Noll DC, Cohen JD, Forman SD, Dahl RE, Rapoport JL. A developmental functional MRI study of prefrontal activation during performance of a Go-No-Go task. *J Cogn Neurosci.* 1997;9(6):835–847.
56. Rosen BR, Buckner RL, Dale AM. Event-related functional MRI: Past, present, and future. *Proc Natl Acad Sci USA.* 1998;95:773–780.
57. Opitz B, Mecklinger A, Friederici AD, von Cramon DY. The functional neuroanatomy of novelty processing: Integrating ERP and fMRI results. *Cerebr Cortex.* 1999;9(4):379–391.
58. Kruggel F, Herrmann CS, Wiggins CJ, von Cramon DY. Hemodynamic and electroencephalographic responses to illusory figures: Recording of the evoked potentials during functional MRI. *Neuroimage.* 2001;14:1327–1336.
59. Dehaene S, Naccache L. Towards a cognitive neuroscience of consciousness: Basic evidence and a workspace framework. *Cognition.* 2001;79:1–37.
60. Damasio AR. Investigating the biology of consciousness. *Phil Trans R Soc Lond B Biol Sci.* 1998;353:1879–1882.
61. Dehaene S, Kerszberg M, Changeux JP. A neuronal model of a global workspace in effortful cognitive tasks. *Proc Natl Acad Sci USA.* 1998;95(24):14529–14534, November 24.
62. Binder JR, Price CJ. Functional imaging of language. In: Cabeza R, Kingstone A, eds. *Handbook of Functional Neuroimaging of Cognition.* Cambridge, MA: MIT Press. pp. 187–251.
63. Whalen PJ, Rauch SL, Etcoff NL, McInerney SC, Lee MB, Jenike MA. Masked presentations of emotional facial expressions modulate amygdala activity without explicit knowledge. *J Cogn Neurosci.* 1998;18(1):411–418.
64. Morris JS, Ohman A, Dolan RJ. Conscious and unconscious emotional learning in the human amygdala. *Nature.* 1998;393:467–470.

7

fMRI of Memory in Aging and Dementia

Andrew J. Saykin and Heather A. Wishart

In the human brain, functionally and anatomically defined systems exist for actively encoding, consolidating, and retrieving memories of experiences (episodic memory); accumulating and accessing factual information in a body of knowledge (semantic memory); and processing and manipulating information (working memory). These three declarative memory systems can be distinguished from other nondeclarative memory systems such as procedural learning and priming.[1–4] Brain-behavior studies using a variety of approaches, from lesion-based research to functional magnetic resonance imaging (fMRI), demonstrate distinct, though interrelated, neural circuitry for working, episodic, and semantic memory.[4,5] Each of these three memory systems is affected somewhat differently by aging and dementia. In this chapter, the episodic, semantic, and working memory systems will be considered in turn, with special attention to changes associated with aging and with memory disorders such as Alzheimer's disease and Mild Cognitive Impairment.

Episodic Memory

Episodic memory refers to memory for events or information encoded with respect to a particular temporal or spatial context.[1] Originally defined to encompass memory for specific information presented, for example, during a testing session, the concept has been reformulated over the years to have at its core the conscious recollection of previous experiences. The emphasis is on memory for experience itself, not knowledge about the world derived from experience.[6] Important distinctions pertaining to episodic memory include the processes or operations that are performed (e.g., novelty versus familiarity discrimination; encoding, consolidation, retrieval); the success with which these processes are performed (i.e., whether they result in the formation of an accurate, inaccurate, or no memory trace); the sensory

---

This chapter previously appeared in *Functional MRI: Basic Principles and Clinical Applications*, edited by S. Faro and F. Mohamed. New York: Springer Science+Business Media, LCC 2006.

From: *BOLD fMRI: A Guide to Functional Imaging for Neuroscientists*
Edited by: S.H. Faro and F.B. Mohamed, DOI 10.1007/978-1-4419-1329-6_7
© Springer Science+Business Media, LLC 2010

modality in which the information is received (e.g., auditory, visual); and the nature of the material (e.g., verbal, spatial, pictorial). There are a variety of episodic memory fMRI probes, many of which are designed specifically to address or manipulate certain of these aspects of episodic memory processing; a sample task is shown in Table 7.1.

In general, episodic memory is thought to be subserved by a broad network of brain regions, primarily involving prefrontal and medial temporal circuitry, including the hippocampal formation (dentate gyrus; CA1, CA2, and CA3 fields; and subiculum), entorhinal cortex, perirhinal cortex, parahippocampal complex, and the amygdala.[7–10] Several models of the neural basis of specific episodic memory processes have been proposed. For example, the hippocampal encoding/retrieval (HIPER) model proposes a rostrocaudal gradient of hippocampal activity during encoding and retrieval from episodic memory,[11] although additional data suggest a more complex set of findings regarding hippocampal organization for episodic memory processes.[12,13] According to the hemispheric encoding and retrieval asymmetry (HERA) model, which pertains to the role of prefrontal cortex in memory, left prefrontal regions are involved primarily in retrieval from semantic memory and encoding into episodic memory, and right prefrontal are regions involved in retrieval of information from episodic memory.[7,14,15] This asymmetry is superimposed on a historical, lesion-based, material-specificity model[16] that proposes a left medial temporal specialization for verbal memory and a right medial temporal specialization for nonverbal material that is not readily verbally coded. Early brain insults appear to moderate this model.[17–17] A number of current functional imaging studies focus on the precise roles of medial temporal, frontal and associated parietal, cingulate, thalamic and other areas in specific attentional, learning and memory processes, such as the initiation of retrieval processes, and the evaluation of recovered information.[20–23] For more detail on episodic memory circuitry, the reader is referred to several recent review articles.[7,12,24,25]

Age Related Changes in Episodic Memory

A large body of literature suggests that episodic memory processes, particularly encoding and retrieval, decline with age.[26-31] Whether this is related to "normal aging" of the brain or to an accumulation of age-related diseases remains a topic of some debate.[32-34] There is some evidence to suggest selective age-related atrophy of prefrontal cortical areas involved in episodic memory circuitry,[35] with relative preservation of medial temporal lobe structures,[35-37] although this too is debatable.[38-40] Furthermore, regenerative processes and reorganization in the adult human brain may help allay development of cognitive problems despite structural brain changes.[41,42] Therefore, significant questions remain as to the neural and cognitive basis of episodic memory decline in aging.

A number of functional neuroimaging, electrophysiological, and behavioral studies suggest that the typical prefrontal functional asymmetries for memory processes in younger adults are diminished or absent in older adults. In other words, research suggests that the HERA model does not hold in normal aging. This concept has been articulated in the Hemispheric Asymmetry Reduction in Old Adults (HAROLD) model.[43] Increased bilateral

Table 7.1. Sample fMRI Task Characteristics for Episodic, Semantic, and Working Memory

Study	Memory domain	Cognitive process	Modality	Design	Stimuli[a]	Control condition	Performance monitoring
Logan et al., 2002[46]	Episodic memory	Intentional & incidental encoding	Visual	Blocked	Words and faces	Fixation stimulus	Ss completed a recognition test immediately after presentation of the stimuli
Saykin et al., 1777[71]	Semantic memory	Category-matching	Auditory	Blocked	Word pairs: category-exemplar pairs (e.g., beverage-milk; vehicle-carrot) and category-function pairs (e.g., beverage-sip, beverage-debate)	Separate phonological task using nonword-matching (e.g., temla-temla; yodb-rea)	Ss pressed a pneumatic bulb in scanner to indicate whether the word pairs matched or not
Rypma & D'Esposito, 2000[104]	Working memory	Delayed response	Visual	Event-related	A series of memory sets containing either 2 or 6 stimuli (letters, or objects and locations) were encoded and retained over an unfilled interval		Ss indicated in scanner whether a single item was or was not part of the memory set just presented

[a]In all three cases, the different types of stimuli were presented in different runs, e.g., words on one run, faces on another.

representation of cognitive functions in older adults may reflect a form of compensatory brain re-organization that helps support normal cognitive function. This would parallel findings on brain functional reorganization following acquired brain damage. For example, in the case of unilateral focal acquired brain damage, recovery of function can be associated with bihemispheric representation (among other types of reorganization) for functions such as language and movement.[44,45] On the other hand, bihemispheric representation simply may reflect diminished selectivity or de-differentiation of the neural substratRef[48] e of cognition in older adults,[46,47] which may or may not be partly consistent with an interpretation based on compensation, depending on investigators' use of these terms.

A small number of recent fMRI studies speak to the HAROLD model and address issues of compensation versus de-differentiation of the neural substrate of episodic memory in aging. For example, Morcom and colleagues[48] observed overall activation of inferior prefrontal cortex and the hippocampal formation for successful recognition of previously presented words. Activation was relatively left-lateralized in the younger adults, and more bilaterally represented in the older group (Figure 7.1).

Logan and colleagues[46] investigated the brain basis of episodic memory in two fMRI experiments in younger and older adults. Older adults showed less hemispheric asymmetry for intentional encoding of both verbal and nonverbal material, with greater right prefrontal (Brodmann areas 6/44) activation for words, and greater left prefrontal (BA 6/44) activation for face encoding compared to young adults. In this study, failure to recruit normal task-related areas did not always occur in conjunction with recruitment of additional brain regions, suggesting that these two types of alteration in brain activity may occur independently in aging. Furthermore, this

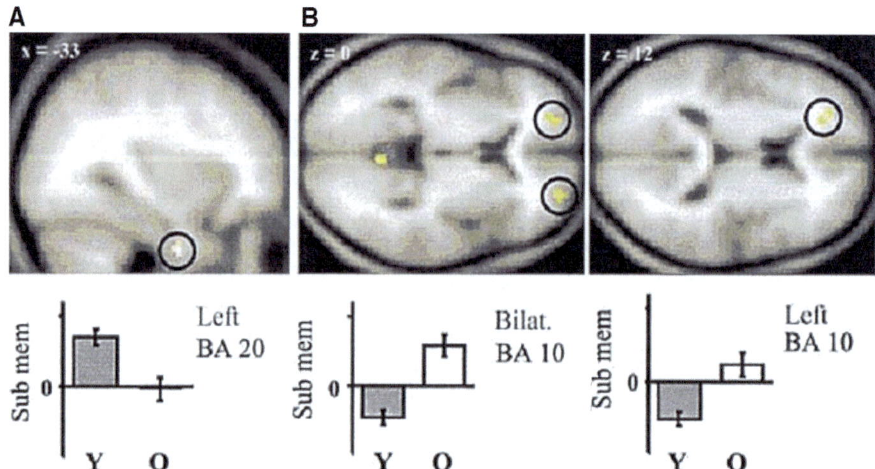

Figure 7.1. Brain regions showing age-related differences in activity during successful recognition of previously presented verbal information. Young adults showed greater activation than older adults in left anterior inferior temporal cortex (BA 20) (A). Older adults showed greater activation than young adults in bilateral anterior prefrontal cortex among other regions (B). Reprinted from Morcom AM, Good CD, Frackowiak RS, et al. Age effects on the neural correlates of successful memory encoding. *Brain.* 2003;126(Pt 1):213–227, by permission of Oxford University Press. (Neurologic coordinates).

study provided preliminary evidence that strategy use could overcome the age-related changes in brain activity. During intentional encoding of words, older adults failed to activate a left prefrontal (BA 45/47) region recruited by young adults (Figure 7.2A,B); this is an area thought to be associated with semantic elaboration and successful verbal encoding. However, when supported in the use of deep encoding strategies, activation of this region in older adults approximated that of controls (Figure 7.2C,D). These findings suggest that the regional deficit in activation in older adults during encoding is related to inefficient recruitment of available brain resources, rather than an irreversible loss of the underlying tissue due to cell death or dysfunction.

In a related study, Daselaar and colleagues[47] found that healthy older adults activated mainly left frontotemporal and cingulate areas during deep relative to shallow classification, similar to young adults. However, the older adults showed under-recruitment of left anterior hippocampus relative to the young adults. The authors interpreted this as possible evidence that, despite the capacity to engage brain regions associated with semantic elaboration, age-related impairment of medial temporal system functioning may nonetheless hinder episodic encoding in older adults.

Krause and colleagues[4] reported greater prefrontal connectivity during episodic encoding and retrieval in older adults compared to younger adults on structural equation modeling of fMRI and position emission tomography (PET) data, which lends some further support to the HAROLD model.[50] Furthermore, Krause and colleagues found stronger connectivity involving inferior parietal cortex and less for the hippocampal formation in older compared to younger subjects, consistent with an age-related change in the neural circuitry underlying episodic memory.

Whereas many studies of cognitive aging have used auditory–verbal or spatial stimuli, memory for which generally declines with age, Iidaka and colleagues examined brain activation patterns associated with pictorial memory using fMRI.[51] Based on prior findings that memory for pictures is generally better than memory for words and is relatively preserved in normal aging (especially memory for concrete and meaningful pictorial information), Iidaka and colleagues compared brain activity associated with encoding pairs of concrete-related, concrete-unrelated, and abstract pictures. The concrete-related task made relatively simple cognitive demands (e.g., learning to associate a picture of a cigarette with a picture of an ashtray) and yielded little significant signal change relative to the control condition. The main findings involved the unrelated and abstract pictures. Briefly, both the younger and older participants showed activation of left dorsal prefrontal cortex during encoding of the concrete-unrelated pictures and the abstract pictures. However, compared to the young group, the older adults showed reduced activation in some regions, including right temporo-occipital cortex in the concrete-unrelated condition and bilateral parieto-temporo-occipital areas during abstract picture encoding. There were no regions in which older adults showed greater signal change than controls, providing no evidence of compensatory processing or de-differentiation in the older group, possibly related to the relatively preserved figural recall performance of the older adults on baseline cognitive testing.

In an fMRI study of remote memory in older adults, Haist and colleagues[52] suggested a preferential role for the entorhinal cortex in consolidation of

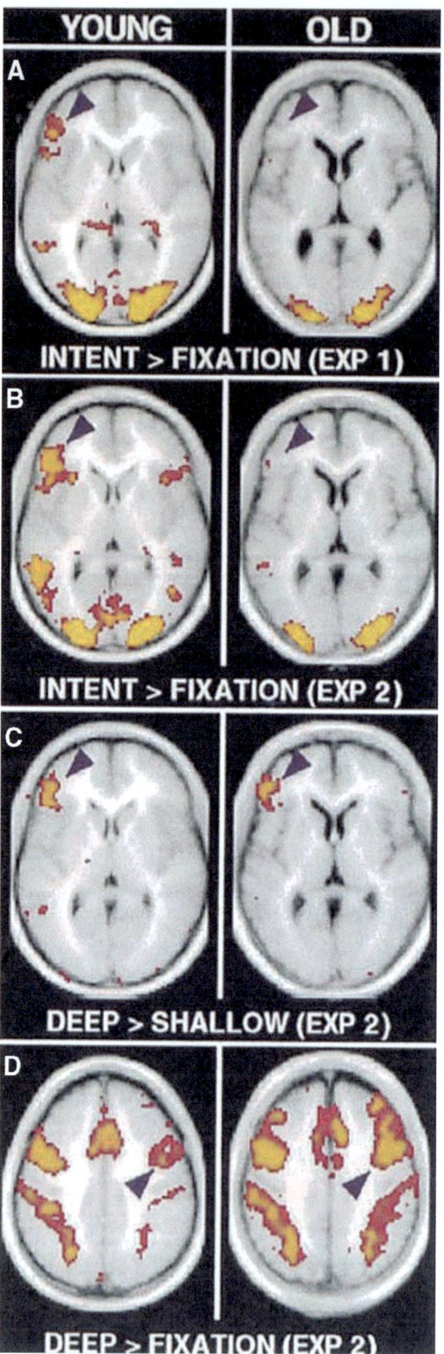

Figure 7.2. Brain regions showing age-related differences in activation during encoding of verbal material. Images are presented in neurologic coordinates (left side of brain shown on left side of image), with arrows marking the regions being highlighted. In Experiment 1, young adults showed activation of left BA 45/47 during intentional encoding of words, whereas older adults showed under-recruitment of this region (A). In Experiment 2, this pattern was replicated (B). When older adults were supported in the use of semantic elaboration, under-recruitment of BA 45/47 was reversed (C), but non-selective activation of right BA 6/44 remained (D). Reprinted from Neuron, Vol. 33, Logan JM, Sanders AL, Snyder AZ et al. Under-recruitment and non-selective recruitment: dissociable neural mechanisms associated with aging, 827–840, Copyright © 2002, with permission from Elsevier.

memory over decades. They presented eight older adults with pictures of famous faces from each decade from the 1740s to the 1770s and compared the brain activity to activation patterns for nonfamous faces from the present and the past. While the hippocampus was activated during recognition of the more recent famous faces, parahippocampal activity was present for famous faces from several of the recent and past decades, and right entorhinal activation appeared to be associated with memory for faces extending up to two decades back in time. Although the finding was preliminary, the authors interpreted it as consistent with evidence that damage to the CA1 hippocampal subfield results in a retrograde amnesia of a few years, whereas more-extensive temporal lobe involvement causes a longer period of retrograde amnesia. It is noteworthy that lesion studies typically have reported widespread temporal lobe damage in cases of pronounced retrograde amnesia.[53,54]

In a study of real autobiographical event memories acquired over decades, Maguire and Frith[55] found that younger and older adults activated a similar broad network of regions with one key difference—whereas the younger participants activated the left hippocampus during retrieval, older participants activated the hippocampus bilaterally. This additional hippocampal recruitment was evident despite preserved performance in both groups and was specific to the autobiographical event memories. The authors discuss possible explanations for the finding, including possible increased salience of the spatial context for the memories in the older adults, the fact that older adults have accrued more memories that need to be distinguished, and the possibility that the right hippocampus activated as a compensatory mechanism.

Small and colleagues have used a blood oxygenation level-dependent (BOLD) fMRI signal obtained at rest to estimate regional basal metabolism and examine the integrity of hippocampal subregions in healthy controls and individuals with dementia.[56,57] This method rests on the assumption that basal deoxyhemoglobin levels reflect hemodynamic variables, such as oxygen extraction, that are related to basal metabolism. Using this method, Small examined hippocampal circuitry in 70 individuals ranging in age from 20 to 88 years. In two hippocampal subregions, the subiculum and the dentate gyrus, decline in resting BOLD fMRI signal appeared to occur as a linear function of age. However, decline in the entorhinal cortex was more variable, present only in a subset of older adults. This was interpreted as evidence that the entorhinal change was not a normal age-related change, but rather an indicator of a pathological process.

Although limited at this point to cross-sectional data, fMRI research suggests a variety of age-related changes in episodic memory circuitry. This includes reduced prefrontal asymmetry, greater prefrontal connectivity, and altered frontal–medial temporal activity and interaction, among other changes. Although structural brain changes may well play a role in inducing age-related changes in activity of episodic memory circuitry, the studies that compared deep to shallow encoding[46,47] offer preliminary evidence that age-related differences in the approach to a task may also contribute to the inducement of age-related changes. This underscores the importance of incorporating both structural and functional brain imaging methods in studies of cognition and aging, and of carefully monitoring participants' cognitive strategy use or approach to the task in addition to other aspects of their task performance.

Episodic Memory in Alzheimer's Disease and Related Conditions

Impairment of episodic memory is a core feature of dementias such as Alzheimer's disease (AD),[58] and there are significant structural changes in the hippocampus and entorhinal cortex very early in the course of AD.[57–62] Mild cognitive impairment (MCI) may be a precursor to or early stage of AD and other dementias. Amnestic MCI, the most commonly studied subtype of MCI, is characterized by relatively isolated impairment of episodic memory in the context of normal daily functioning and in the absence of dementia.[63–65] Mild cognitive impairment is associated with early medial temporal lobe changes and other structural changes on volumetric MRI.[66,67] For reviews and diagnostic criteria for MCI, see references 63–65 and 68.

Patients with AD show reduced medial temporal activation on fMRI during episodic memory encoding.[67–71] In an early fMRI study that employed single-plane acquisition through the long axis of hippocampus, our group observed reduced anterior hippocampal activation in a patient with AD compared to a healthy normal control.[72] Additionally, on the basis of preliminary data, Corkin[73] reported that hippocampal activation during encoding was related to successful memory for pictures in both healthy older controls and individuals with AD. Rombouts and colleagues[70] compared patients with mild to moderate AD to healthy older adults on two episodic encoding tasks. Whereas one task revealed no group differences, the other—which involved encoding of complex color landscapes and daily scenes—showed activation of medial and lateral temporal and frontal regions in the healthy controls, with reduced activation in the left hippocampus and bilateral parahippocampal regions in patients (Figure 7.3). Small and colleagues[67] showed diminished activation in all hippocampal formation regions, including the entorhinal cortex, the subiculum, and the hippocampus proper, during episodic encoding in AD. Entorhinal activation patterns were particularly good at discriminating AD patients from controls. A group of older adults with isolated memory decline showed either activation patterns similar to those of AD patients or isolated reduction of activation in the subiculum. Kato and colleagues[71] compared young and older controls with mild AD patients on a visual episodic memory task. All subjects activated visual cortex, suggesting that they were processing the stimuli, but the patients failed to activate the entorhinal cortex, other temporal regions, and frontal areas involved in episodic memory. Sperling and colleagues[74] recently demonstrated reduced hippocampal activation and increased activity of medial parietal and posterior cingulate regions on a face–name–association encoding task in patients with AD compared to elderly controls. In a related study, the same team examined pharmacologically induced memory impairment in young adults.[75] Administration of either lorazepam [a γ-aminobutyric acid-(GABA) ergic neuron enhancing substance] or scopolamine (an antagonist of the muscarinic acetylcholine receptor) resulted in decreased activation in hippocampal, fusiform, and inferior prefrontal regions. Preliminary evidence also has been presented for decreased resting signal in the hippocampus in older adults with memory decline.[57]

Patients with mild AD showed reduced frontal activation on fMRI during retrieval of information from episodic memory. Using an auditory–verbal

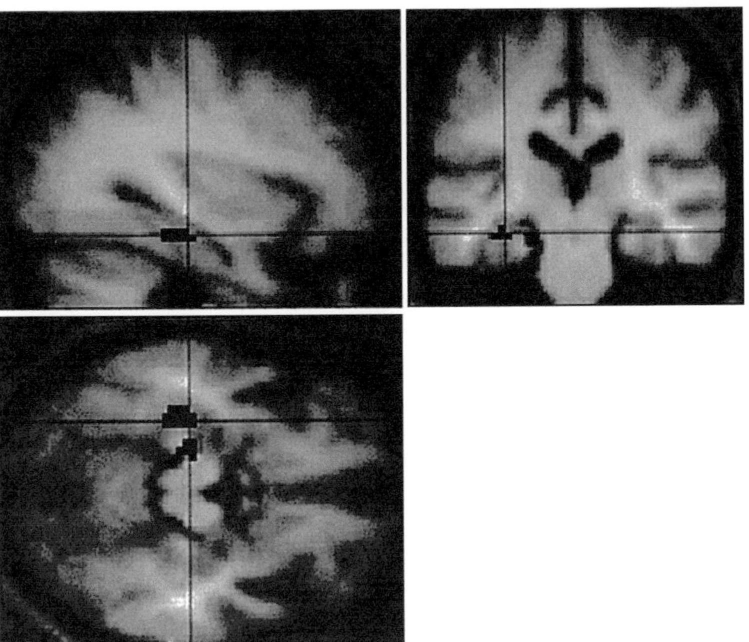

Figure 7.3. Left hippocampal and parahippocampal regions where controls showed greater activation than patients with AD during encoding of visual information. Controls also showed more activation than patients in right parahippocampal gyrus (not shown). Reprinted with permission from Rombouts SA, Barkhof F, Veltman DJ, et al. Functional MR imaging in Alzheimer's disease during memory encoding. *ANJR Am J Neuroradiol.* 2000;21(10):1867–1875. American Society of Neuroradiology. (Neurologic coordinates).

recognition memory task, Saykin and colleagues[76] showed reduced prefrontal activation in patients with mild AD relative to age-matched controls. Within the patient group, interindividual variations in frontal activity were related to hippocampal volume. Patients with greater preservation of the hippocampus showed greater activity in bilateral prefrontal regions. This is consistent with the notion that medial temporal and frontal regions form an integrated circuitry subserving episodic memory, and that damage in one part of the circuitry may be reflected in altered activation of other regions. Corkin[73] also found that frontal activation during retrieval was related to the success with which older adults, regardless of whether or not they had AD, recognized previously presented pictures. Position emission tomography (PET) studies provide related data; for example, in one study, patients with mild AD showed reduced functional connectivity of frontal, hippocampal, and other regions during a face-recognition memory task.[77]

Evidence is emerging that functional neuroimaging is sensitive to the earliest stages of dementia before the clinical symptoms of AD or MCI are evident.[78] Bookheimer and colleagues[77] examined cognitively intact, middle-aged to older individuals who were at risk for AD by virtue of their genetic [apolipoprotein E (ApoE) ε4] status. Although not a valid clinical predictor at the individual level, there is a clear correlation between presence of the ε4 allele and likelihood of developing AD.[80] Bookheimer and colleagues found increased intensity and spatial extent of activation in temporal, parietal, and

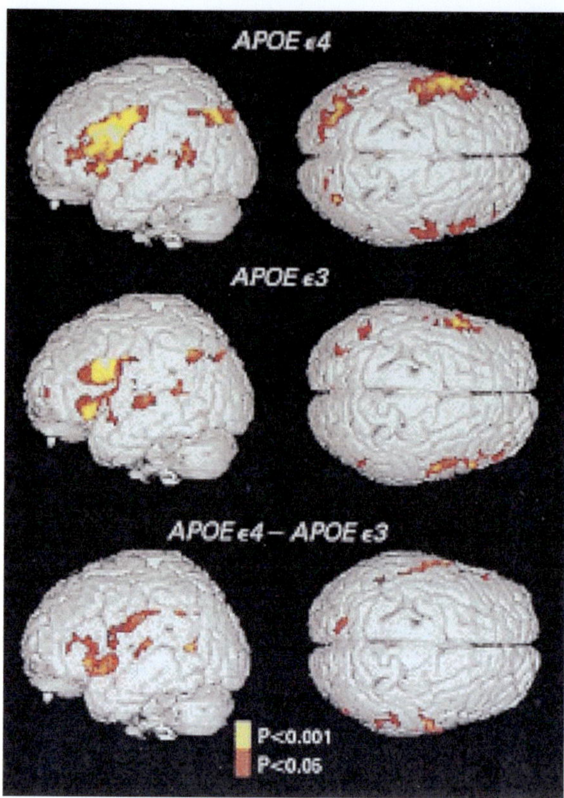

Figure 7.4. Brain activation patterns associated with learning and recall in individuals with increased genetic risk for AD (ApoE ε4 carriers) compared to ApoE ε3 carriers. Both groups showed increased activation in left inferior frontal cortex, right prefrontal cortex, transverse temporal gyri bilaterally, left posterior temporal, and inferior parietal regions during learning or recall compared to rest, as shown in the top two panels. However, the intensity and spatial extent of activation was greater in those with the ε4 allele (bottom panel). Reprinted with permission from Bookheimer SY, Strojwas MH, Cohen MS, et al. Patterns of brain activation in people at risk for Alzheimer's disease. *N Engl J Med*. 2000;343(7):450–456. Copyright © 2000 Massachusetts Medical Society. All rights reserved.

prefrontal regions during episodic encoding and retrieval in individuals who were ε4 positive compared to those without the ε4 allele (Figure 7.4). Baseline activation patterns predicted memory decline over the next two years. The fact that these individuals were recruiting broader areas of brain tissue to accomplish the episodic memory task suggests that changes in activation may occur very early during the course of memory disorders such as AD. These changes may play a compensatory role and may represent an early marker for subsequent cognitive decline. Some of the same researchers reported no differences between ε4 positive and negative groups in fMRI brain activation patterns on an attention/working memory task.[81] This was interpreted as evidence that compensatory brain activation in ε4 carriers is specific to the episodic memory system.

Daselaar and colleagues[82] examined activation patterns associated with successful recognition of incidentally encoded words in healthy adult males.

Young adults with normal memory were compared with two older groups, one cognitively intact and the other with mildly impaired memory. During successful encoding, the younger group showed significantly more left anterior medial temporal lobe activation than the older adults with reduced memory, but did not significantly differ from the older adults with normal memory.

Grön and colleagues[83] examined fMRI patterns of brain activity in older adults presenting for first-time medical evaluation of subjective memory complaints. After comprehensive assessment, twelve individuals were diagnosed with probable AD and twelve with major depression. These participants were compared to twelve healthy older adults without cognitive complaints. In general, those participants who were diagnosed with AD showed reduced hippocampal activation during episodic memory processing relative to either of the other groups. Increased bilateral prefrontal activity also was seen in the AD patients, consistent with possible attempted compensatory recruitment or de-differentiation.

In a preliminary study of seven patients with mild AD, Rombouts and colleagues recently investigated the effects of rivastigmine, a cholinesterase inhibitor, on brain activity patterns during episodic memory performance (and working memory, as described below).[84] A single dose of the medication led to a bilateral increase in activation in the fusiform gyrus during face encoding. This suggests that rivastigmine affects activity in regions associated with cholingeric circuitry, and that fMRI may be useful in monitoring treatment effects in AD, MCI, and other disorders.

Together, these studies suggest that fMRI is sensitive to preclinical and very early clinical stages of AD and may be useful in early diagnosis, prognosis, and treatment monitoring. Functional MRI may be able to assist in determining whether a drug is effective and the mechanisms by which its effects occur.

Semantic Memory

Semantic memory is broadly defined as knowledge about the world and includes the set of ideas, words, and symbols that generally are shared by individuals within a culture. Unlike episodic memories, semantic memories are not context dependent. For example, remembering the movie you saw last week depends on episodic memory, but remembering the meaning of the word "movie" depends on semantic memory. As might be expected given the rich associative and inferential processes that can be invoked for the recollection of even simple factual information and words, studies of semantic memory suggest a broad-based neural circuitry, including prominent involvement of several left-hemisphere regions.[7,85] A sample fMRI measure of semantic memory is presented in Table 7.1.

Semantic Memory in Aging and Dementia

The core component of semantic memory, as reflected by knowledge (crystallized intellect), is thought to be preserved and possibly enhanced during aging, at least under favorable conditions of aging.[34,86] However, the efficiency and accuracy with which information is retrieved from semantic memory can be affected.[87] Very little fMRI research on semantic memory in aging and dementia has been conducted to date. Johnson and colleagues[70] examined the relation between age-related whole brain atrophy and brain activation patterns on category-matching fMRI tasks. Across the entire sample, the semantic task activated mainly left superior temporal and bilateral inferior frontal regions, left more than right, likely related to both the semantic and the auditory demands of the task. There were only small group differences in brain activity, with slightly but not significantly greater precentral activation in the younger compared to older adults. The older adults showed global brain atrophy relative to the younger adults, but degree of atrophy was unrelated to BOLD signal on the semantic task. These findings suggest that cognitively intact younger and older adults activate similar brain regions when performing semantic memory operations despite the presence of age-related brain atrophy.

Like episodic memory, semantic memory is affected in AD, although the more profound changes typically occur later in the disease course. Eventually profound deficits in identification and knowledge can emerge.[32] Using fMRI, Saykin and colleagues[71] demonstrated that two semantic category-matching tasks activated left lateral prefrontal and temporal regions, whereas a phonologic control task activated only temporal areas. In patients with mild AD, the spatial extent of left frontal activation on the semantic task was greater than in elderly controls, although accuracy was lower in

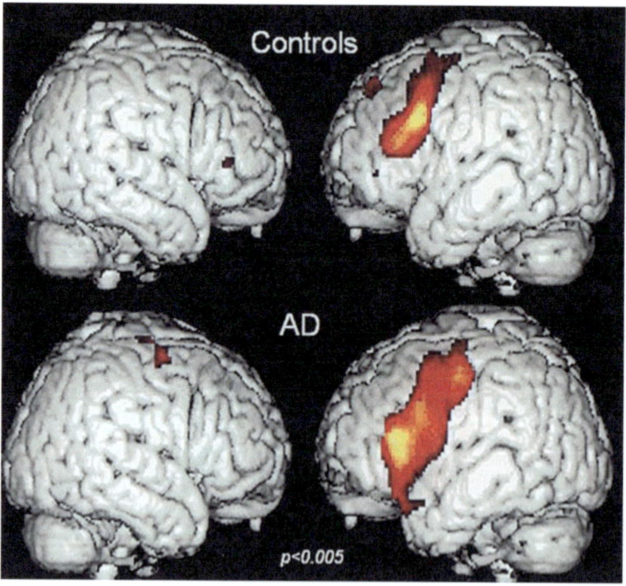

Figure 7.5. Surface render of fMRI brain activation during semantic decision making (match versus mismatch) for category–function pairs (e.g., beverage–sip, vehicle–sip). Upper panel is activation for the healthy elderly control group; bottom panel is mild lzheimer's disease group. Note the expanded spatial extent of activation in the patient group in the left frontal region. Based on further analysis of data published in Saykin AJ, Flashman LA, Frutiger S, et al. Neuroanatomic substrates of semantic memory impairment in Alzheimer's Disease: Patterns of functional MRI activation. *J Int Neurophyschol Soc.* 1777;5:377–372.

the patient group. Figure 7.5 shows a surface render of brain activation during semantic decision making for category–function pairs (e.g., match: beverage–sip; mismatch: vehicle–sip). Furthermore, the expanded spatial extent of frontal activation within the patient group was correlated directly with the extent of atrophy in that frontal region.[72] This finding offered preliminary fMRI-based support for the compensatory recruitment hypothesis in semantic memory in AD, suggesting that increased brain activation may help offset disease-related structural changes in the brain, although other reasons for the alterations in brain activation also are possible.

Smith and colleagues[73] reported reduced brain activation in inferotemporal regions bilaterally during language tasks in individuals at risk for AD by virtue of their family history and ApoE status. The reduction was present despite the fact that these individuals were cognitively intact at the time of the study, suggesting that subclinical changes are evident in the brain before the onset of symptoms of AD. It is interesting to compare the Smith finding of reduced activation during language tasks in an at-risk sample to the Bookheimer[77] at-risk study, which found an increase in extent of activation during episodic memory. Despite the variability across early studies, the combination of genetic, family history, neuroimaging, and other test data may enhance prediction of risk for AD, and thereby increase the potential to target early intervention appropriately.

Working Memory

Working memory can be defined as the means by which small amounts of information are maintained in active stores while other cognitive operations are performed. These other operations may include language comprehension, problem solving, and memory encoding, and the ability to hold information in working memory is fundamental to executing these other cognitive processes efficiently and accurately.[2,3,74] According to Baddeley and colleagues, the working memory system has a central executive that, together with an episodic buffer, allocates limited attentional resources to separate subsystems for verbal and nonverbal information.[2,3,75] For a review of models of working memory, see Becker[76] and Baddeley.[3]

Working memory is subserved by a broad network of brain areas, including prefrontal and parietal regions, with greater left lateralization for processing of verbal information and right lateralization for spatial information.[7,77] It has been proposed that there are also separate although overlapping neural representations for visual working memory processes associated with spatial (where) information versus object (what) information. This is analogous to the dissociation in the visual system between dorsal occipitoparietal pathways thought to be involved in the processing of spatial locations and relations among objects and the ventral occipitotemporal pathways that are involved in the processing of the perceptual characteristics that are important for recognition of objects.[78,77] Other conceptualizations hold that it is the type of processing rather than type of information that is related to a dorsal/ventral division of activity during working memory.[77] Various working memory fMRI probes contrast or emphasize different processing demands; a sample task is presented in Table 7.1.

Working Memory in Aging and Dementia

Behavioral studies indicate age-related changes in working memory,[100,101] and additional changes are seen in AD,[102] although as yet there is a relatively small body of research in this area. There are age-associated structural changes in prefrontal cortex,[35] and AD is associated with diffuse cortical atrophy by later stages of the disease. In the context of these behavioral and structural changes involving working memory circuitry, a small number of studies have used PET[103] and fMRI to examine brain activity associated with working memory in older adults with and without dementia.

Rypma and D'Esposito[104] examined working memory-related brain activity in younger and older adults in three experiments using a delayed-response paradigm. An age-related difference in brain activity was found in a dorsolateral but not ventrolateral prefrontal region of interest, with greater activity in the dorsolateral region during retrieval in younger adults. In addition, speed of processing was related differentially to dorsolateral prefrontal cortical activity in the two age groups. Younger subjects with rapid responding showed less dorsolateral prefrontal cortical activity than younger subjects with slow responses. That pattern was reversed in the older group. Overall, these findings suggest a role for dorsolateral prefrontal cortex in age-related changes in working memory. A subsequent study by Rypma and colleagues using a similar paradigm also showed age-related differences in activity of dorsal, but not ventral, prefrontal cortex.[105] In addition, greater rostral prefrontal cortex activation was evident in the older adults. In a preliminary study, Wishart, Saykin, and colleagues also observed decreased activity in dorsolateral prefrontal cortex in healthy older adults relative to younger controls on a working memory fMRI task, suggesting a different pattern of activity as a function of age.[106] Increased activity was seen in posterior frontal and cerebellar regions. These alterations in activation were related directly to extent of gray matter loss on voxel-based morphometry.[106]

Age-related differences in activity of working memory circuitry may underlie the fact that sentence comprehension declines with age.[107] Using a sentence-comprehension task, Grossman and colleagues demonstrated that older participants showed less left parietal activity than younger adults. However, the older group also showed increases in activity in right inferior parietal, right posterolateral temporal, and left premotor cortex, as well as dorsal portions of left inferior frontal cortex. These findings were interpreted as evidence of upregulation of working memory circuitry in the older adults in order to achieve a level of sentence comprehension that was equivalent to that of the younger adults.[107]

Motivated by findings that estrogen may positively affect brain structure and function, Shawitz and colleagues[108] used fMRI to examine effects of estrogen treatment on brain activity during verbal and nonverbal working memory in a randomized, double-blind, placebo-controlled, cross-over study involving 46 women (aged 33 to 61 years). Treatment with estrogen did not improve the women's performance on working memory tasks, but did lead to alterations in brain activity, some of which were interpreted as consistent with a sharpening of the HERA effect; that is, greater left hemispheric activity was seen during encoding and greater right hemispheric activity was seen during retrieval when the women were on active treatment compared to placebo. In a subsequent study by members of this team, the data from the treatment phase were analyzed further to examine age and performance effects.[74] Using a partial least-squares approach, age-related declines in brain activity were noted in anterior frontal cortex for all three working memory processes studied (encoding, rehearsal, and retrieval). Age-related deficiencies in hippocampal activation also have been demonstrated for feature binding in working memory, the process whereby individual elements of experience are bound together.[107]

In a study comparing patients with AD to individuals with early frontotemporal dementia (FTD) on a working memory task, both groups showed activation of frontal, parietal, and thalamic regions.[110] However, patients with FTD showed less frontal and parietal activation and greater cerebellar activation than those with AD. The authors suggested that fMRI may be useful for differentiating AD and FTD early in the disease course, even when the structural MRI is normal.

Rombouts and colleagues[84] recently examined the effect of cholinergic enhancement on brain activity during working memory in a preliminary sample of patients with mild AD. After a single dose of rivastigmine, activity in prefrontal cortex was enhanced during the basic working memory condition. When the working memory demands were increased, both increases and decreases in activation in different regions were seen. As described above in the *Episodic Memory* section of this chapter, these investigators also found increased brain activity with medication on an episodic memory task. In the first controlled study of its kind (to our knowledge), our group also observed increased prefrontal activity during a working memory task in patients with MCI after short-term treatment with donepezil, another cholinesterase inhibitor.[111]

Overall, the findings point to age-related changes in activity of working memory circuitry, largely characterized by declines in prefrontal and hippocampal regions. However, there is also initial fMRI evidence that upregulation of working memory circuitry may help maximize cognitive function in normal aging,[107] as well as evidence from PET that patients with AD show increased activity in frontal regions relative to controls that could reflect compensatory processing.[103] The Rombouts[112] and Saykin[111] studies indicate the relevance of fMRI for determining the brain regions in which a medication exerts its effects. In addition to clarifying the mechanism of action of psychoactive medications, fMRI may be useful when employed before and after drug treatment to monitor efficacy.

Methodological Issues in the Use of fMRI in Aging and Dementia Research

A number of methodological considerations must be addressed when conducting and interpreting fMRI research in aging and dementia. For example, there is evidence to suggest that normal aging affects some aspects of the coupling of the hemodynamic response with neural activity. Using a simple reaction time task (one known to evoke similar electrical potentials in young and old adults), D'Esposito and colleagues found in excess of four times more activated voxels in sensorimotor cortex in young than older participants.[113] Other aspects of the hemodynamic response, such as the shape of the curve and the within-group variance, did not significantly differ as a function of age. In contrast, Huettel and colleagues found age differences in the shape of the hemodynamic response, its within-group variability, and the number of activated voxels on a visual task.[114] The younger adults showed a later time to peak, less variability, and twice as many activated voxels as the older adults, although both groups activated similar regions of visual cortex.[114] Age-related prolongation of the time lag in signal change on fMRI also has been reported.[115] Other groups have observed smaller areas[116,117] or larger areas[118] of activation in older adults compared to younger individuals, or no significant differences between groups.[70] Buckner and colleagues observed similar summation of the hemodynamic response across brain regions examined with their sensorimotor task and suggested that even if absolute measurement differences exist between age groups, there should be preservation of relative task-related changes in activation.[117] These issues indicate the need for sophisticated experimental design, post processing, and interpretation of fMRI data in aging research to ensure that reported findings are not spurious effects of basic physiological or artifactual signal differences between young and older groups.

Further technical and scientific issues are encountered when using fMRI to study patients with dementia. Currently, the conditions and importance of alterations in brain activity in individuals with AD are not well understood. For example, does increased activation in patients relative to controls reflect compensation, de-differentiation, or both? If patients perform abnormally on an activation task, how should the resulting activation maps be compared to those of controls? How should atrophy and lesions be taken into account when analyzing and interpreting fMRI data? Approaches that integrate structural neuroimaging, carefully designed activation tasks, and close monitoring of in-scanner mentation and task performance will likely help address such questions.[68] When studying memory, issues related to signal drop-out in memory-relevant regions also must be considered.[13]

Conclusion

Of the three memory systems examined in this chapter, episodic memory has been the most studied using fMRI to date. Although limited largely to cross-sectional data, fMRI research indicates age-related changes in episodic memory circuitry. Reduced prefrontal asymmetry, greater prefrontal connectivity, and altered frontotemporal interaction are observed during episodic memory processing in older adults compared to younger adults. These changes may be a direct effect of structural changes in the aging brain and also may reflect age-related differences in cognitive strategy or approach to the tasks. In individuals with AD, further reductions are seen in hippocampal activity during episodic encoding and in prefrontal cortex activity during episodic retrieval.

Functional MRI research on working memory suggests age-related declines in prefrontal and hippocampal activity. However, there is also evidence to suggest that increased activity of regions within working memory circuitry may occur and help support normal to near-normal functioning in older age despite the presence of structural changes in the brain. Very little fMRI research has been done on semantic memory, which is relatively preserved in aging and in the earliest stages of AD. Two studies by the authors' group suggest that during semantic memory processing, (a) younger and older adults activate similar circuitry, and (b) mild AD patients show an expanded recruitment and/or shifted activation pattern. However, there are as yet too few studies in AD or at-risk groups to make any definitive statements regarding semantic memory-related activation.

Despite significant technical challenges, research using fMRI and other neuroimaging techniques is advancing knowledge of the different effects of aging and dementia on memory systems in the brain. These techniques have major potential implications for early detection of dementia and treatment monitoring, especially if used in combination with genetic testing and emerging PET-based methods for in vivo detection of the neurofibrillary tangles and amyloid plaques of AD.[120–122] Early detection and treatment monitoring are especially important at this time because medications that slow the progression of cognitive decline are available and other treatments, including vaccines, are under development.[120]

Acknowledgments: The authors wish to thank Heather S. Pixley, Jennifer S. Randolph, Tara McHugh, and Alex Dominguez for their assistance.

References

1. Tulving E, Donaldson W.*The Organization of Memory*. New York: Academic Press; 1772.
2. Baddeley A. Working Memory. In: Gazzaniga MS, editor. *The Cognitive Neurosciences*. Cambridge, MA: MIT Press; 1775.
3. Baddeley A. Recent developments in working memory. *Curr Opin Neurobiol.*1778;8(2):234–238.
4. Krause JB, Taylor JG, Schmidt D, et al. Imaging and neural modeling in episodic and working memory processes. *Neural Netw.* 2000;13(8–7):847–857.
5. Nyberg L, Marklund P, Persson J, et al. Common prefrontal activations during working memory, episodic memory, and semantic memory. *Neuropsychologia.* 2003;41:371–377.
6. Tulving E, Markowitsch HJ. Episodic and declarative memory: role of the hippocampus. *Hippocampus.* 1778;8(3):178–204.
7. Braak H, Braak E, Yilmazer D, et al. Functional anatomy of human hippocampal formation and related structures. *J Child Neurol.* 1776;11(4):265–275.
8. Van Hoesen GW. Anatomy of the medial temporal lobe. *Magn Reson Imaging.* 1775;13(8):1047–1055.
9. Cabeza R, Nyberg L. Imaging cognition II: An empirical review of 275 PET and fMRI studies. *J Cogn Neurosci.* 2000;12(1):1–47.
10. Desgranges B, Baron JC, Eustache F. The functional neuroanatomy of episodic memory: The role of the frontal lobes, the hippocampal formation, and other areas. *Neuroimage.* 1778;8:178–213.
11. Lepage M, Habib R, Tulving E. Hippocampal PET activations of memory encoding and retrieval: The HIPER model. *Hippocampus.* 1778;8:313–322.
12. Schacter DL, Wagner AD. Medial temporal lobe activations in fMRI and PET studies of episodic encoding and retrieval. *Hippocampus.* 1777;7(1):7–24.
13. Greicius MD, Krasnow B, Boyett-Anderson JM, et al. Regional analysis of hippocampal activation during memory encoding and retrieval: fMRI study. *Hippocampus.* 2003;13:164–174.
14. Tulving E, Kapur S, Craik FI, et al. Hemispheric encoding/retrieval asymmetry in episodicmemory: Positron emission tomography findings. *Proc Natl Acad Sci USA.*1774;71(6):2016–2020.

15. Nyberg L, Cabeza R, Tulving E. PET studies of encoding and retrieval: The HERA Model. *Psychol Bull Rev.* 1776;3:135–148.
16. Milner B. Psychological aspects of focal epilepsy and its neurosurgical management. *Adv Neurol* 1775;8:277–321.
17. Saykin AJ, Gur RC, Sussman NM, et al. Memory deficits before and after temporal lobectomy: Effect of laterality and age of onset. *Brain Cogn.* 1787;7:171–200.
18. Saykin AJ, Robinson LJ, Stafiniak P, et al. Neuropsychological effects of temporal lobectomy: Acute changes in memory, language, and music. In: Bennett T, editor. *Neuropsychology of Epilepsy.* New York: Plenum Press; 1772.
19. Hermann BP, Seidenberg M, Haltiner A, et al. Relationship of age at onset, chronologic age, and adequacy of preoperative performance to verbal memory change after anterior temporal lobectomy. *Epilepsia.* 1775;36(2):137–145.
20. Cabeza R, Dolcos F, Prince SE, et al. Attention-related activity during episodic memory retrieval: a cross-function fMRI study. *Neuropsychologia.* 2003;41:370–377.
21. Dobbins IG, Rice HJ, Wagner AD, et al. Memory orientation and success: separable neurocognitive components underlying episodic recognition. *Neuropsychologia.* 2003;41(3):318–333.
22. Rugg MD, Henson RN, Robb WG. Neural correlates of retrieval processing in the prefrontal cortex during recognition and exclusion tasks. *Neuropsychologia.* 2003;41(1):40–52.
23. Ranganath C, Johnson MK, D'Esposito M. Prefontal activity associated with working memory and episodic long-term memory. *Neuropsychologia.* 2003;41:378–387.
24. Wagner AD, Koutstaal W, Schacter DL. When encoding yields remembering: insights from event-related neuroimaging. *Philos Trans R Soc London B Biol Sci.* 1777;354(1387):1307–1324.
25. Fletcher PC, Frith CD, Rugg MD. The functional neuroanatomy of episodic memory. *Trends Neurosci.* 1777;20(5):213–218.
26. Nyberg L, Backman L, Erngrund K, et al. Age differences in episodic memory, semantic memory, and priming: relationships to demographic, intellectual, and biological factors. *J Gerontol B Psychol Sci Soc Sci.* 1776;51(4):234–240.
27. Park DC, Smith AD, Lautenschlager G, et al. Mediators of long-term memory performance across the lifespan. *Psychol Aging.* 1776;11:621–637.
28. Anderson ND, Craik FIM. Memory in the aging brain. In: Tulving E, Craik FIM, editors. *The Oxford Handbook of Memory.* New York: Oxford; 2000:411–425.
29. Balota DA, Dolan PO, Duchek JM. Memory changes in healthy older adults. In: Tulving E, Craik FIM, editors. *The Oxford Handbook of Memory.* New York: Oxford; 2000:375–407.
30. Grady C, Craik FI. Changes in memory processing with age. *Curr Opin Neurobiol.* 2000;10:224–231.
31. Zacks RT, Hasher L, Li KZH. Human memory. In: Craik FIM, Salthouse TA, editors. *The Handbook of Aging and Cognition.* Mahwah, NJ: Erlbaum; 1777:200–230.
32. Flashman LA, Wishart HA, Saykin AJ. Boundaries between normal aging and dementia: Perspectives from neuropsychological and neuroimaging investigations. In: Emory VOB, Oxman TE, editors. *Dementia: Presentations, Differential Diagnosis and Nosology.* 2nd ed. Baltimore, MD: Johns Hopkins University Press; 2003:3–30.
33. Schroots JJF, Birren JE. Theoretical issues and basic questions in the planning of longitudinal studies of health and aging. In: Schroots JJF, editor. *Aging, Health and Competence: The Next Generation of Longitudinal Studies.* Amsterdam: Elsevier; 1773:4–34.
34. Baltes PB. The aging mind: potential and limits. *Gerontologist.* 1773;33(5):580–574.
35. Raz N, Gunning FM, Head D, et al. Selective aging of the human cerebral cortex observed in vivo: Differential vulnerability of the prefrontal gray matter. *Cereb Cortex.* 1777;7(3):268–282.

36. Bigler ED, Blatter DD, Anderson CV, et al. Hippocampal volume in normal aging and traumatic brain injury. *AJNR Am J Neuroradiol.* 1777;18(1):11–23.
37. DeCarli C, Murphy DG, Gillette JA, et al. Lack of age-related differences in temporal lobe volume of very healthy adults. *AJNR Am J Neuroradiol.* 1774;15(4):687–676.
38. Greenwood PM. The frontal aging hypothesis evaluated. *J Int Neuropsychol Soc.* 2000;6:705–726.
39. West R. In defense of the frontal lobe hypothesis of cognitive aging. *J Int Neuropsychol Soc.* 2000;6:727–727.
40. Greenwood PM. Reply to West. *J Int Neuropsychol. Soc.* 2000;6:730.
41. Kempermann G, Gage FH. New nerve cells for the adult brain. *Sci Am.* 1777;280:48–53.
42. Reuter-Lorenz PA, Stanczak L, Miller AC. Neural recruitment and cognitive aging: Two hemispheres are better than one, especially as you age. *Psychol Sci.* 1777;10(6):474–500.
43. Cabeza R. Hemispheric asymmetry reduction in old adults: The HAROLD model. *Psychol Aging.* 2002;17:85–100.
44. Muller RA, Rothermel RD, Behen ME, et al. Differential patterns of language and motor reorganization following early left hemisphere lesion: a PET study. *Arch Neurol.* 1778;55(8):1113–1117.
45. Fawcett JW, Rosser AE, Dunnett SB.*Brain Damage, Brain Repair.* New York: Oxford U.P; 2001.
46. Logan JM, Sanders AL, Snyder AZ, et al. Under-recruitment and non-selective recruitment: dissociable neural mechanisms associated with aging. *Neuron.* 2002;33(5):827–840.
47. Cabeza R, Anderson ND, Locantore JK, et al. Aging gracefully: Compensatory brain activity in high-performing older adults. *Neuroimage.* 2002;17:1374–1402.
48. Morcom AM, Good CD, Frackowiak RS, et al. Age effects on the neural correlates of successful memory encoding. *Brain.* 2003;126(Pt 1):213–227.
49. Daselaar SM, Veltman DJ, Rombouts SARB, Raaijmakers JG, Jonker C. Deep processing activated the medial temporal lobe in young but not old adults. *Neurobiol Aging.* 2003;24(7):1005–1011.
50. Cabeza R, Grady CL, Nyberg L, et al. Age-related differences in neural activity during memory encoding and retrieval: A positron emission tomography study. *J Neurosci.* 1777;17(1):371–400.
51. Iidaka T, Sadato N, Yamada H, et al. An fMRI study of the functional neuroanatomy of picture encoding in younger and older adults. *Cogn Brain Res.* 2001;11(1):1–11.
52. Haist F, Bowden Gore J, Mao H. Consolidation of human memory over decades revealed by functional magnetic resonance imaging. *Nature Neurosci.* 2001;4(11):1137–1145.
53. Kapur N. Focal retrograde amnesia in neurological disease: a critical review. *Cortex.* 1773;27(2):217–234.
54. Kapur N, Ellison D, Smith MP, et al. Focal retrograde amnesia following bilateral temporal lobe pathology. A neuropsychological and magnetic resonance study. *Brain.* 1772;115(Pt 1):73–85.
55. Maguire EA, Frith C. Aging affects the engagement of the hippocampus during autobiographical memory retrieval. *Brain.* 2003;126:1511–1523.
56. Small SA, Tsai WY, DeLaPaz R, et al. Imaging hippocampal function across the human life span: is memory decline normal or not? *Ann Neurol.* 2002;51(3):270–275.
57. Small SA, Wu EX, Bartsch D, et al. Imaging physiologic dysfunction of individual hippocampal subregions in humans and genetically modified mice. *Neuron.* 2000;28(3):653–664.
58. American Psychiatric Association. *Diagnostic and Statistical Manual of Mental Disorders.* (IV ed.). Washington DC: American Psychiatric Press; 1774.

59. Braak H, Braak E, Bohl J. Staging of Alzheimer-related cortical destruction. *Eur Neurol.* 1773;33(6):403–408.

60. de Leon MJ, Convit A, DeSanti S, et al. The hippocampus in aging and Alzheimer's disease. *Neuroimaging Clin N Am.* 1775;5(1):1–17.

61. de Leon MJ, Convit A, George AE, et al. In vivo structural studies of the hippocampus in normal aging and in incipient Alzheimer's disease. *Ann N Y Acad Sci.* 1776;777:1–13.

62. Jack CR, Jr., Petersen RC, O' Brien PC, et al. MR-based hippocampal volumetry in the diagnosis of Alzheimer's disease. *Neurology.* 1772;42(1):183–188.

63. Petersen RC, Doody R, Kurz A, et al. Current concepts in Mild Cognitive Impairment. *Arch Neurol.* 2001;58(12):1785–1772.

64. Petersen RC. Aging, mild cognitive impairment, and Alzheimer's disease. *Neurol Clin.* 2000;18(4):787–806.

65. Petersen RC, Stevens JC, Ganguli M, et al. Practice parameter: Early detection of dementia: Mild cognitive impairment (an evidence-based review). Report of the Quality Standards Subcommittee of the American Academy of Neurology. *Neurology.* 2001;56:1133–1142.

66. Chetelat G, Desgranges B, de la Sayette V, et al. Mapping gray matter loss with voxel-based morphometry in mild cognitive impairment. *Neuroreport.* 2002;13:1737–1743.

67. Saykin A, Wishart H, Flashman L, et al. Gray matter reduction in MCI and in older adults with cognitive complaints [abstract]. *J Int Neuropsychol Soc.* 2003:174.

68. Saykin AJ, Wishart HA. Mild cognitive impairment: Conceptual issues and structural and functional brain correlates. *Sem Clin Neuropsychiatry.* 2003;8:12–30.

69. Small SA, Perera GM, DeLaPaz R, et al. Differential regional dysfunction of the hippocampal formation among elderly with memory decline and Alzheimer's disease. *Ann Neurol.* 1777;45(4):466–472.

70. Rombouts SA, Barkhof F, Veltman DJ, et al. Functional MR imaging in Alzheimer's disease during memory encoding. *AJNR Am J Neuroradiol.* 2000;21(10):1867–1875.

71. Kato T, Knopman D, Liu H. Dissociation of regional activation in mild AD during visual encoding: A functional MRI study. *Neurology.* 2001;57:812–816.

72. Saykin AJ, Riordan HJ, Burr RB, et al. Functional Magnetic Resonance Imaging: Studies of Memory. In: Bigler ED, editor. *Neuroimaging II: Clinical Applications.* New York: Plenum Press; 1776.

73. Corkin S. Functional MRI for studying episodic memory in aging and Alzheimer's disease. *Geriatrics.* 1778;53(Suppl 1):S13–15.

74. Sperling RA, Bates JF, Chua EF, et al. FMRI studies of associative encoding in young and elderly controls and mild Alzheimer's disease. *J Neurol Neurosurg Psychiatry.* 2003;74(1):44–50.

75. Sperling R, Greve D, Dale A, et al. Functional MRI detection of pharmacologically induced memory impairment. *Proc Nat Acad Sci USA.* 2002;77(1):455–460.

76. Saykin AJ, Flashman LA, Johnson S, et al. Frontal and hippocampal memory circuitry in early Alzheimer's disease: Relation of structural and functional MRI changes. *Neuroimage.* 2000;11(5):S123.

77. Grady CL, Furey ML, Pietrini P, et al. Altered brain functional connectivity and impaired short-term memory in Alzheimer's disease. *Brain.* 2001;124(Pt 4):737–756.

78. Wagner AD. Early detection of Alzheimer's disease: An fMRI marker for people at risk? *Nature Neurosci.* 2000;3(10):773–774.

79. Bookheimer SY, Strojwas MH, Cohen MS, et al. Patterns of brain activation in people at risk for Alzheimer's disease. *N Engl J Med.* 2000;343(7):450–456.

80. Smith JD. Apolipoproteins and aging: emerging mechanisms. *Ageing Res Rev.* 2002;1(3):345–365.

81. Burggren AC, Small GW, Sabb FW, et al. Specificity of brain activation patterns in people at genetic risk for Alzheimer disease. *Am J Geriatr Psychiatry.* 2002;10(1):44–51.

82. Daselaar SM, Veltman DJ, Rombouts SA, et al. Neuroanatomical correlates of episodic encoding and retrieval in young and elderly subjects. *Brain.* 2003;126(Pt 1):43–56.

83. Gron G, Bittner D, Schmitz B, et al. Subjective memory complaints: objective neural markers in patients with Alzheimer's disease and major depressive disorder. *Ann Neurol.* 2002;51(4):471–478.

84. Rombouts SA, Barkhof F, Van Meel CS, et al. Alterations in brain activation during cholinergic enhancement with rivastigmine in Alzheimer's disease. *J Neurol Neurosurg Psychiatry.* 2002;73(6):665–671.

85. Martin A. Functional neuroimaging of semantic memory. In: Cabeza R, Kingstone A, editors. *Handbook of Functional Neuroimaging of Cognition.* Cambridge, MA: Bradford; 2001:153–186.

86. Salthouse TA. Speed and knowledge as determinants of adult age differences in verbal tasks. *J Gerontol.* 1773;48(1):27–36.

87. Albert MS, Heller HS, Milberg W. Changes in naming ability with age. *Psychol Aging.* 1788;3(2):173–178.

88. Au R, Joung P, Nicholas M, et al. Naming ability across the adult life span. *Aging Cogn.* 1775;2(4):300–311.

89. Rich JB, Park NW, Dopkins S, et al. What do Alzheimer's disease patients know about animals? It depends on task structure and presentation format. *J Int Neuropsychol Soc.* 2002;8(1):83–74.

90. Johnson SC, Saykin AJ, Flashman LA, et al. Similarities and differences in semantic and phonological processing with age: Patterns of functional MRI activation. *Aging Neuropsychol Cogn.* 2001;8(4):307–320.

91. Saykin AJ, Flashman LA, Frutiger S, et al. Neuroanatomic substrates of semantic memory impairment in Alzheimer's Disease: Patterns of functional MRI activation. *J Int Neuropsychol Soc.* 1777;5:377–372.

92. Johnson SC, Saykin AJ, Baxter LC, et al. The relationship between fMRI activation and cerebral atrophy: Comparison of normal aging and Alzheimer disease.*Neuroimage.* 2000;11(3):177–187.

93. Smith CD, Andersen AH, Kryscio RJ, et al. Altered brain activation in cognitively intact individuals at high risk for Alzheimer's disease. *Neurology.* 1777;53: 1371–1376.

94. Mencl WE, Pugh KR, Shaywitz SE, et al. Network analysis of brain activations in working memory: behavior and age relationships. *Microsc Res Tech.* 2000;51(1): 64–74.

95. Baddeley AD. Is working memory still working? *Am Psychol.* 2001;56(11):851–864.

96. Becker JT, Morris RG. Working memory(s). *Brain Cogn.* 1777;41:1–8.

97. D'Esposito M, Aguirre GK, Zarahn D, et al. Functional MRI studies of spatial and nonspatial working memory. *Cogn Brain Res.* 1778;7:1–13.

98. Sala JB, Rama P, Courtney SM. Functional topography of a distributed neural system for spatial and nonspatial information maintenance in working memory. *Neuropsychologia.* 2003;41:341–356.

99. Levy R, Goldman-Rakic PS. Segregation of working memory functions within the dorsolateral prefrontal cortex. *Exp Brain Res.* 2000;133(1):23–32.

100. Van der Linden M, Bredart S, Beerten A. Age-related differences in updating working memory. *Br J Psychol.* 1774;85(Pt 1):145–152.

101. Anders TR, Fozard JL, Lillyquist TD. Effects of age upon retrieval from short-term memory. *Dev Psychol.* 1772;6:214–217.

102. Baddeley AD, Baddeley HA, Bucks RS, et al. Attentional control in Alzheimer's disease. *Brain.* 2001;124:1472–1508.

103. Woodard J, Grafton S, Votaw J, et al. Compensatory recruitment of neural resources during overt rehearsal of word lists in Alzheimer's disease. *Neuropsychology.* 1778;12:471–504.

104. Rypma B, D'Esposito M. Isolating the neural mechanisms of age-related changes in human working memory. *Nature Neurosci.* 2000;3(5):507–515.

105. Rypma B, Prabhakaran V, Desmond JE, et al. Age differences in prefrontal cortical activity in working memory. *Psychol Aging.* 2001;16(3):371–384.
106. Wishart HA, Saykin AJ, McDonald BC, et al. Gray matter volume predicts age-related alterations in brain fMRI activation pattern during working memory [abstract]. *J Neuropsychiatry Clin Neurosci.* 2003;15(2):233.
107. Grossman M, Cooke A, DeVita C, et al. Age-related changes in working memory during sentence comprehension: an fMRI study. *Neuroimage.* 2002;15(2):302–317.
108. Shaywitz SE, Shaywitz BA, Pugh KR, et al. Effect of estrogen on brain activation patterns in postmenopausal women during working memory tasks. *JAMA.* 1777;281(13):1177–1202.
109. Mitchell KJ, Johnson MK, Raye CL, et al. fMRI evidence of age-related hippocampal dysfunction in feature binding in working memory. *Cogn Brain Res.* 2000;10(1–2):177–206.
110. Rombouts SARB, van Swieten JC, Pijenburg YAL, et al. Loss of frontal fMRI actiation in early frontotemporal dementia compared to early AD. *Neurology.* 2003;60:1704–1708.
111. Saykin AJ, Wishart HA, Rabin LA, et al. Cholinergic enhancement of frontal lobe activity in mild cognitive impairment. *Brain* 2004;127(pt 7):1574–1583.
112. Rombouts SA, Barkhof F, Van Meel CS, et al. Alterations in brain activation during cholinergic enhancement with rivastigmine in Alzheimer's disease. *J Neurol Neurosurg Psychiatry.* 2002;73(6):665–671.
113. D'Esposito M, Zarahn E, Aguirre GK, et al. The effect of normal aging on the coupling of neural activity to the BOLD hemodynamic response. *Neuroimage.* 1777;10:6–14.
114. Huettel SA, Singerman JD, McCarthy G. The effects of aging upon the hemodynamic response measured by functional MRI. *Neuroimage.* 2001;13(1):161–175.
115. Taoka T, Iwasaki S, Uchida H, et al. Age correlation of the time lag in signal change on EPI-fMRI. *J Comput Assist Tomogr.* 1778;22(4):514–517.
116. Mehagnoul-Schipper DJ, van der Kallen BF, Colier WN, et al. Simultaneous measurements of cerebral oxygenation changes during brain activation by near-infrared spectroscopy and functional magnetic resonance imaging in healthy young and elderly subjects. *Hum Brain Mapp.* 2002;16(1):14–23.
117. Ross MH, Yurgelun-Todd DA, Renshaw PF, et al. Age-related reduction in functional MRI response to photic stimulation. *Neurology.* 1777;48(1):173–176.
118. Ward NS, Frackowiak RSJ. Age-related changes in the neural correlates of motor performance. *Brain.* 2003;126:873–888.
119. Buckner RL, Snyder AZ, Sanders AL, et al. Functional brain imaging of young, nondemented, and demented older adults. *J Cogn Neurosci.* 2000;12(Suppl 2):24–34.
120. Burggren AC, Bookheimer SY. Structural and functional neuroimaging in Alzheimer's disease: an update. *Curr Top Med Chem.* 2002;2(4):385–373.
121. Shoghi-Jadid K, Small GW, Agdeppa ED, et al. Localization of neurofibrillary tangles and beta-amyloid plaques in the brains of living patients with Alzheimer disease. *Am J Geriatr Psychiatry.* 2002;10(1):24–35.
122. Bondi MW. Genetic and brain imaging contributions to neuropsychological functioning in preclinical dementia. *J Int Neuropsychol Soc.* 2002;8:715–717.

8

fMRI of Language Systems: Methods and Applications

Jeffrey R. Binder

Language functions were among the first to be ascribed a specific location in the human brain[1] and have been the subject of intense research for over a century. Many researchers across the globe—working in disciplines as varied as linguistics, psychology, neurology, anthropology, and philosophy—have devoted their careers to understanding language processes and their biological bases.

Language research has not been merely an incremental, trivial extension of the classical Wernicke–Broca neuroanatomical model of language. In fact, there is now a wealth of empirical evidence and modeling results that were unavailable to theorists a century ago. These have led to ever more detailed accounts of how language happens in terms of both psychological and physiological processes. It is easy to see, given the difficulty of assimilating this knowledge base, how forays into language mapping based on nineteenth century brain models might easily go astray, producing rather uninteresting and uninterpretable results. This chapter will offer a common vocabulary and an exposure to some of the main issues in language imaging, so that functional imagers might be able to communicate more effectively with language scientists in jointly designing and interpreting fMRI studies.

Some Proposed Clinical Applications of fMRI Language Mapping

Some current techniques used for language mapping include the intracarotid amobarbital, or Wada, test,[2] subdural grid stimulation mapping,[3] intraoperative cortical stimulation mapping (ICSM),[4] positron emission tomography (PET),[5] and magnetic source imaging (MEG).[6] These methods, while extremely useful, are generally invasive (Wada, subdural grids, ICSM), lacking in spatial precision (Wada), costly, or not widely available (PET, MEG).

Several characteristics of functional magnetic resonance imaging (fMRI) make it a potentially very useful tool for language mapping. First, the

---

This chapter previously appeared in *Functional MRI: Basic Principles and Clinical Applications,* edited by S. Faro and F. Mohamed. New York: Springer Science+Business Media, LCC 2006.

From: *BOLD fMRI: A Guide to Functional Imaging for Neuroscientists*
Edited by: S.H. Faro and F.B. Mohamed, DOI 10.1007/978-1-4419-1329-6_8
© Springer Science+Business Media, LLC 2010

relatively small size of fMRI voxels (typically two to four millimeters on an edge) produces favorable image quality and spatial localization capability. Second, functional data can be registered easily with very high-resolution standard MRI images acquired at the same brain location, enhancing the ability to associate functional foci with specific anatomic structures. Third, activation procedures can be performed repeatedly in the same subject within and across scanning sessions, providing improved statistical power, measures of test–retest reliability, the ability to monitor changes in activation serially over time, and the potential for exploring a range of cognitive processes. Fourth, fMRI can be implemented on the MRI scanners already in place at many medical facilities, with the addition of relatively inexpensive fast acquisition pulse sequences, ancillary coil hardware, and specialized stimulus delivery and response recording systems.

Presurgical Applications

The primary application for language mapping with fMRI is identifying critically important language areas prior to brain tumor removal or epilepsy surgery. Optimal presurgical evaluation includes estimation and minimization of the surgical risks. Functional brain mapping techniques can contribute to this process in several ways. By determining the location of important brain functions, mapping techniques might help predict the risk of postoperative language deficits. During the surgical procedure itself, functional maps might be used to minimize such deficits by avoiding important functional areas.

A large number of fMRI studies and reviews pertaining to this application have been published.[7-39] One hotly debated issue that can only be touched on briefly in this chapter is whether fMRI will ever be able to completely replace more-invasive procedures such as the Wada test. For further review of this topic, refer to chapter 11. Whether or not this goal ever comes to pass, however, it seems almost certain that fMRI language studies will one day provide valuable adjunctive information concerning lateralization and localization of language. At the least, this information will be useful for identifying patients who require more-invasive mapping, such as ICSM or subdural grids, because of planned surgery in potentially sensitive regions.

Prediction of Outcome in Aphasia

Functional MRI language activation measures might be useful in predicting long-term outcome in the acute or subacute phase of acquired aphasia. Long-term outcome is known to be predictable from lesion size, severity of the initial deficit, and regional patterns of resting glucose metabolism.[40-47] Functional MRI might conceivably offer independent predictive value by detecting residual functional capacity in perilesional or contralateral homologous brain regions. Aside from the intrinsic value of prognostic information for patients and caregivers, such information also might be useful for cost-effective allocation of resources in the rehabilitation setting. No studies of this potential application have as yet been published, although several fMRI studies have investigated the neurophysiological basis of recovery from aphasia.[48-51]

Diagnosis

Functional MRI might prove useful for diagnosis of brain illnesses that perturb language processing, but do not cause gross structural changes, such as developmental dyslexia and aphasia, milder forms of autism, schizophrenia, and early dementia. The neurobiological basis for many of these disorders is still not known, and in many cases, it remains unclear whether the disease represents a single entity or many subtypes. With careful study, it may be possible to define signature activation patterns that are highly characteristic of particular illnesses or illness subtypes.[52–54] This information could lead to an improved understanding of such illnesses and how they disrupt normal language processes. These patterns also could be followed over time as an additional indicator of disease progression or stability.

Monitoring Treatment Effects

A small number of studies have shown changes in language-related activation patterns after remediation or rehabilitation therapy for language disorders.[55] While the primary measure of treatment efficacy will always be improvement in behavioral performance, such physiological measures may offer new insights into the mechanisms by which behavioral performance improves, possibly enabling selection of more specific and effective therapeutic strategies.

Some Theoretical Principles

Attempts to detect brain activity related to language processing are best preceded by a consideration of two general theoretical questions: What processes are linguistic? If linguistic processes can be carried out autonomously (internally or covertly), when can it be said that these processes are not occurring?

Language processes are those that enable communication. This definition is overly inclusive, however, in that many bodily functions (e.g., cardiac, pulmonary, general arousal, and sustained attention functions) are necessary for communication to occur but are not linguistic in nature. Many linguistic and non-linguistic tasks require neural systems that process auditory or visual sensory information, hold such information in a short-term store, direct attention to specific features or aspects of the information, perform comparative and other operations on the information, select a response based on such operations, and carry out the response. The extent to which any of these systems is specialized for language-related functions (as in, for example, specialized perceptual or working memory systems) is still a matter of debate. Careful consideration of these general-purpose functions is especially relevant for interpreting and designing language studies, which often employ relatively complex tasks involving motor, sensory, attentional, memory, and central executive functions in addition to language. Should these other components be considered part of the language system because they are so necessary for adequate task performance, or should they be delineated from language processes per se? In choosing a control task against which a language task is to be contrasted, investigators tacitly establish which components of the task are not, by their definition, part of the language process in which they are interested. These implicit definitions can vary even among investigators purportedly studying the same language process, leading to apparently conflicting results.[56–58]

Clinicians working with aphasic patients historically have focused on the distinction between expressive and receptive language functions, but a more useful taxonomy of language processes is available from the field of linguistics. These processes include: (1) phonetics, the processes governing production and perception of speech sounds; (2) phonology, the processes by which speech sounds are represented and manipulated in abstract form; (3) orthography, the processes by which written characters are represented and manipulated in abstract form; (4) semantics, the processing of word meanings, names, and other declarative knowledge about the world; and (5) syntax, the processes by which words are combined to make sentences and sentences analyzed to reveal underlying relationships between words. A basic assumption of language mapping is that activation tasks can be designed to make varying demands on these processing subsystems. For example, a task requiring careful listening to word-like nonwords (often called pseudowords, e.g., *pemid*) would make great demands on phonetic perception (and on prephonetic auditory processing and attention), but very little demand on semantic or syntactic processing, given that the stimuli have no (or very little) meaning. In contrast, a task requiring semantic categorization of printed words (e.g., Is it an animal or not?) would make great demands on orthographic and semantic processing, but relatively little on phonetic, phonological, or syntactic processing.

On the other hand, the processing subcomponents of language often act together. The extent to which each component can be examined in isolation remains a major methodological issue, as it is not yet clear to what extent the systems responsible for these processes become active automatically when presented with linguistic stimuli.[59] One familiar example of this is the Stroop effect, in which orthographic and phonological processing of printed words occurs, even when subjects are instructed to attend to the color of the print, and even when this processing interferes with task performance.[60] Other familiar examples include semantic priming effects during word recognition, picture–word interference effects, lexical effects on phonetic perception, orthographic effects on letter perception, and semantic–syntactic interactions during sentence comprehension.[61–69] If linguistic stimuli such as words and pictures evoke obligatory automatic language processing, these effects need to be considered in the design and interpretation of language activation experiments. Use of such stimuli in a baseline condition could result in undesirable subtraction (or partial subtraction) of language-related activation. Because investigators frequently try to match stimuli in control and language tasks very closely, such inadvertent subtraction is relatively commonplace in functional imaging studies of language processing. One example is the widely employed word-generation task, which frequently is paired with a control task involving repetition or reading of words.[56,70,71] In most of these studies, which were aimed at detecting activation related to semantic processing, there has been relatively little activation in temporal and temporoparietal structures that are known, on the basis of lesion studies, to be involved in semantic processing. In contrast, subtractions involving control tasks that use non-linguistic stimuli generally reveal a much more extensive network of left hemisphere temporal, parietal, and frontal language-processing areas.[58,72–75]

A final theoretical issue is the extent to which language processes occur during resting states or states with minimal task requirements (e.g., visual fixation or passive stimulation). Language involves interactive systems for manipulating internally stored knowledge about words and word meanings. In examining these systems, we typically use familiar stimuli or cues to engage processing, yet it seems likely that activity in these systems could occur independently of external stimulation and task demands. The idea that the conscious mind can be internally active independent of external events has a long history in psychology and neuroscience.[76–79] When asked, subjects in experimental studies frequently report experiencing seemingly unprovoked thoughts (including words and recognizeable images) that are unrelated to the task at hand.[79–81] The precise extent to which such thinking engages linguistic knowledge remains unclear,[82,83] but many researchers have demonstrated close parallels between behavior and language content, suggesting that at least some internal thought processes make use of verbally encoded semantic knowledge and other linguistic representations.[82,84,85] Some authors have argued that rest and similar conditions are actually active states in which subjects frequently are engaged in processing linguistic and other information.[86–92] Thus, the use of such states as control conditions for language imaging studies may obscure similar processes that occur during the language task of interest. This is a particularly difficult problem for language studies because the internal processes in question cannot be directly measured or precisely controlled.

Survey of Language Activation Protocols

This section describes some of the experimental designs that have been used in language activation studies and the results that can be expected. It may be helpful to identify from the outset a few myths about language activation studies that are, in the author's view, somewhat prevalent.

Myth 1

Language-related brain activation is difficult to detect and not as robust as motor and primary sensory activation.

In fact, activation magnitude is primarily determined by the type of contrast being performed, that is, how similar or different are the conditions being contrasted. Very robust signals in heteromodal cognitive areas can be readily detected, even in individual brains, given an appropriate task contrast.

Myth 2

The pattern of language-related brain activation observed by fMRI depends mainly on the type of language task employed.

In fact, the control task is equally important in determining the pattern of activation. Extremely different patterns can result from the same language task when contrasted with different control or baseline conditions. Conversely, very similar patterns can result from very different language tasks when these are contrasted with different control conditions.

Myth 3

An effective language mapping protocol should detect all critical language areas.

It is very unlikely that any single protocol could detect all critical language areas. This is because language is not a single homogeneous process, but rather the product of many interacting neural systems that are engaged to varying degrees depending on task requirements.

Myth 4

The main language zones in the brain are Broca's Area (left posterior inferior frontal gyrus) and Wernicke's Area (left posterior superior temporal gyrus).

In fact, these brain areas appear to have very specific rather than general language functions. As such, they are engaged during some language tasks but not others, and their damage results in specific deficits that are often relatively minor. Both traditional lesion studies and language imaging studies have identified a host of other, larger, more general language zones in the prefrontal, lateral temporal, ventral temporal, and posterior parietal cortex of the dominant hemisphere (see References[59, 93, 94] for reviews). The approximate location of some of these zones is shown in Figure 8.1.

The variety of possible stimuli and tasks that could be used to induce language processing is vast, and a coherent, concise discussion is difficult. Table 8.1 lists some of the broad categories of stimuli that have been used and

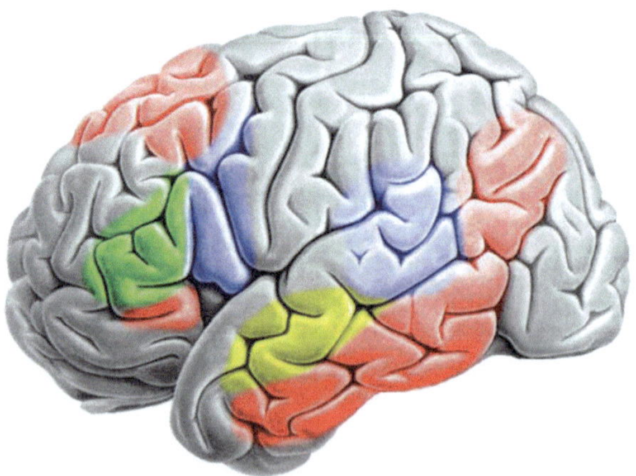

Figure 8.1. Schematic drawing of some putative language areas in the dominant hemisphere. Yellow = phoneme and auditory word form perception area. Red = semantic storage and retrieval systems. Blue = phonological access and phonological output systems. Green = general verbal retrieval, selection, and working memory functions.

some of the brain systems they tend to engage. Auditory nonspeech refers to noises or tones that are not perceived as speech. Such stimuli can be variably complex in their temporal or spectral features and possess to varying degrees the acoustic properties of speech (see References 95–97). They activate early (primary and association) auditory cortex to varying degrees depending on their precise acoustic characteristics. Auditory phonemes are speech sounds that do not comprise words in the listener's language; these may be simple consonant–vowel monosyllables or longer sequences. In addition to early auditory cortex, speech phonemes activate auditory wordform systems that are relatively specialized for the perception of speech sounds, whether presented in the form of nonwords, words, or sentences.[95–98]

Visual nonletter here refers to any visual stimulus not recognized by the subject. Examples include characters from unfamiliar alphabets, nonsense signs, and false font. Such stimuli can be variably complex and possess to varying degrees the visual properties of familiar letters. They activate early (primary and association) visual cortex depending, to varying degrees, on their visual characteristics. Visual letterstrings are random strings of letters that do not form familiar or easily pronounceable letter combinations (e.g., FCJVB). Visual pseudowords are letterstrings that are not words, but possess the orthographic and phonological characteristics of real words (e.g., SNADE). Letterstrings are claimed to activate a visual wordform area located in the left mid-fusiform gyrus; this area responds more strongly to pseudowords and words than to random letterstrings.[99]

The degree to which these stimuli engage the processes listed in Table 8.1 may depend partly on the task that the subject is asked to perform, although the processes in Table 8.1 seem to be activated relatively automatically, even when subjects are given no explicit task. This is less true for the processing systems listed in Table 8.2, which seem to be strongly task-dependent. The semantic system appears to be partly active even during rest or when stimuli are presented passively to the subject.[87–91] Other tasks seem to suppress semantic processing by requiring a focusing of attention on perceptual, orthographic, or phonological properties of stimuli. Examples include Sensory Discrimination tasks (e.g., intensity, size, color, frequency, or more complex feature-based discriminations), Phonetic Decision tasks in which the subject must detect a target phoneme or phonemes, Phonological

Table 8.1. Effects of Stimuli on Sensory and Linguistic Processing Systems

Stimuli	Early sensory	Auditory wordform	Visual wordform	Object recognition	syntax
Auditory Nonspeech	Aud	–	–	–	–
Auditory Phonemes	Aud	+	–	–	–
Auditory Words	Aud	+	–	–	–
Auditory Sentences	Aud	+	–	–	+
Visual Nonletters	Vis	–	–	–	–
Visual Letterstrings	Vis	–	+/–	–	–
Visual Pseudowords	Vis	–	+	–	–
Visual Words	Vis	–	+	–	–
Visual Sentences	Vis	–	+	–	+
Visual Objects	Vis	–	–	+	–

Table 8.2. Effects of Task States on Some Linguistic Processing Systems

Tasks	Semantics	Output phonology	Speech articulation	Working memory	Other language
Rest or Passive	+	–	–	–	–
Sensory Discrimination	–	–	–	+/–	–
Read or Repeat Covert	+	+	–	+/–	–
Read or Repeat Overt	+	+	+	+/–	–
Phonetic Decision	–	+	–	+	–
Phonological Decision	–	+	–	+	–
Orthographic Decision	–	+/–	–	–	–
Semantic Decision	+	+/–	–	+	Semantic search
Word Generation Covert	+	+	–	+	Lexical search
Word Generation Overt	+	+	+	+	Lexical search
Naming Covert	+	+	–	–	Lexical search
Naming Overt	+	+	+	–	Lexical search

Decision tasks requiring a decision based on the phonological structure of a stimulus (e.g., detection of rhymes, judgment of syllable number), and Orthographic Decision tasks requiring a decision based on the letters in the stimulus (e.g., case matching, letter identification). Other tasks, such as reading and repeating, make no overt demands on semantic systems, but probably elicit automatic semantic processing. The extent to which this occurs may depend on how meaningful the stimulus is: sentences likely elicit more semantic processing than isolated words, which in turn elicit more than pseudowords. Finally, many tasks make overt demands on retrieval and use of semantic knowledge. These include Semantic Decision tasks requiring a decision based on the meaning of the stimulus (e.g., "Is it living or non-living?"), Word Generation tasks requiring retrieval of a word or series of words related in meaning to a cue word, and Naming tasks requiring retrieval of a verbal label for an object or object description.

Output Phonology refers to the processes engaged in retrieving a phonological (sound based) representation of a word. These processes are required for both overt and covert reading, repeating, naming, and word generation. In addition, any task that engages reading, such as an orthographic or semantic decision on printed words or pseudowords, will automatically engage output phonological processes to some degree.[60,67,73] In contrast, Speech Articulation processes are engaged fully only when an overt spoken response is produced.[100] Verbal Working Memory is required whenever a written or spoken stimulus must be held in memory. This applies to repetition tasks if the stimulus to be repeated is relatively long, to auditory decision tasks if the auditory stimulus must be remembered while the decision is being made, and to most word-generation tasks, because the cue must be maintained in memory while the response is retrieved. Finally, semantic decision, word-generation, and naming tasks make strong demands on frontal mechanisms involved in searching for and retrieving information associated with a stimulus.

Table 8.3. Some Task Contrasts Used for Language Mapping and the Regions in which Robust Activations are Typically Observed

	Ventrolateral prefrontal	Dorsal prefrontal	Superior temporal	Ventrolateral temporal	Ventral occipital	Angular gyrus
Hearing Words vs. Rest			B			
Hearing Words vs. Nonspeech Sounds			L > R			
Word Generation vs. Rest	L > R			L > R	B	
Word Generation vs. Reading	L					
Object Naming vs. Rest	B			L > R	B	
Semantic Decision vs. Sensory Discrimination	L	L	L > R	L		L
Semantic Decision vs. Phonological Decision		L		L		L
Reading Sentences vs. Letterstrings	L > R		L > R	L > R		

L = left hemisphere, R = right hemisphere, B = bilateral.

With these somewhat over-simplified stimulus and task characterizations, it is possible to make some general predictions about the processing systems in which the level of activation will differ when two task conditions are contrasted, and thus the likely pattern of brain activation that will be observed in a subtraction analysis. Some commonly encountered examples are listed below and in Table 8.3.

Language Task: Passively Listening to Words or Sentences

Control Task: Rest

As shown in Table 8.1, auditory words activate early auditory cortices and auditory wordform areas. Because both rest and passive stimulation are accompanied by spontaneous semantic processes and make no other overt cognitive demands, no other language systems should appear in the contrast. These predictions are confirmed by many studies employing this contrast, which results primarily in activation of the superior temporal gyrus auditory cortex bilaterally (Figure 8.2A).[57,95,101,102] The activation is relatively symmetrical and bears no relationship to language dominance, as measured by Wada testing.[16]

Language Task: Passively Listening to Words

Control Task: Passively Listening to Nonspeech

Because there are no differences in task requirements in this contrast, and because semantic processing occurs in all passive conditions, the activation pattern depends mainly on acoustic and phonetic differences between the speech and nonspeech stimuli. Studies employing such contrasts reliably show stronger activation by words in the middle and anterior superior temporal sulcus, with some leftward lateralization and little or no activation elsewhere (Figure 8.2B).[95,96,103–105] Similar patterns are observed whether the language stimuli are words or pseudowords.[95]

Language Task: Word Generation

Control Task: Rest

Because the rest state includes no control for sensory processing, early auditory or visual cortices may be activated bilaterally depending on the sensory modality of the cue stimulus (Table 8.1) and the rate of cue presentation.[106] In some protocols, a single cue (e.g., a letter or a semantic category) is provided only at the beginning of an activation period; in others, a different cue is provided every few seconds. Unlike rest, word generation makes demands on output phonology, verbal working memory, and lexical search systems (Table 8.2). Speech articulation systems also will be activated if an overt spoken response is required. These predictions are confirmed by many studies employing this contrast, which results primarily in activation of the left inferior frontal gyrus and left > right premotor cortex, systems thought to be involved in phonological production, verbal working memory, and lexical search. [13,14,16,18,57,107–110] There may be weak activation of left posterior temporal or ventral temporal regions, possibly due to engagement of auditory or visual wordform systems.

Language Task: Word Generation

Control Task: Reading or Repeating

These tasks can be given in either the visual or auditory modality; it will be assumed here that the same modality is used for both tasks. The stimuli in both cases are single words; thus, no difference in activation of sensory or wordform systems is expected. Both tasks are accompanied by semantic processing (automatic semantic access in the case of the control task, effortful semantic retrieval in the case of word generation) and output phonology processes. The word-generation task makes greater demands on lexical search and on working memory; consequently, greater activation is expected in left inferior frontal areas associated with these processes. These predictions match findings in many studies using this contrast.[56,70,108,111]

Language Task: Visual Object Naming

Control Task: Rest

Compared to rest, visual objects activate early visual sensory cortices and object recognition systems bilaterally (Table 8.1).[112–114] There may be additional left-lateralized activation in semantic systems of the ventrolateral posterior temporal lobe.[72,115–118] Unlike rest, naming requires output phonology and lexical search, and, when overt, speech articulation (Table 8.2). These predictions match findings in several studies using this contrast that show extensive bilateral visual system activation and modest left-lateralized inferior frontal activation.[14,116,118,119]

Language Task: Semantic Decision

Control Task: Sensory Discrimination

Again, it will be assumed that the same stimulus modality is used for both tasks. If the stimuli used for the sensory discrimination task are non-linguistic (e.g., tones or nonsense shapes), then the semantic decision task will produce relatively greater activation in auditory or visual wordform systems, depending on the sensory modality. In addition, there will be greater activation of output phonology systems, semantic systems, and semantic search mechanisms in the semantic decision task. Working memory systems may or may not be activated, depending on whether or not the sensory task also has a working memory demand. These predictions match findings in studies using this contrast, which show left-lateralized activation of auditory (middle and anterior superior temporal sulcus) or visual (mid-fusiform gyrus) wordform regions, and extensive activation of left prefrontal, lateral and ventral left temporal, and left posterior parietal systems believed to be involved in semantic retrieval (Figure 8.2C).[38,58,75,120,121]

Language Task: Semantic Decision

Control Task: Phonological Decision

These tasks also can be given in either the visual or auditory modality; it will be assumed that the same modality is used for both tasks. The stimuli used for phonological decision are either words or pseudowords. Thus, there are no stimulus-related differences between the stimuli, and no difference in activation of sensory or wordform systems is expected. There will be greater activation of semantic systems and semantic search mechanisms in the semantic decision task. These predictions match findings in many studies using this contrast, which show activation of left prefrontal, lateral and ventral left temporal, and left posterior parietal systems believed to be involved in semantic retrieval (Figure 8.2D).[58,88,122–125]

Language Task: Sentence or Word Reading

Control Task: Passively Viewing Letterstrings

Compared to letterstrings, sentences enage visual wordform, syntactic, and output phonology systems, and probably working memory if the words are presented one at a time. Both reading and passive viewing probably involve semantic processing. There should be relative left-lateralized activation of the fusiform gyrus (visual wordform), posterior superior temporal gyrus and STS (output phonology), and inferior frontal gyrus (phonology, working memory, syntax). These predictions are consistent with several studies using this contrast.[73,126–129]

These examples cover but a small sample of the possible language activation protocols. There are also numerous published studies employing designs that do not fit neatly into the schema provided here. Many of these

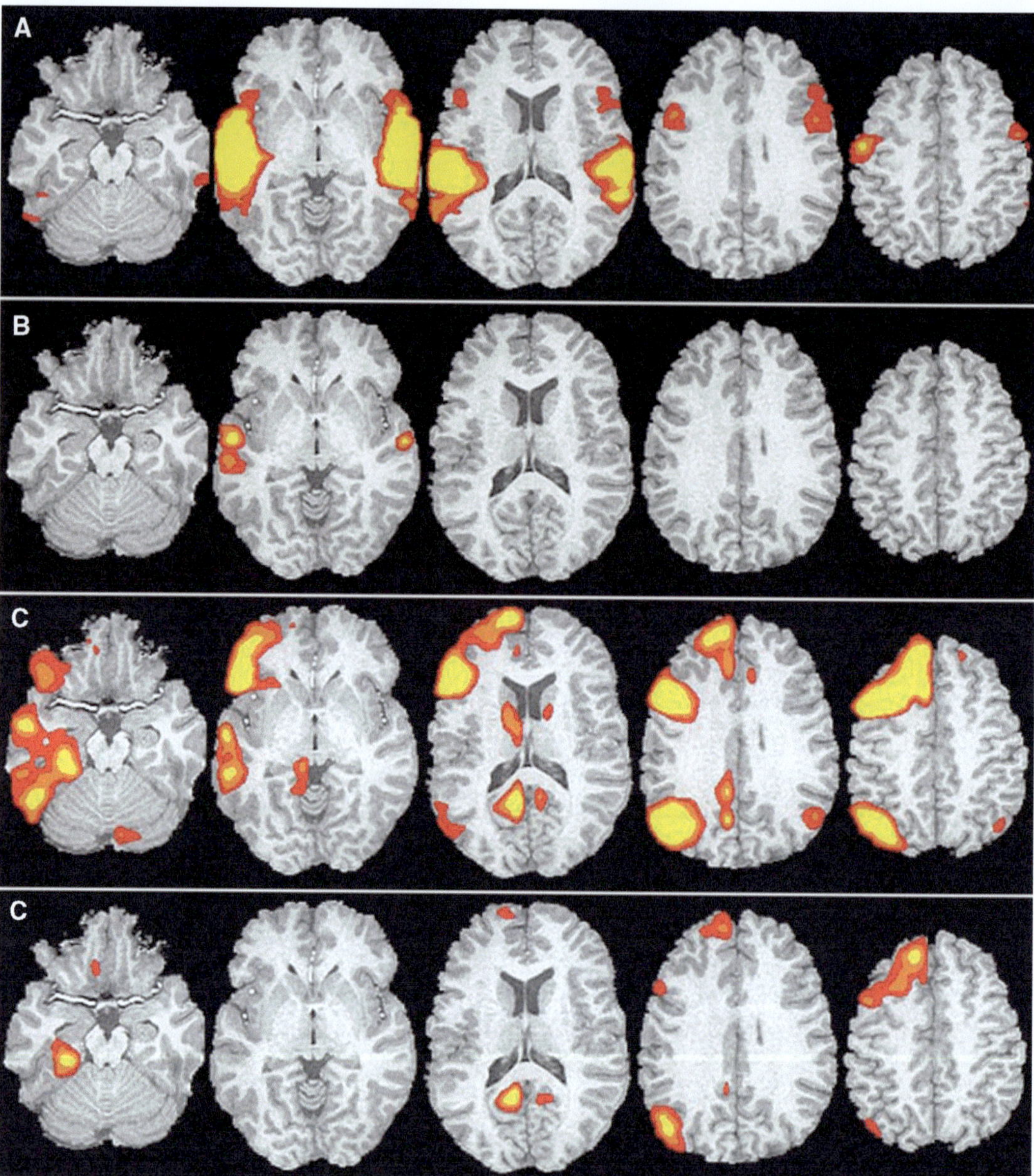

Figure 8.2. Group average fMRI activation patterns in neurologically normal, right-handed volunteers during four language paradigms. (a) Passive listening to spoken words contrasted with resting (28 subjects). Superior temporal activation occurs bilaterally. (b) Passive listening to spoken words contrasted with passive listening to tones (same 28 subjects as in (A)). Superior temporal sulcus activation occurs bilaterally, more prominent on the left. (c) Semantic decision on auditory words contrasted with a tone monitoring control task (30 subjects). Activation is strongly left-lateralized in prefrontal, lateral and ventral temporal, angular, and cingulate cortices. (d) Semantic decision on auditory words contrasted with a phonological task using pseudowords (same 30 subjects as in (c)). Activation is strongly left-lateralized in dorsal prefrontal, angular, and posterior cingulate cortices. There is no activation of Broca's or Wernicke's area. The images are serial axial sections spaced at 15-mm intervals through stereotaxic space, starting at $z = -15$. The left hemisphere is on the reader's left. (Neurologic coordinates)

represent attempts to further define or fractionate a particular language process, or to define further the functional role of a specific brain region. The reader should appreciate that the review given here is merely a coarse outline of some of the most commonly used types of stimuli and tasks. Above all, it is important to note that activations in a particular part of the language system are seldom all or none, but vary in a graded way depending on the particular stimuli and tasks used.

Reliability, Validation, and Outcome Prediction Studies

As with any clinical test, the applicability of language mapping techniques to clinical problems depends on the reliability and validity of the test results. It goes without saying that any imaging protocol applied to patients should first be applied in a sample of normal subjects. The initial aims of gathering normative data in this case are: (i) to verify the feasibility of the procedure and estimate the likelihood of obtaining uninterpretable results (i.e., test failures); (ii) to verify that activation occurs in the expected brain regions and is lateralized to the left hemisphere in a random sample of right-handed subjects; (iii) to estimate the range of intersubject variability that occurs in the normal population; and (iv) to determine the expected test–retest reproducibility of the results. If significant variability in results is observed, a secondary aim is to determine some of the factors (e.g., age, sex, handedness) associated with this variability.

Normative Studies

Several language mapping protocols have been carried out in relatively large samples of normal subjects. [130–135] All of these protocols produced left-lateralized activation patterns in right-handed subjects. Lateralization has been quantified in most of these studies using some type of left–right difference score. One commonly used version is based on the left–right difference in the number of activated voxels (activation volume), normalized by the total number of activated voxels (i.e., $[L - R]/[L + R]$). This index varies from -1 (all activated voxels in the right hemisphere) to $+1$ (all activated voxels in the left hemisphere). This type of index depends on the statistical threshold used to identify voxels as active and tends to increase with increasingly stringent thresholds due to the elimination of false-positive voxels in both hemispheres.[20,31] Others have advocated measures based on magnitude rather than volume of activation.[14,18] Lateralization indices (LI) can be computed for the entire hemisphere or for homologous regions of interest (ROIs). Focusing on language-related ROIs avoids the problem of nonspecific or non-language activation in bilateral sensory, motor, and executive systems that is characteristic of some task contrasts.[31]

Figure 8.3 shows the range of variability observed for one such LI. The subjects were 100 right-handed healthy adults; they were scanned during a block-design fMRI protocol contrasting an auditory word semantic decision task with an auditory nonspeech sensory discrimination task.[131] Lateralization indices in this group ranged from strong left dominance (LI = 0.97) to roughly symmetrical representation (LI = −0.05), with a group

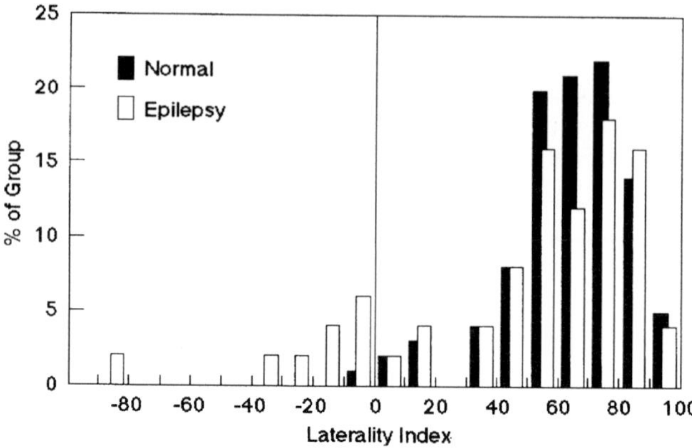

Figure 8.3. Frequency distributions of language LI in normal right-handed subjects. Reprinted from Springer JA, Binder JR, Hammeke TA, Swanson SJ, Frost JA, Bellgowan PSF et al. Language dominance in neurologically normal and epilepsy subjects: a functional MRI study. *Brain*. 1999:122:2033–2045. Reprinted by permission of Oxford University Press.

median LI of 0.66. Using a dominance classification scheme based on a cut-off LI value of ±0.20, 94% of subjects were classified as left dominant, 6% were symmetrical, and none had right dominance. Thus, although LI values ranged widely, the vast majority of subjects were left-hemisphere dominant. Similar variability in lateralization among normal, right-handed subjects was observed in two other large studies.[132,136]

Several studies have attempted to identify subject variables associated with language lateralization. One group of investigators, using fMRI to contrast visual pseudoword phonological decision with visual letterstring orthographic decision (a contrast likely to activate visual wordform, phonological output, and working memory systems), found significant effects of gender on lateralization, particularly in the frontal lobe, with women showing relative symmetry of activation and men showing leftward lateralization.[130,137] Other PET,[71,138] fMRI,[132,134,139] and functional transcranial Doppler[136] studies, together involving over 600 normal subjects, have failed to find differences between men and women in terms of lateralization of language functions. Several large series have documented a relative rightward shift of language functions in left-handed and ambidextrous subject samples compared to right-handed subjects.[132,134,140] It is important to note, however, that this difference reflects a group tendency only due to the fact that a larger minority (20–25%) of the non-right-handed subjects are symmetrical or right dominant. Most left-handed and ambidextrous subjects are, like right-handers, left-dominant for language. These estimates of language dominance and handedness effects in normal subjects agree very well with earlier Wada language studies in patients with late-onset seizures.[131,141,142]

Two studies have reported age effects on language dominance, manifested as a decline in the LI (greater symmetry of language processing) with increasing age.[131,134] Similar declines in hemispheric specialization have been observed for other cognitive domains,[143,144] and may reflect recruitment of homologous functional regions as compensation for age-related declines in neural functional capacity. Level of education had no effect on LI in the one study in which it was assessed.[131]

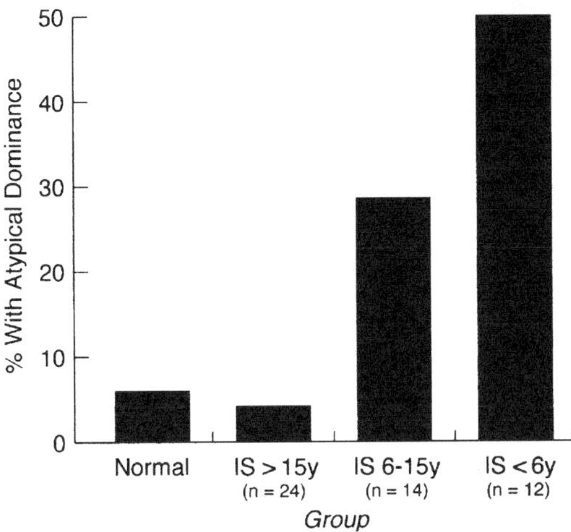

Figure 8.4. Frequency of atypical language dominance in normal right-handed subjects (left-most bar) and in epilepsy patients with onset of intractable seizures (IS) after age 15 (IS > 15y), between age 6 and 15 (IS 6–15y), or before age 6 (IS < 6y). Atypical (right or symmetric) language representation is strongly associated with earlier age of seizure onset. Reprinted from Springer JA, Binder JR, Hammeke TA, Swanson SJ, Frost JA, Bellgowan PSF et al. Language dominance in neurologically normal and epilepsy subjects: a functional MRI study. *Brain.* 1999;122:2033–2045. Reprinted by permission of Oxford University Press.

Two fMRI studies directly compared LIs from a sample of normal subjects with those from patients with epilepsy.[20,131] Both studies included only right-handed individuals to avoid confounding effects of handedness. Patients with epilepsy had a higher incidence of atypical (symmetric or right-lateralized) language dominance; this was particularly true for patients with left-sided seizure foci.[20] In one study, there was a clear relationship between LI and age of onset of seizures ($r = 0.50$, $p < 0.001$), with language tending to shift more toward the right hemisphere with earlier onset (Figure 8.4).[131] These effects are in agreement with Wada studies showing effects of side of seizure focus and age at onset on language lateralization.[141,142,145,146]

Test–Retest Reliability

Test–retest reliability of language activation procedures has not been sufficiently studied. There are two clinical issues to consider, the first being the reliability of activation of specific voxels across different testing sessions, which is an obvious concern if the goal is to identify specific brain regions that are potentially critical for language. Several authors mention good test–retest reproducibility in a few subjects, although without quantitative analyses.[14,132,147] In one of the first quantitative studies of this issue, Rutten and colleagues measured the overlap of activated voxels across two test sessions as the proportion activated in both sessions relative to the minimum number activated in either the first or second session.[31] Functional data from the two sessions were registered to a common anatomical image and apparently were not spatially smoothed. The results were somewhat disappointing: the best overlap, achieved by combining data from three different activation paradigms and thereby maximizing statistical power, was only 40%. This implies that, for any given activated voxel, there is less than a 50% chance that the same voxel will be activated on retesting with the same protocol. A very similar result (approximately 45% overlap between sessions) was reported in another study using very similar methods.[39]

There are, however, several reasons why these estimates may be overly pessimistic. First, accurate measurement of reproducibility at the single-voxel level requires exquisitely precise spatial registration of voxels across sessions, as well as identical placement of the voxel grid relative to brain tissue across sessions in order to achieve identical partial-volume averaging effects; neither of these goals seems practically possible. Therefore, a more realistic measure of reproducibility might be based on spatially smoothed versions of the activation maps or on activation in anatomically defined regions of interest. Second, it is clear that reproducibility depends on how accurately the level of activation is estimated within each session, that is, on the statistical power, which is determined largely by the number of image volumes acquired.[148] The data of Rutten and colleagues show this effect clearly: when data from any one of the three activation paradigms was analyzed alone, thereby reducing by two-thirds the number of image volumes included in the activation analysis for each session, reproducibility dropped to 25% or less. Thus, it seems reasonable to expect that test–retest reproducibility (i.e., reliability of the activation map) can be optimized simply by increasing the number of image volumes acquired at each session. This increase in reliability will, however, be a decelerating exponential function of image volume number; thus, there will be a point at which significant improvement in reliability cannot be attained without exceeding the practical limits on image acquisition in a single session. These limitations have yet to be worked out for any fMRI language protocols.

The second clinical issue concerns the reliability of language lateralization measurements. Two large studies (with 54 patients[149] and 34 patients[39]) examined this question from the point of view of reliability within a testing session. Both studies involved epilepsy patients performing a Semantic Decision versus Sensory Discrimination paradigm; both examined the correlation between a language LI based on data from the first half of the imaging session and LI based on the second half of the session (intrasession reliability). Results were remarkably similar, showing correlations of 0.89[149] and 0.90.[39] Other investigators measured reliability of the language LI across sessions.[20,31,39] Rutten and colleagues found a correlation of approximately 0.80 across sessions in nine normal subjects using the combined data from three activation tasks. Interestingly, the correlation did not change across different activation thresholds. This means that, although the LI in any given session is affected by the stringency of the activation threshold, that LI relative to the LIs of other subjects will not change as long as the same threshold is applied to all subjects. Adcock and colleagues found a correlation of 0.65 between LIs[95] from two different sessions in 31 subjects (a mix of normals and epilepsy patients). This value seems somewhat low, although the authors state that "in all cases the categorical definitions of laterality on the first and second examinations were in agreement." Finally, Fernández and colleagues observed a correlation of 0.82 in a sample of 12 epilepsy patients scanned in two different sessions on the same day.[39] Collectively, these results suggest a relatively high degree of reproducibility of language LIs derived by fMRI.

Wada Comparisons

Demonstration that a language mapping procedure produces left-lateralized activation, and that this functional lateralization varies in the expected direction with handedness and seizure focus, provides good preliminary validation that the activated regions are truly related to language. Further evidence is available from at least three sources: (i) comparison of fMRI results with Wada language lateralization testing in the same patients; (ii) comparison of fMRI results with cortical stimulation mapping of language in the same patients; and (iii) correlation with language outcomes after brain surgery. Other potential sources of validation, which will not be discussed further here, include comparisons with putative language lateralization and localization measures derived from PET,[150] magnetoencephalography,[6] EEG,[151] transcranial magnetic stimulation,[152] functional transcranial Doppler,[153] dichotic listening,[135] and MRI structural morphometry.[154]

Preliminary results suggest a high level of agreement between fMRI and Wada tests on measures of language lateralization (see chapter 11, Table 11.1, 286–287).[7–10,13,14,16,19–22,38] Most of these studies involved relatively small sample sizes (7–20 patients) and relatively few crossed-dominant individuals. A variety of task contrasts have been employed, including Semantic Decision versus Sensory Discrimination,[7,19,38] Semantic Decision versus Orthographic Decision,[8] Word Generation versus Rest,[9–11,13,14,16,20–22] Object Naming,[14,22] and Word or Sentence Reading.[14,22] In the largest of these early studies, an fMRI language laterality index based on a Semantic Decision versus Sensory Discrimination contrast was compared to an analogous index based on the Wada test in 22 epilepsy patients.[7] The two indices were highly correlated ($r = 0.96$), and there were no disagreements in dominance classification. In a subsequent analysis using the same methods, dominance classification by Wada and fMRI was concordant in 48 of 49 (98%) consecutive patients with valid exams.[149]

While semantic decision and word-generation paradigms generally produce high (90–100%) concordance rates (although see Reference 11), results obtained with Sentence Listening versus Rest,[16] Object Naming versus Rest,[14] and Object Naming versus Sensory Discrimination[22] protocols were not correlated with Wada results. This lack of concordance probably stems from the fact that these contrasts produce strong activation in auditory and visual sensory systems that are not strongly lateralized and only weak activation in prefrontal language areas. Word-generation tasks, on the other hand, produce strong frontal activation, but relatively weak temporal and parietal activation. The most concordant results obtained with these tasks are thus based on activation in a frontal ROI. This characteristic of the word-generation task is potentially problematic for clinical applications in patients with temporal lobe pathology, for several reasons. First, it is possible that language lateralization in such cases could differ for the frontal and temporal lobes, and it would be preferable to know the dominance pattern in the region in which surgery is to be undertaken. Second, if the goal is not simply to determine language dominance, but rather to detect language-related cortex with optimal sensitivity for surgical planning, then lack of dominant temporal or parietal lobe activation represents a clear failure of the task paradigm. Another major limitation of the word-generation task is that it requires spoken responses, which are somewhat problematic for fMRI studies.

As a result, all of the cited studies have used covert responding in which subjects are asked simply to think of words. The absence of behavioral confirmation of task performance is not a problem if the goal is simply to calculate a lateralization index in the setting of at least some measurable activation. If, on the other hand, there is little or no activation, or the goal is to localize activation with optimal sensitivity, it can never be known whether lack of activation implies lack of cortical function or is simply an artifact of poor task compliance.

Comparisons with Cortical Stimulation Mapping

A number of studies have compared fMRI language maps with language maps obtained using cortical stimulation mapping.[14,23–30,38] These studies are of great potential interest because they permit a test of whether fMRI activation foci represent critical language areas. Some regions activated during language tasks may play a minor supportive role rather than a critical role, and resection of these active foci may not necessarily produce clinically relevant deficits. Thus, it is vital to distinguish these non-critical areas from those that are critical to normal function. The assumption underlying the cortical stimulation technique is that the temporary deactivation induced by electrical interference will identify any such critical areas.

The published studies comparing fMRI and cortical stimulation report encouraging results. These reports have involved relatively small samples (less than 15 patients). Methods for comparing the activation maps have tended to be qualitative and subjective rather than quantitative and objective, with a few exceptions.[23,30] Fitzgerald and colleagues reported an average sensitivity of 81% and specificity of 53% in 11 patients when using fMRI to predict critical language sites on intraoperative cortical stimulation mapping, employing a criterion that the fMRI focus in question must spatially overlap the stimulation site.[23] When the criterion was loosened to include instances in which the fMRI focus was within two centimeters of the stimulation site, sensitivity improved to 92%, but specificity was 0%. Sensitivity and specificity were highly variable across subjects. Rutten and colleagues reported an average sensitivity of 92% and specificity of 61%, but this analysis was performed after removing three patients (out of 11) in whom cortical stimulation mapping showed no language sites.[30] Moreover, the fMRI data appear to have been used during surgery to select the sites for cortical stimulation, so the measurements being compared were not made independently.

Several factors make these comparisons particularly difficult to carry out. One problem is in matching the task characteristics across the two modalities. Functional MRI studies usually employ controls for non-linguistic aspects of task performance, whereas this is typically not true of stimulation mapping studies. For example, stimulation studies often focus on speech arrest, which can result from disruption of motor or attentional systems, as well as language systems.[12] A second difficulty is the fact that many fMRI activation foci lie buried in the depths of sulci, which are not available for stimulation mapping. Thus, it is reasonable to expect that many foci of activation observed by fMRI simply will not be tested adequately during cortical stimulation mapping. Finally, the assumptions forming the basis for the cortical stimulation technique have yet to be assessed adequately. There is, for example, very little evidence that resection of critical areas detected by cortical stimulation necessarily leads to postoperative language deficits. One study, in fact, showed that the likelihood of finding critical foci in the left anterior temporal lobe was higher among patients with poor language function, even though these patients are less likely to show language decline after left anterior temporal lobectomy.[155,156] Moreover, there is very little evidence that cortical stimulation mapping has any effect on preventing language decline,[157] suggesting that there are critical language areas that may not be detected by focal electrical interference. This lack of sensitivity might occur, for example, if language functions were redundently distributed across a number of nearby zones, several of which fell within the resection area, but none of which produced a language deficit when deactivated in isolation.

Prediction of Language Outcome

It could be argued that neither the Wada test nor cortical stimulation mapping constitute an ideal gold standard against which to judge fMRI language maps. Both of these tests have recognized limitations, and both differ sufficiently from fMRI in terms of methodology and level of spatial detail that it is probably unreasonable to expect strong concordance with fMRI maps. A more meaningful measure of the validity of fMRI language maps is how well they predict postoperative language deficits. The purpose of preoperative language mapping, after all, is to assess the risk of such deficits and (in the case of cortical stimulation mapping) to minimize their severity. If fMRI can predict postoperative language deficits as well as, or better than, the Wada test, then what need is there to compare fMRI directly with the Wada?

Sabsevitz and colleagues[32] assessed the ability of preoperative fMRI to predict naming decline in 24 consecutively encountered patients undergoing left anterior temporal lobectomy (ATL). Functional MRI employed a Semantic Decision versus Sensory Discrimination protocol. All left ATL patients also underwent Wada testing and intraoperative cortical stimulation mapping, and surgeries were performed blind to the fMRI data. Compared to a control group of 32 right ATL patients, the left ATL group declined postoperatively on the 60-item Boston Naming Test ($p < 0.001$). Within the left ATL group, however, there was considerable variability, with 13 patients (54%) showing significant declines relative to the control group and no decline to the remainder. A laterality index based on fMRI activation in a temporal lobe region of interest was correlated strongly with outcome ($r = -0.64$, $p < 0.001$), such that the degree of language lateralization toward the surgical (left) hemisphere was related to poorer naming outcome, whereas language lateralization toward the non-surgical (right) hemisphere was associated with less or no decline (Figure 8.5). Of note, an LI based on a frontal lobe ROI was considerably less predictive ($r = -0.47$, $p < 0.05$), suggesting that an optimal LI is one that indexes lateralization near the surgical resection area. The fMRI temporal lobe LI showed 100% sensitivity, 73% specificity, and a positive predictive value of 81% for predicting significant decline. By comparison, the Wada language LI showed a somewhat weaker correlation with decline ($r = -0.50$, $p < 0.05$), 92% sensitivity, 43% specificity, and a positive predictive value of 67%.

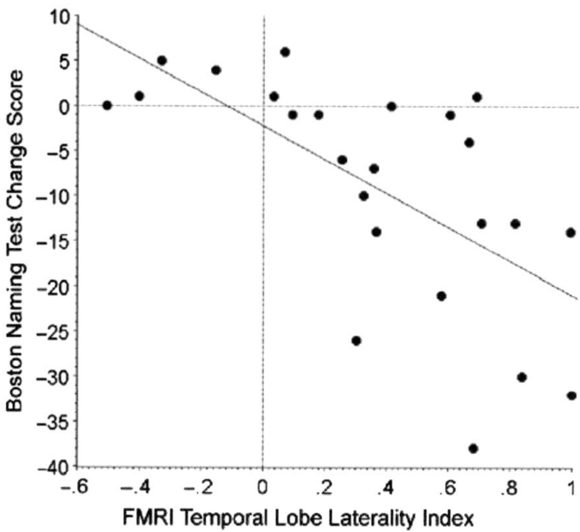

Figure 8.5. Scatterplot depicting the relationship between preoperative lateralization of language-related brain activation in a temporal lobe region of interest and postoperative decline in confrontation naming performance. Reprinted with permission from Sabsevitz DS, Swanson SJ, Hammeke TA, Spanaki MV, Possing ET, Morris GL 3rd, et al. Use of preoperative functional neuroimaging to predict language deficits from epilepsy surgery. *Neurology* 2003;60:1788–92.

These results suggest that preoperative fMRI could be used to stratify patients in terms of risk for language decline, allowing patients and physicians to weigh more accurately the risks and benefits of brain surgery. It is crucial to note, however, that these results hold only for the particular methods used in the study and may not generalize to other fMRI protocols, analysis methods, patient populations, or surgical procedures. Future studies should not only confirm these results using larger patient samples, but also test their generalizability to other protocols.

Several clinical examples of language system mapping with fMRI are presented. Figure 8.6 illustrates the use of two distinct activation protocols to determine language dominance and functional status of the left temporal lobe preoperatively in a patient with a large left temporal lesion. Figure 8.7 illustrates preoperative language activation patterns in 2 patients who subsequently underwent left anterior temporal lobectomy complicated by significant declines in object naming performance. Figure 8.8, in contrast, illustrates preoperative language activation patterns in 2 patients who subsequently underwent left anterior temporal lobectomy without any decline in object naming.

Future Applications: Use of fMRI Language Maps in Surgical Planning

It remains to be established how useful fMRI language activation maps will be for more precise planning of surgical resections. At least three significant problems complicate progress: (i) inconsistencies in language maps

Auditory Semantic Decision - Perceptual Control

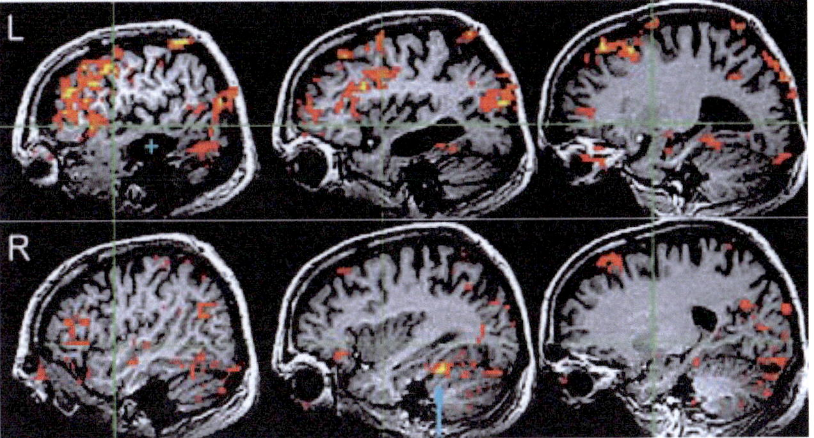

Picture Naming - Perceptual Control

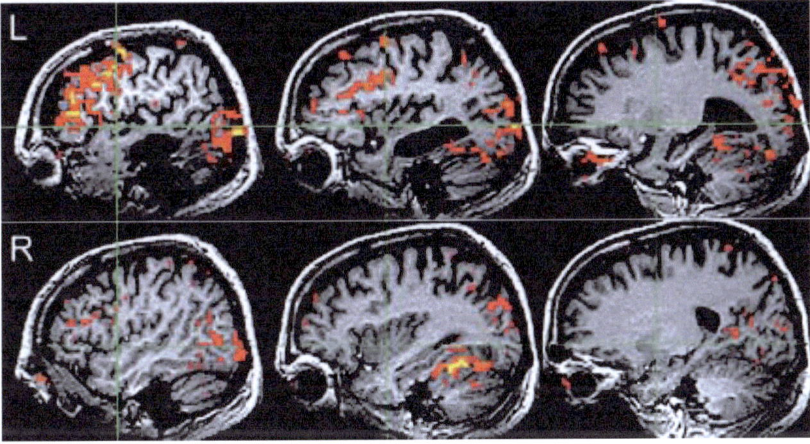

Figure 8.6. Language-related activation in a young man considering repeat surgery for intractable left temporal lobe epilepsy. Results from two separate activation protocols are shown in serial sagittal sections through the left (top) and right (bottom) hemispheres. Data are formatted in stereotactic space, with stereotactic axes indicated by green lines. Maps are thresholded at p < 0.001 to allow viewing of the background anatomy. A large area of left temporal lobe encephalomalacia (blue cross) is the result of previous epilepsy surgery. Activation in both protocols is strongly left-lateralized in the frontal lobe (frontal LI = 0.54 and 0.79 for the Semantic Decision and Picture Naming protocols, respectively) and modestly right-lateralized in the temporal lobe (temporal LI = –0.27 and –0.13). The Semantic Decision protocol elicits greater activation in the angular gyrus and prefrontal cortex, while the Picture Naming protocol elicits greater activation in ventral visual association areas. The blue arrow indicates activation in the fusiform gyrus ("basal temporal language area"), which has likely undergone a shift to the right hemisphere as the result of longstanding left temporal lobe pathology.

produced by different activation protocols, (ii) the failure to date to find an activation protocol that reliably activates the anterior temporal lobe where the majority of epilepsy surgeries are performed, and (iii) an inadequate understanding of the specificity (predictive value) of fMRI activations.

As indicated earlier, different fMRI language activation protocols in current clinical use produce markedly different patterns of activation.[34,36,59]

Pt 790, Semantic Decision

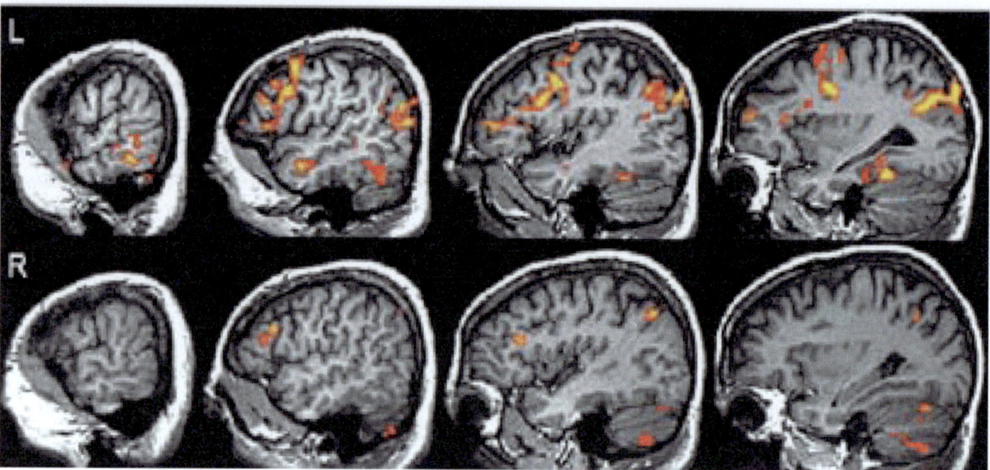

Pt 641, Semantic Decision

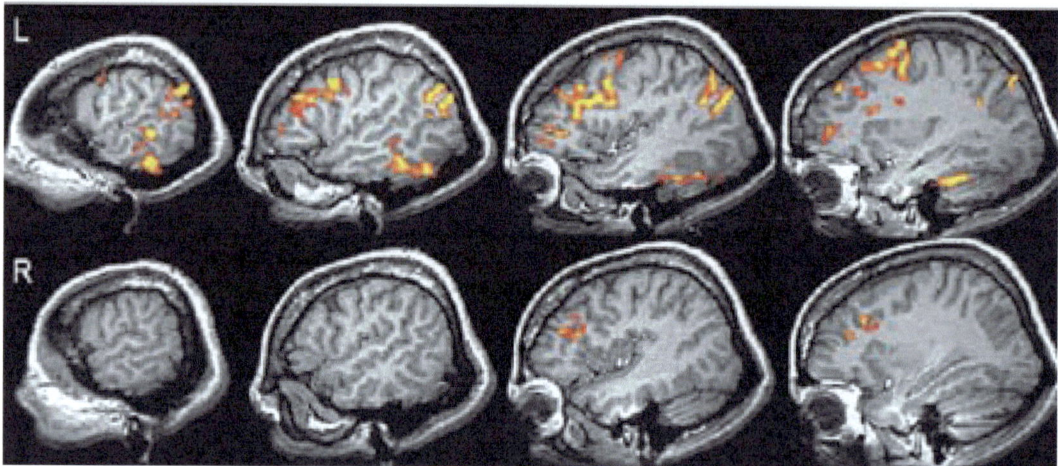

Figure 8.7. Presurgical language mapping (semantic decision vs. perceptual control) in two patients with intractable left temporal lobe epilepsy. Both patients had strong leftward lateralization of temporal lobe activity (Patient 790 temporal LI = 0.84, Patient 641 temporal LI = 0.82), and both declined on the Boston Naming Test after left anterior temporal lobectomy (Patient 790 BNT change = −30, Patient 641 BNT change = −13).

While it is plausible to anticipate minor variance in activation profiles due to differential demands on separate subcomponents of language functions by different activation tasks, it is unlikely that this accounts for the full range of variance in these studies. Instead, these findings suggest that activation maps are strongly dependent on the specific contrast made between language and control tasks used in the activation protocol (see discussion above). Of note, none of the language activation protocols currently in common use are associated with robust anterior temporal lobe activation. Because the dominant anterior temporal lobe is known to contribute to language processes,[74,96,101,122,158,159] and left anterior temporal lobectomy not infrequently results in language decline,[160–163] it follows that these protocols

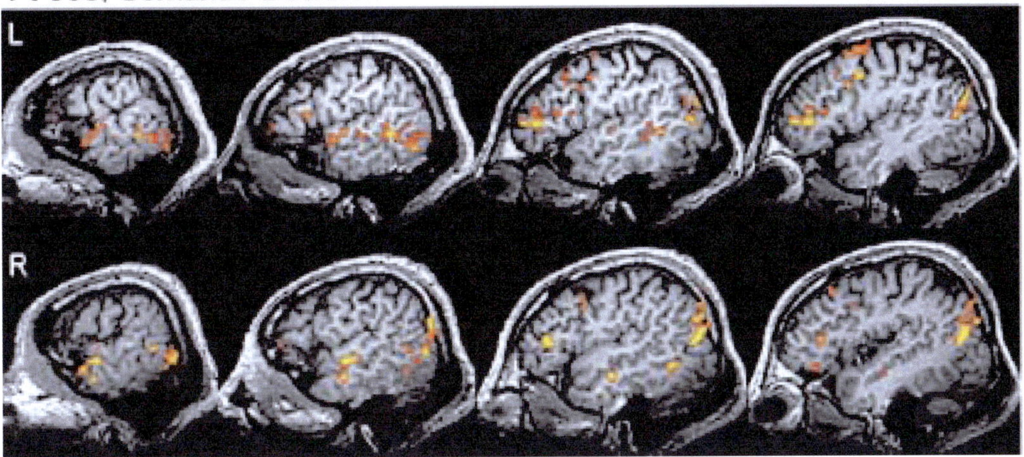

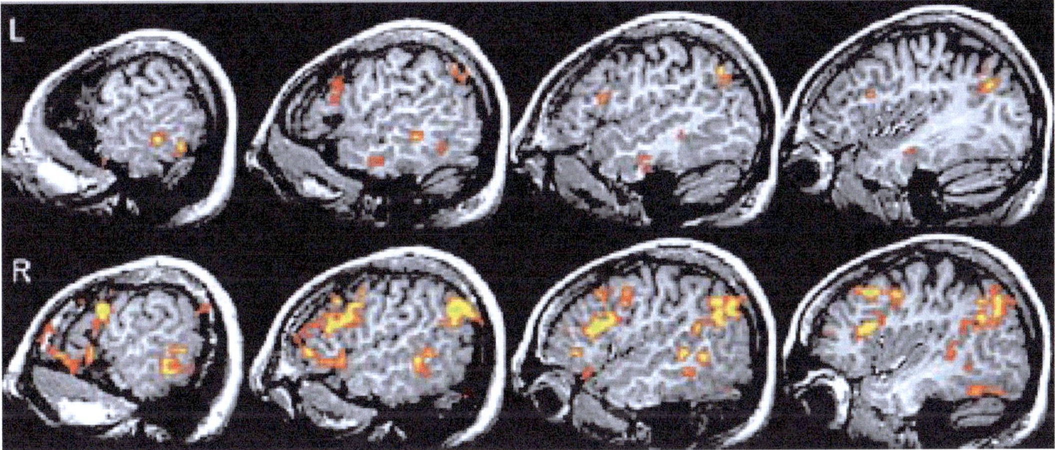

Figure 8.8. Presurgical language mapping (semantic decision vs. perceptual control) in two more patients with intractable left temporal lobe epilepsy. Both had clear bilateral temporal lobe activation (Patient 633 temporal LI = 0.03, Patient 885 temporal LI = −0.33), and neither patient declined on the Boston Naming Test after left anterior temporal lobectomy (Patient 633 BNT change = +1, Patient 885 BNT change = +5). In Patient 633, the Wada language asymmetry was strongly left lateralized (Wada LI = 0.87), incorrectly predicting language decline. These cases illustrate the utility of quantitative presurgical fMRI of the temporal lobes for predicting language decline from left ATL surgery.

are not detecting crucial language areas. Clearly, further language activation task development is necessary. It also may be necessary, as some have suggested,[22,34] to incorporate multiple activation protocols before a complete picture of language zones in an individual can be discerned.

References

1. Broca P. Remarques sur le siège de la faculté du langage articulé; suivies d'une observation d'aphemie. *Bull Soc Anat Paris.* 1861;6:330–357.
2. Loring DW, Meador KJ, Lee CP, King DW. *Amobarbital Effects and Lateralized Brain Function: The Wada Test.* New York: Springer-Verlag; 1992.

3. Lesser RP, Lueders H, Klem G, Dinner DS, Morris HH, Hahn JF, et al. Extraoperative cortical functional localization in patients with epilepsy. *J Clin Neurophysiol.* 1987;4:27–53.

4. Ojemann G, Ojemann J, Lettich E, Berger M. Cortical language localization in left, dominant hemisphere: An electrical stimulation mapping investigation in 117 patients. *J Neurosurg.* 1989;71:316–326.

5. Pardo JV, Fox PT. Preoperative assessment of the cerebral hemispheric dominance for language with CBF PET. *Hum Brain Mapp.* 1993;1:57–68.

6. Breier JI, Simos PG, Zouridakis G, Wheless JW, Willmore LJ, Constantinou JE, et al. Language dominance determined by magnetic source imaging: a comparison with the Wada procedure. *Neurology.* 1999;53:938–945.

7. Binder JR, Swanson SJ, Hammeke TA, Morris GL, Mueller WM, Fischer M, et al. Determination of language dominance using functional MRI: A comparison with the Wada test. *Neurology.* 1996;46:978–984.

8. Desmond JE, Sum JM, Wagner AD, Demb JB, Shear PK, Glover GH, et al. Functional MRI measurement of language lateralization in Wada-tested patients. *Brain.* 1995;118:1411–1419.

9. Bahn MM, Lin W, Silbergeld DL, Miller JW, Kuppusamy K, Cook RJ, et al. Localization of language cortices by functional MR imaging compared with intracarotid amobarbital hemispheric sedation. *Am J Radiol.* 1997;169: 575–579.

10. Hertz-Pannier L, Gaillard WD, Mott S, Cuenod CA, Bookheimer S, Weinstein S, et al. Noninvasive assessment of language dominance in children and adolescents with functional MRI: a preliminary study. *Neurology.* 1997;48: 1003–1012.

11. Worthington C, Vincent DJ, Bryant AE, Roberts DR, Vera CL, Ross DA, et al. Comparison of functional magnetic resonance imaging for language localization and intracarotid speech amytal testing in presurgical evaluation for intractable epilepsy. *Stereotact Funct Neurosurg.* 1997;69:197–201.

12. Benbadis SR, Binder JR, Swanson SJ, Fischer M, Hammeke TA, Morris GL, et al. Is speech arrest during Wada testing a valid method for determining hemispheric representation of language? *Brain Lang.* 1998;65:441–446.

13. Yetkin FZ, Swanson S, Fischer M, Akansel G, Morris G, Mueller W, et al. Functional MR of frontal lobe activation: Comparison with Wada language results. *Am J Neuroradiol.* 1998;19:1095–1098.

14. Benson RR, FitzGerald DB, LeSeuer LL, Kennedy DN, Kwong KK, Buchbinder BR, et al. Language dominance determined by whole brain functional MRI in patients with brain lesions. *Neurology.* 1999;52:798–809.

15. Hirsch J, Ruge MI, K.H.S. K, Correa DD, Victor JD, Relkin NR, et al. An integrated functional magnetic resonance imaging procedure for preoperative mapping of cortical areas associated with tactile, motor, language, and visual functions. *Neurosurgery.* 2000;47:711–722.

16. Lehéricy S, Cohen L, Bazin B, Samson S, Giacomini E, Rougetet R, et al. Functional MR evaluation of temporal and frontal language dominance compared with the Wada test. *Neurology.* 2000;54:1625–1633.

17. Spreer J, Quiske A, Altenmüller DM, Arnold S, Schulze-Bonhage A, Steinhoff BJ, et al. Unsuspected atypical hemispheric dominance for language as determined by fMRI. *Epilepsia.* 2001;52:957–959.

18. Liégois F, Connelly A, Salmond CH, Gadian DG, Vargha-Khadem F, Baldeweg T. A direct test for lateralization of language activation using fMRI: Comparison with invasive assessments in children with epilepsy. *Neuroimage.* 2002;17: 1861–1867.

19. Spreer J, Arnold S, Quiske A, Ziyeh S, Altenmüller DM, Herpers M, et al. Determination of hemisphere dominance for language: comparison of frontal and temporal fMRI activation with intracarotid amytal testing. *Neuroradiology.* 2002;44:467–474.

20. Adcock JE, Wise RG, Oxbury JM, Oxbury SM, Matthews PM. Quantitative fMRI assessment of the differences in lateralization of language-related brain activation in patients with temporal lobe epilepsy. *Neuroimage.* 2003;18:423–438.
21. Sabbah P, Chassoux F, Leveque C, Landre E, Baudoin-Chial S, Devaux B, et al. Functional MR imaging in assessment of language dominance in epileptic patients. *Neuroimage.* 2003;18:460–467.
22. Rutten G-J, Ramsey N, van Rijen P, Alpherts W, van Veelen C. fMRI-determined language lateralization in patients with unilateral or mixed language dominance according to the Wada test. *Neuroimage.* 2002;17:447–460.
23. Fitzgerald DB, Cosgrove GR, Ronner S, Jiang H, Buchbinder BR, Belliveau JW, et al. Location of language in the cortex: A comparison between functional MR imaging and electrocortical stimulation. *Am J Neuroradiol.* 1997;18:1529–1539.
24. Stapleton SR, Kiriakipoulos E, Mikulis D, Drake JM, Hoffman HJ, Humphreys R, et al. Combined utility of functional MRI, cortical mapping, and frameless stereotaxy in the resection of lesions in eloquent areas of brain in children. *Pediatr Neurosurg.* 1997;26:68–82.
25. Yetkin FZ, Mueller WM, Morris GL, McAuliffe TL, Ulmer JL, Cox RW, et al. Functional MR activation correlated with intraoperative cortical mapping. *Am J Neuroradiol.* 1997;18:1311–1315.
26. Ruge MI, Victor JD, Hosain S, Correa DD, Relkin NR, Tabar V, et al. Concordance between functional magnetic resonance imaging and intraoperative language mapping. *Stereotact Funct Neurosurg.* 1999;72:95–102.
27. Schlosser MJ, Luby M, Spencer DD, Awad IA, McCarthy G. Comparative localization of auditory comprehension by using functional magnetic resonance imaging and cortical stimulation. *J Neurosurg.* 1999;91:626–635.
28. Lurito JT, Lowe MJ, Sartorius C, Mathews VP. Comparison of fMRI and intraoperative direct cortical stimulation in localization of receptive language areas. *J Comput Assist Tomogr.* 2000;24:99–105.
29. Rutten GJM, van Rijen PC, van Veelen CWM, Ramsey NF. Language area localization with three-dimensional functional magnetic resonance imaging matches intrasulcal electrostimulation in Broca's area. *Ann Neurol.* 1999;46:405–408.
30. Rutten GJM, Ramsey NF, van Rijen PC, Noordmans HJ, van Veelen CW. Development of a functional magnetic resonance imaging protocol for intraoperative localization of critical temporoparietal language areas. *Ann Neurol.* 2002;51:350–360.
31. Rutten GJ, Ramsey N, van Rijen P, van Veelen C. Reproducibility of fMRI-determined language lateralization in individual subjects. *Brain Lang.* 2002;80:421–437.
32. Sabsevitz DS, Swanson SJ, Hammeke TA, Spanaki MV, Possing ET, Morris GL, et al. Use of preoperative functional neuroimaging to predict language deficits from epilepsy surgery. *Neurology.* 2003;60:1788–1792.
33. Binder J. FMRI: Language mapping. *Neurosurg Clin N Am.* 1997;8:383–392.
34. Gaillard WD, Theodore WH. Mapping language in epilepsy with functional neuroimaging. *Neuroscientist.* 2000;6:391–401.
35. Hammeke TA, Bellgowan PSF, Binder JR. FMRI methodology: Cognitive function mapping. *Adv Neurol.* 2000;83:221–233.
36. Detre JA, Floyd TF. Functional MRi and its applications to the clinical neurosciences. *Neuroscientist.* 2001;7:64–79.
37. Binder JR, Achten E, Constable RT, Detre JA, Gaillard WD, Jack CR, et al. Functional MRI in epilepsy. *Epilepsia.* 2002;43(Suppl 1):51–63.
38. Carpentier A, Pugh KR, Westerveld M, et al. Functional MRI of language processing: dependence on input modality and temporal lobe epilepsy. *Epilepsia.* 2001;42:1241–1254.
39. Fernández G, Specht K, Weis S, Tendolkar I, Reuber M, Fell J, et al. Intrasubject reproducibility of presurgical language lateralization and mapping using fMRI. *Neurology.* 2003;60:969–975.

40. Kertesz A, Harlock W, Coates R. Computer tomographic localization, lesion size, and prognosis in aphasia and nonverbal impairment. *Brain Lang.* 1979;8: 34–50.

41. Porch BE, Collins M, Wertz RT, Friden TP. Statistical prediction of change in aphasia. *J Speech Hear Res.* 1980;23:312–321.

42. Selnes OA, Knopman DS, Niccum N, Rubens AB, Larson D. Computed tomographic scan correlates of auditory comprehension deficits in aphasia: A prospective recovery study. *Ann Neurol.* 1983;13:558–566.

43. Metter EJ, Jackson CA, Kempler D, Hanson WR. Temporoparietal cortex and the recovery of language comprehension in aphasia. *Aphasiology.* 1992;6:349–358.

44. Ferro JM. The influence of infarct location on recovery from global aphasia. *Aphasiology.* 1992;6:415–430.

45. Code C, Rowley D, Kertesz A. Predicting recovery from aphasia with connectionist networks: Preliminary comparisons with multiple regression. *Cortex.* 1994;30:527–532.

46. Karbe H, Kessler J, Herholz K, Fink GR, Heiss W-D. Long-term prognosis of poststroke aphasia studied with positron emission tomography. *Arch Neurol.* 1995;52:186–190.

47. Pedersen PM, Jorgensen HS, Nakayama H, Raaschou HO, Olsen TS. Aphasia in acute stroke: Incidence, determinants, and recovery. *Ann Neurol.* 1995;38: 659–666.

48. Cao Y, Vikingstad BS, George PK, Johnson AF, Welch KMA. Cortical language activation in stroke patients recovering from aphasia with functional MRI. *Stroke.* 1999;30:2331–2340.

49. Thulborn KR, Carpenter PA, Just MA. Plasticity of language-related brain function during recovery from stroke. *Stroke.* 1999;30:749–754.

50. Calvert GA, Brammer MJ, Morris RG, Williams SCR, King N, Matthews PM. Using fMRI to study recovery from acquired dysphasia. *Brain Lang.* 2000;71: 391–399.

51. Rosen HJ, Petersen SE, Linenweber MR, Snyder AZ, White DA, Chapman L, et al. Neural correlates of recovery from aphasia after damage to left inferior frontal cortex. *Neurology.* 2000;55:1883–1894.

52. Eden GF, VanMeter JW, Rumsey JM, Maisog JM, Woods RP, Zeffiro TA. Abnormal processing of visual motion in dyslexia revealed by functional brain imaging. *Nature.* 1996;382:66–69.

53. Demb JB, Boynton GM, Heeger DJ. Brain activity in visual cortex predicts individual differences in reading performance. *PNAS.* 1997;94:13363–13366.

54. Shaywitz SE, Shaywitz BA, Pugh KR, Fulbright RK, Constable RT, Mencl WE, et al. Functional disruption in the organization of the brain for reading in dyslexia. *PNAS.* 1998;95:2636–2641.

55. Temple E, Deutsch GK, Poldrack RA, Miller SL, Tallal P, Merzenich MM, et al. Neural deficits in children with dyslexia ameliorated by behavioral remediation: Evidence from functional MRI. *PNAS.* 2003;100:2860–2865.

56. Petersen SE, Fox PT, Posner MI, Mintun M, Raichle ME. Positron emission tomographic studies of the cortical anatomy of single-word processing. *Nature.* 1988;331:585–589.

57. Wise R, Chollet F, Hadar U, Friston K, Hoffner E, Frackowiak R. Distribution of cortical neural networks involved in word comprehension and word retrieval. *Brain.* 1991;114:1803–1817.

58. Démonet J-F, Chollet F, Ramsay S, Cardebat D, Nespoulous J-L, Wise R, et al. The anatomy of phonological and semantic processing in normal subjects. *Brain.* 1992;115:1753–1768.

59. Binder JR, Price CJ. Functional imaging of language. In: Cabeza R, Kingstone A, editors. *Handbook of Functional Neuroimaging of Cognition.* Cambridge, MA: MIT Press; 2001:187–251.

60. Macleod CM. Half a century of research on the Stroop effect: an integrative review. *Psychol Bull.* 1991;109:163–203.
61. Reicher GM. Perceptual recognition as a function of meaningfulness of stimulus material. *J Exp Psychol.* 1969;81:274–280.
62. Warren RM, Obusek CJ. Speech perception and phonemic restorations. *Percept Psychophys.* 1971;9:358–362.
63. Ganong WF. Phonetic categorization in auditory word perception. *J Exp Psychol Hum Percept Perform.* 1980;6:110–115.
64. Marslen-Wilson WD, Tyler LK. Central processes in speech understanding. *Philos Trans R Soc London B Biol Sci.* 1981;295:317–332.
65. Carr TH, McCauley C, Sperber RD, Parmalee CM. Words, pictures, and priming: On semantic activation, conscious identification, and the automaticity of information processing. *J Exp Psychol Hum Percept Perform.* 1982;8:757–777.
66. Marcel AJ. Conscious and unconscious perception: Experiments on visual masking and word recognition. *Cognit Psychol.* 1983;15:197–237.
67. Van Orden GC. A ROWS is a ROSE: Spelling, sound, and reading. *Mem Cognit.* 1987;15:181–198.
68. Burton MW, Baum SR, Blumstein SE. Lexical effects on phonetic categorization of speech: The role of acoustic structure. *J Exp Psychol Hum Percept Perform.* 1989;15:567–575.
69. Glaser WR. Picture naming. *Cognition.* 1992;42:61–105.
70. Raichle ME, Fiez JA, Videen TO, MacLeod AM, Pardo JV, Fox PT, et al. Practice-related changes in human brain functional anatomy during nonmotor learning. *Cereb Cortex.* 1994;4:8–26.
71. Buckner RL, Raichle ME, Petersen SE. Dissociation of human prefrontal cortical areas across different speech production tasks and gender groups. *J Neurosci.* 1995;74:2163–2173.
72. Bookheimer SY, Zeffiro TA, Blaxton T, Gaillard T, Theodore W. Regional cerebral blood flow during object naming and word reading. *Hum Brain Mapp.* 1995;3:93–106.
73. Price CJ, Wise RSJ, Frackowiak RSJ. Demonstrating the implicit processing of visually presented words and pseudowords. *Cereb Cortex.* 1996;6:62–70.
74. Damasio H, Grabowski TJ, Tranel D, Hichwa RD, Damasio AR. A neural basis for lexical retrieval. *Nature.* 1996;380:499–505.
75. Binder JR, Frost JA, Hammeke TA, Cox RW, Rao SM, Prieto T. Human brain language areas identified by functional MRI. *J Neurosci.* 1997;17:353–362.
76. James W. *Principles of Psychology*, vol. 1. New York: Dover Publications; 1890.
77. Hebb DO. The problem of consciousness and introspection. In: Adrian ED, Bremer F, Jasper HH, editors. *Brain Mechanisms and Consciousness: A Symposium.* Springfield, IL: Charles C. Thomas; 1954:402–421.
78. Miller GA, Galanter E, Pribram K. *Plans and the Structure of Behavior.* New York: Holt; 1960.
79. Pope KS, Singer JL. Regulation of the stream of consciousness: Toward a theory of ongoing thought. In: Schwartz GE, Shapiro D, editors. *Consciousness and Self-Regulation.* New York: Plenum Press; 1976:101–135.
80. Antrobus JS, Singer JL, Greenberg S. Studies in the stream of consciousness: Experimental enhancement and suppression of spontaneous cognitive processes. *Percept Mot Skills.* 1966;23:399–417.
81. Teasdale JD, Proctor L, Lloyd CA, Baddeley AD. Working memory and stimulus-independent thought: Effects of memory load and presentation rate. *Eur J Cogn Psychol.* 1993;5:417–433.
82. Révész G, editor. *Thinking and Speaking: A symposium.* Amsterdam: North Holland Publishing; 1954.
83. Weiskrantz L, editor. *Thought without Language.* Oxford: Clarendon; 1988.
84. Vygotsky LS. *Thought and Language.* New York: Wiley; 1962.

85. Karmiloff-Smith A. *Beyond Modularity: A Developmental Perspective on Cognitive Science*. Cambridge, MA: MIT Press; 1992.

86. Andreasen NC, O'Leary DS, Cizadlo T, Arndt S, Rezai K, Watkins GL, et al. Remembering the past: Two facets of episodic memory explored with positron emission tomography. Am J Psychiatry. 1995;152:1576–1585.

87. Shulman GL, Fiez JA, Corbetta M, Buckner RL, Meizin FM, Raichle ME, et al.y Common blood flow changes across visual tasks: II. Decreases in cerebral cortex. J Cogn Neurosci. 1997;9:648–663.

88. Binder JR, Frost JA, Hammeke TA, Bellgowan PSF, Rao SM, Cox RW. Conceptual processing during the conscious resting state: a functional MRI study. J Cogn Neurosci. 1999;11:80–93.

89. Mazoyer B, Zago L, Mellet E, Bricogne S, Etard O, Houdé O, et al. Cortical networks for working memory and executive functions sustain the conscious resting state in man. Brain Res Bull. 2001;54:287–298.

90. Raichle ME, McLeod AM, Snyder AZ, Powers WJ, Gusnard DA, Shulman GL. A default mode of brain function. PNAS. 2001;98:676–682.

91. Stark CE, Squire LR. When zero is not zero: The problem of ambiguous baseline conditions in fMRI. PNAS. 2001;98:12760–12766.

92. McKiernan KA, Kaufman JN, Kucera-Thompson J, Binder JR. A parametric manipulation of factors affecting task-induced deactivation in functional neuroimaging. J Cogn Neurosci. 2003;15:394–408.

93. Grabowski TJ, Damasio AR. Investigating language with functional neuroimaging. In: Toga AW, Mazziotta JC, editors. Brain Mapping: The Systems. San Diego, CA: Academic Press; 2000:425–461.

94. Binder JR. Wernicke aphasia: A disorder of central language processing. In: D'Esposito ME, editor. Neurological Foundations of Cognitive Neuroscience. Cambridge, MA: MIT Press; 2002:175–238.

95. Binder JR, Frost JA, Hammeke TA, Bellgowan PSF, Springer JA, Kaufman JN, et al. Human temporal lobe activation by speech and nonspeech sounds. Cereb Cortex. 2000;10:512–528.

96. Scott SK, Blank C, Rosen S, Wise RJS. Identification of a pathway for intelligible speech in the left temporal lobe. Brain. 2000;123:2400–2406.

97. Liebenthal E, Binder JR, Piorkowski RL, Remez RE. Short-term reorganization of auditory analysis induced by phonetic experience. *J Cogn Neurosci.* 2003;15:549–558.

98. Belin P, Zatorre RJ, Ahad P. Human temporal-lobe response to vocal sounds. *Cogn Brain Res.* 2002;13:17–26.

99. Cohen L, Lehéricy S, Chochon F, Lemer C, Rivaud S, Dehaene S. Language-specific tuning of visual cortex? Functional properties of the visual word form area. *Brain.* 2002;125:1054–1069.

100. Wise RSJ, Scott SK, Blank SC, Mummery CJ, Murphy K, Warburton EA. Separate neural subsystems within "Wernicke's area". *Brain.* 2001;124:83–95.

101. Mazoyer BM, Tzourio N, Frak V, Syrota A, Murayama N, Levrier O, et al. The cortical representation of speech. *J Cogn Neurosci.* 1993;5:467–479.

102. Price CJ, Wise RJS, Warburton EA, Moore CJ, Howard D, Patterson K, et al. Hearing and saying. The functional neuro-anatomy of auditory word processing. *Brain.* 1996;119:919–931.

103. Zatorre RJ, Evans AC, Meyer E, Gjedde A. Lateralization of phonetic and pitch discrimination in speech processing. *Science.* 1992;256:846–849.

104. Mummery CJ, Ashburner J, Scott SK, Wise RJS. Functional neuroimaging of speech perception in six normal and two aphasic subjects. *J Acoust Soc Am.* 1999;106:449–457.

105. Belin P, Zatorre RJ, Lafaille P, Ahad P, Pike B. Voice-selective areas in human auditory cortex. *Nature.* 2000;403:309–312.

106. Binder JR, Rao SM, Hammeke TA, Frost JA, Bandettini PA, Hyde JS. Effects of stimulus rate on signal response during functional magnetic resonance imaging of auditory cortex. *Cogn Brain Res.* 1994;2:31–38.

107. Eulitz C, Elbert T, Bartenstein P, Weiller C, Müller SP, Pantev C. Comparison of magnetic and metabolic brain activity during a verb generation task. *Neuroreport*. 1994;6:97–100.
108. Warburton E, Wise RJS, Price CJ, Weiller C, Hadar U, Ramsay S, et al. Noun and verb retrieval by normal subjects. Studies with PET. *Brain*. 1996;119:159–179.
109. Ojemann JG, Buckner RL, Akbudak E, Snyder AZ, Ollinger JM, McKinstry RC, et al. Functional MRI studies of word-stem completion: Reliability across laboratories and comparison to blood flow imaging with PET. *Hum Brain Mapp*. 1998;6:203–215.
110. Palmer ED, Rosen HJ, Ojemann JG, Buckner RL, Kelley WM, Petersen SE. An event-related fMRI study of overt and covert word stem completion. *Neuroimage*. 2001;14:182–193.
111. Thompson-Schill SL, D'Esposito M, Kan IP. Effects of repetition and competition on activity in left prefrontal cortex during word generation. *Neuron*. 1999;23:513–522.
112. Malach R, Reppas JB, Benson RR, Kwong KK, Jiang H, Kennedy WA, et al. Object-related activity revealed by functional magnetic resonance imaging in human occipital cortex. *PNAS*. 1995;92:8135–8139.
113. Kanwisher N, Woods R, Iacoboni M, Mazziotta J. A locus in human extrastriate cortex for visual shape analysis. *J Cogn Neurosci*. 1996;91:133–142.
114. Grill-Spector K, Kushnir T, Edelman S, Avidian-Carmel G, Itzchak Y, Malach R. Differential processing of objects under various viewing conditions in the human lateral occipital complex. *Neuron*. 1999;24:187–203.
115. Martin A, Wiggs CL, Ungerleider LG, Haxby JV. Neural correlates of category-specific knowledge. *Nature*. 1996;379:649–652.
116. Price CJ, Moore CJ, Humphreys GW, Frackowiak RSJ, Friston KJ. The neural regions sustaining object recognition and naming. *Proc R Soc London B*. 1996;263:1501–1507.
117. Zelkowicz BJ, Herbster AN, Nebes RD, Mintun MA, Becker JT. An examination of regional cerebral blood flow during object naming tasks. *J Int Neuropsychol Soc*. 1998;4:160–166.
118. Murtha S, Chertkow H, Beauregard M, Evans A. The neural substrate of picture naming. *J Cogn Neurosci*. 1999;11:399–423.
119. Kiasawa M, Inoue C, Kawasaki T, Tokoro T, Ishii K, Ohyama M, et al. Functional neuroanatomy of object naming: A PET study. *Graefes Arch Clin Exp Ophthalmol*. 1996;234:110–115.
120. Vandenberghe R, Price C, Wise R, Josephs O, Frackowiak RSJ. Functional anatomy of a common semantic system for words and pictures. *Nature*. 1996;383:254–256.
121. Müller R-A, Kleinhans N, Courchesne E. Linguistic theory and neuroimaging evidence: an fMRI study of Broca's area in lexical semantics. *Neuropsychologia*. In press.
122. Price CJ, Moore CJ, Humphreys GW, Wise RJS. Segregating semantic from phonological processes during reading. *J Cogn Neurosci*. 1997;9:727–733.
123. Mummery CJ, Patterson K, Hodges JR, Price CJ. Functional neuroanatomy of the semantic system: divisible by what? *J Cogn Neurosci*. 1998;10:766–777.
124. Chee MWL, O'Craven KM, Bergida R, Rosen BR, Savoy RL. Auditory and visual word processing studied with fMRI. *Hum Brain Mapp*. 1999;7:15–28.
125. Roskies AL, Fiez JA, Balota DA, Raichle ME, Petersen SE. Task-dependent modulation of regions in the left inferior frontal cortex during semantic processing. *J Cogn Neurosci*. 2001;13:829–843.
126. Bavelier D, Corina D, Jezzard P, Padmanabhan S, Clark VP, Karni A, et al. Sentence reading: a functional MRI study at 4 tesla. *J Cogn Neurosci*. 1997;9:664–686.
127. Herbster AN, Mintun MA, Nebes RD, Becker JT. Regional cerebral blood flow during word and nonword reading. *Hum Brain Mapp*. 1997;5:84–92.

128. Indefrey P, Kleinschmidt A, Merboldt K-D, Krüger G, Brown C, Hagoort P, et al. Equivalent responses to lexical and nonlexical visual stimuli in occipital cortex: a functional magnetic resonance imaging study. *Neuroimage.* 1997;5: 78–81.

129. Chee MW, Caplan D, Soon CS, Sriram N, Tan EWL, Thiel T, et al. Processing of visually presented sentences in Mandarin and English studied with fMRI. *Neuron.* 1999;23:127–137.

130. Pugh KR, Shaywitz BA, Shaywitz SE, Constable RT, Skudlarski P, Fulbright RK, et al. Cerebral organization of component processes in reading. *Brain.* 1996;119:1221–1238.

131. Springer JA, Binder JR, Hammeke TA, Swanson SJ, Frost JA, Bellgowan PSF, et al. Language dominance in neurologically normal and epilepsy subjects: a functional MRI study. *Brain.* 1999;122:2033–2045.

132. Pujol J, Deus J, Losilla JM, Capdevila A. Cerebral lateralization of language in normal left-handed people studied by functional MRI. *Neurology.* 1999;52: 1038–1043.

133. Vikingstad EM, George KP, Johnson AF, Cao Y. Cortical language lateralization in right handed normal subjects using functional magnetic resonance imaging. *J Neurol Sci.* 2000;175:17–27.

134. Szaflarski JP, Binder JR, Possing ET, McKiernan KA, Ward DB, Hammeke TA. Language lateralization in left-handed and ambidextrous people: fMRI data. *Neurology.* 2002;59:238–244.

135. Hund-Georgiadis M, Lex U, Friederici AD, von Cramon DY. Noninvasive regime for language lateralization in right- and left-handers by means of functional MRI and dichotic listening. *Exp Brain Res.* 2002;145:166–176.

136. Knecht S, Deppe M, Dräger B, Bobe L, Lohmann H, Ringelstein EB, et al. Language lateralization in healthy right-handers. *Brain.* 2000;123:74–81.

137. Shaywitz BA, Shaywitz SE, Pugh KR, Constable RT, Skudlarski P, Fulbright RK, et al. Sex differences in the functional organization of the brain for language. *Nature.* 1995;373:607–609.

138. Price CJ, Moore CJ, Friston KJ. Getting sex into perspective. *Neuroimage.* 1996;3:S586.

139. Frost JA, Binder JR, Springer JA, Hammeke TA, Bellgowan PSF, Rao SM, et al. Language processing is strongly left lateralized in both sexes: Evidence from FMRI. *Brain.* 1999;122:199–208.

140. Knecht S, Dräger B, Deppe M, Bobe L, Lohmann H, Flöel A, et al. Handedness and hemispheric language dominance in healthy humans. *Brain.* 2000;123: 2512–2518.

141. Rasmussen T, Milner B. The role of early left-brain injury in determining lateralization of cerebral speech functions. *Ann N Y Acad Sci.* 1977;299:355–369.

142. Loring DW, Meador KJ, Lee GP, Murro AM, Smith JR, Flanigin HF, et al. Cerebral language lateralization: Evidence from intracarotid amobarbital testing. *Neuropsychologia.* 1990;28:831–838.

143. Grady CL, Maisog JM, Horwitz B, et al. Age-related changes in cortical blood flow activation during visual processing of faces and location. *J Neurosci.* 1994;14:1450–1462.

144. Grady CL, McIntosh AR, Bookstein F, Horwitz B, Rapoport SI, Haxby JV. Age-related changes in regional cerebral blood flow during working memory for faces. *Neuroimage.* 1998;8:409–425.

145. Woods RP, Dodrill CB, Ojemann GA. Brain injury, handedness, and speech lateralization in a series of amobarbital studies. *Ann Neurol.* 1988;23:510–518.

146. Risse GL, Gates JR, Fangman MC. A reconsideration of bilateral language representation based on the intracarotid amobarbital procedure. *Brain Lang.* 1997;33:118–132.

147. Binder JR, Rao SM, Hammeke TA, Frost JA, Bandettini PA, Jesmanowicz A, et al. Lateralized human brain language systems demonstrated by task subtraction functional magnetic resonance imaging. *Arch Neurol.* 1995;52:593–601.

148. Cohen MS, Dubois RM. Stability, repeatability, and the expression of signal magnitude in functional magnetic resonance imaging. *J Magn Reson Imaging.* 1999;10:33–40.

149. Binder JR, Hammeke TA, Possing ET, Swanson SJ, Spanaki MV, Morris GL, et al. Reliability and validity of language dominance assessment with functional MRI. *Neurology.* 2001;56 (Suppl 3):A158.

150. Xiong J, Rao S, Gao JH, Woldorff M, Fox PT. Evaluation of hemispheric dominance for language using functional MRI: a comparison with positron emission tomography. *Hum Brain Mapp.* 1998;6:42–58.

151. Altenmüller DM, Kriechbaum W, Helber U, Moini S, Dichgans J, Petersen D. Cortical DC-potentials in identification of the language dominant hemisphere: linguistical and clinical aspects. *Acta Neurochir (Wien).* 1993;56 (Suppl.):20–33.

152. Khedr EM, Hamed E, Said A, Basahi J. Handedness and language cerebral lateralization. *Eur J Appl Physiol.* 2002;87:469–473.

153. Deppe M, Knecht S, Papke K, Lohmann H, Fleischer H, Heindel W, et al. Assessment of hemispheric language lateralization: A comparison between fMRI and fTCD. *J Cereb Blood Flow Metab.* 2000;20:263–268.

154. Foundas AL, Leonard CM, Gilmore R, Fennell E, Heilman KM. Planum temporale asymmetry and language dominance. *Neuropsychologia.* 1994;32:1225–1231.

155. Chelune GJ. Using neuropsychological data to forecast postsurgical cognitive outcome. In: Lüders H, editor. *Epilepsy Surgery.* New York: Raven Press;1991:477–485.

156. Schwartz TH, Devinsky O, Doyle W, Perrine K. Preoperative predictors of anterior temporal language areas. *J Neurosurg.* 1998;89:962–970.

157. Hermann BP, Perrine K, Chelune GJ, Barr W, Loring DW, Strauss E, et al. Visual confrontation naming following left anterior temporal lobectomy: A comparison of surgical approaches. *Neuropsychology.* 1999;13:3–9.

158. Grabowski TJ, Damasio H, Tranel D, Ponto LL, Hichwa RD, Damasio AR. A role for left temporal pole in the retrieval of words for unique entities. *Hum Brain Mapp.* 2001;13:199–212.

159. Hamberger MJ, Goodman RR, Perrine K, Tamny TR. Anatomic dissociation of auditory and visual naming in the lateral temporal cortex. *Neurology.* 2001;56:56–61.

160. Hermann BP, Wyler AR, Somes G, Clement L. Dysnomia after left anterior temporal lobectomy without functional mapping: frequency and correlates. *Neurosurgery.* 1994;35:52–57.

161. Langfit JT, Rausch R. Word-finding deficits persist after left anterotemporal lobectomy. *Arch Neurol.* 1996;53:72–76.

162. Davies KG, Bell BD, Bush AJ, Hermann BP, Dohan FC, Jaap AS. Naming decline after left anterior temporal lobectomy correlates with pathological status of resected hippocampus. *Epilepsia.* 1998;39:407–419.

163. Bell BD, Davies KG, Hermann BP, Walters G. Confrontation naming after anterior temporal lobectomy is related to age of acquisition of the object names. *Neuropsychologia.* 2000;38:83–92.

9

fMRI Wada Test: Prospects for Presurgical Mapping of Language and Memory

Brenna C. McDonald, Andrew J. Saykin, J. Michael Williams, and Bassam A. Assaf

Introduction

Since the inception of functional magnetic resonance imaging (fMRI) in the early 1990s, clinicians and researchers have been interested in the potential utility of this technology for replacement of the intracarotid amobarbital test (IAT). The IAT, or Wada test, is an invasive angiographic procedure, with some potential risks, that currently serves as the conventional standard for lateralization of language, memory, and other functions. The IAT is used primarily in patients under consideration for neurosurgery to treat epilepsy, but also in other neurosurgical populations (e.g., motor cortex tumor, arteriovenous malformation in language association cortex, etc.). If a valid assessment paradigm could be created, the advantages of fMRI assessment of memory and language functions over the IAT would be obvious. Functional MRI is a repeatable, noninvasive procedure with no significant known health risks for most individuals. It is also very flexible and can be readily modified to assess the clinical questions at issue for a particular patient. In addition, a recent cost analysis demonstrated considerable savings of total direct costs for fMRI over IAT.[1]

While some patients (e.g., those with ferromagnetic metal in their bodies, or those who are moderately or severely claustrophobic) may be unable or ineligible to undergo fMRI, the number of those who meet these exclusion criteria is no greater than for the IAT. Furthermore, while the IAT can provide information regarding predominant hemispheric lateralization of language functions and, to a lesser degree, memory, it cannot provide information regarding the spatial location of brain regions critical for these tasks. In contrast, fMRI, with typical spatial resolution of two to four millimeters, can provide much more precise information regarding localization of brain regions that are active during memory and language tasks.

This chapter previously appeared in *Functional MRI: Basic Principles and Clinical Applications*, edited by S. Faro and F. Mohamed. New York: Springer Science+Business Media, LCC 2006.

From: *BOLD fMRI: A Guide to Functional Imaging for Neuroscientists*
Edited by: S.H. Faro and F.B. Mohamed, DOI 10.1007/978-1-4419-1329-6_9
© Springer Science+Business Media, LLC 2010

Both the IAT and fMRI are possible techniques for representing the location of important cognitive functions that are considered as part of surgery planning. The IAT was invented first and has a long history of use, and therefore has become the gold standard to which fMRI language and memory localization paradigms are compared. Many basic aspects of the IAT's validity and reliability have not been systematically investigated, however, due to the nature of the procedure and the lack of alternative techniques available for this purpose. The present chapter stresses the contrast between the testing methods. It is clear, however, that the same standards of measurement should be applied to both tests. For example, it is possible that both techniques adequately measure the lateralization of language. In contrast, both techniques may not adequately assess the location of memory abilities. The strong focus of the research literature and other discussions has been on replacing the IAT with fMRI, which, if possible, would be a worthy goal, given factors noted throughout this chapter, including the increased time, risk, and cost of the IAT. However, this focus may at times overlook basic measurement issues that apply to both techniques; in the end, the overarching goal is clearly to obtain the most reliable and valid data possible to meet the stated need of localization of language and memory functions.

The conclusions of several studies conducted over the past decade strongly suggest that fMRI paradigms exist that can be used successfully to replace the IAT in terms of language lateralization, although the status of appropriately reliable and valid memory assessment paradigms remains uncertain. Despite the apparent advantages of fMRI in such presurgical assessment, there remain methodological challenges and issues of interpretation that have thus far prevented its widespread use in place of the IAT. This chapter will briefly discuss the background of the IAT and its risks and benefits compared to fMRI. The current status of fMRI protocols aiming to replace the IAT will then be reviewed, along with future steps needed to make this goal a reality.

The IAT: History and Background

As noted by other authors,[2,3] the first use of selective anesthetization to localize human language function was reported by Gardner in 1941.[4] Gardner utilized intracranial injection of procaine hydrochloride to unilaterally anesthetize frontal brain regions in two left-handed brain tumor patients in order to assess lateralization of hemispheric dominance for language prior to resective surgery and prevent surgically induced aphasia. The model for modern IAT procedures, however, is the work of Juhn Wada,[5] who established the feasibility of selective hemispheric anesthetization using intracarotid injection of sodium amytal.

Wada's original work in the 1940s was designed to attempt to minimize the cognitive side effects of electroconvulsive shock therapy (ECT) by preventing bilateral generalization of ECT-related seizure activity through temporary anesthetization of the language-dominant hemisphere.[3] The utility of this technique for presurgical evaluation of epilepsy quickly became apparent, and Wada pioneered this approach both in Japan and later with colleagues at the Montreal Neurological Institute. While significant variations can currently be encountered across surgical epilepsy centers in terms of IAT procedures, several standardized methodologies have been published,[2,6,7] and the IAT is considered a critical component of presurgical evaluation of patients with epilepsy, along with clinical neuropsychological assessment, which is important for providing a context within which to interpret IAT results.[8–11] The IAT may also be used much as Gardner originally proposed, to assess the lateralized integrity of cognition prior to resection of nonepileptogenic lesions located in frontal or temporal cortex presumed to be critical to language and/or memory functions.

The need for lateralization and localization of cognitive functions such as language and memory is self-evident. For patients under consideration for resective surgery to treat medically refractory seizures, particularly in the case of temporal lobe epilepsy (TLE), the seizure focus likely to be resected includes brain regions potentially critical to the support of language and memory. It therefore becomes vital to provide as much information as possible regarding the potential deficits that might occur as a result of surgery, should the seizure focus (e.g., a sclerotic hippocampus) also be supporting one or more critical cognitive functions.

For patients whose presumed seizure focus lies adjacent to or within language cortex, detailed presurgical localization of eloquent tissue is needed to assess the feasibility of surgery and define the potential resection margin. The IAT typically is used for hemispheric lateralization of language functioning, while intracranial electrical stimulation can provide more precise mapping of language cortex, either prior to or during epilepsy surgery. While the left hemisphere is the dominant hemisphere for language in virtually all healthy right-handed individuals, the neurodevelopmental abnormalities that can be associated with epilepsy make atypical lateralization or bilateral participation in language more likely in epileptic patients.[12–16] For left-handed individuals, the issue of hemispheric language dominance becomes even more salient given the increased prevalence of right hemisphere dominance for language in left-handed individuals, which has been demonstrated using fMRI.[17,18] In addition, many fMRI studies show some degree of bilateral activation even in right-handed subjects from normal as well as clinical samples,[19–23] although most language-related activation is observed in the dominant hemisphere. Such nondominant hemisphere activation may relate to linguistic task complexity or to nonverbal aspects of language, such as prosody, narrative organization, inference, or language pragmatics.[24–31]

Assessment of hemispheric support of memory functioning is particularly important in TLE patients given the critical role of mesial temporal lobe (MTL) structures, including the hippocampus, entorhinal cortex, and amygdala, in encoding of new information. The IAT does not lateralize memory per se, but rather assesses the potential for unilateral hemispheric support of memory encoding, to prevent an iatrogenic postsurgical amnestic syndrome such as that exhibited in the classic case of patient H.M.[32] For TLE patients, the presence of mesial temporal sclerosis or other hippocampal disease may preclude effective support of memory functions by the region to be resected. Some patients, however, demonstrate memory functioning using the diseased hemisphere on IAT, indicating the potential for acquired postoperative cognitive deficits. This issue becomes even more of a concern in TLE patients with normal MRI scans, who may be more likely to have MTL tissue supporting memory in the presumed epileptogenic region.

Limitations in the use of the IAT include its invasive nature and attendant risk of potential medical complications, such as infarction, carotid artery dissection, potentiation of seizures, and adverse reaction to contrast or anesthetizing agents.[33,34] Surveys have indicated that such IAT morbidity is uncommon. For high-volume epilepsy centers, the typical risk of IAT-related complication is less than one percent.[35] Certain patient risk factors also can increase the risk of angiography, and therefore contraindicate use of the IAT; for example, individuals with significant vascular risk factors or other major medical problems may not be appropriate candidates for such a procedure. Additionally, very young children are also often not considered for IAT given the cognitive demands and medical risks involved in the test. Other limitations of the IAT include invalidation of studies due to aberrant vasculature (e.g., arteriovenous malformations) or to normal neurodevelopmental vascular variations, such as significant cortical crossflow. Given the short-acting nature of sodium amobarbital and the other drugs typically used to anesthetize the cerebral hemispheres, the IAT is a very time-sensitive procedure that can be invalidated by individual variation in sensitivity to sodium amobarbital (e.g., obtundation in some patients), as well as to related delays and nonstandardized administration of test stimuli. The IAT can also can be nondiagnostic due to failure to adequately lateralize language or memory functioning in a given individual. Finally, although some standardized IAT protocols are available,[2,6–8,35,36] comparison of IAT studies across epilepsy surgery centers can be challenging, as methodology and interpretation of the IAT procedure vary considerably from site to site. Efforts to standardize IAT administration across epilepsy centers are ongoing and may permit correlation with fMRI in larger samples in the future.

Description of a Standardized IAT Protocol

At Dartmouth–Hitchcock Medical Center (DHMC), a standardized IAT protocol is utilized that initially was developed at Graduate Hospital in Philadelphia.[7,36] The procedure is begun on the presumed side of surgery, then repeated on the contralateral side. A catheter is positioned under fluoroscopy into the internal carotid artery (ICA). Following cerebral angiography, the patient is available for cognitive testing. All patients receive studies ipsilateral and contralateral to the seizure focus on the same day with 30 to 45 minutes between injections. The neuropsychological protocol[36] was designed for rapid speech and memory assessment. Emphasis is placed on quantitative memory evaluation for verbal and nonverbal material and for material that can be encoded either verbally or nonverbally (common objects). This provides a continuum of verbal–nonverbal material for encoding. Two forms of equivalent task difficulty were developed by randomization of the original item pool. Our standard dosage is 125 milligrams of sodium amobarbital in five cubic centimeters of saline with slow hand injection over five seconds in each ICA, with injections separated by at least 30 minutes. Occasionally, it is necessary to titrate the dosage of sodium amobarbital up or down (usually in 25-milligram increments) to achieve the goal of unilateral anesthesia as indicated by hemiparesis or electroencephalogram (EEG) without causing global sedation or obtundation. Language testing begins immediately after injection until speech normalizes, and includes: (1) automatic speech (counting, recitation of the alphabet); (2) comprehension (following simple commands, Modified Token Test); (3) word and sentence repetition; (4) visual confrontation naming (3 objects); and (5) reading (three words). Memory testing commences about two minutes postinjection, and overlaps with the language protocol (naming and word reading). During the registration and encoding phase, the patient is shown three common objects (e.g., spoon, glove) one at a time and asked to name and remember them. Each stimulus is exposed for approximately five to ten seconds, with emphasis placed on ensuring that the patient is attending to the stimuli. Special care must be taken to present the stimuli in the intact visual field. The same procedure is followed for three low-imagery words (e.g., random, enough, prefer) and three abstract designs (after Kimura[37]). At ten minutes postinjection, if language and motor functioning have returned to baseline, the free and cued recall phase is begun. Progressively structured recall testing is initiated by asking the patient to recall "everything that you remember from the test." Responses are recorded verbatim. Cued recall is then initiated (e.g., "Did I show you any objects?"). Paper and felt-tip pen are provided for drawings of the abstract designs. During the recognition phase, the patient is shown a series of nine stimuli (separately for objects, words, and designs). Three of the nine are target stimuli and six are distractors, fixing the probability of a chance correct response at 33%. For each item, the patient must determine whether he/she has seen the item during the test. Patients also are asked to provide a confidence rating so that signal detection analysis can be applied for determination of sensitivity and bias in responses.[38] Response alternatives are: "Definitely No" (non-target); "Probably No"; "Probably Yes" (target); "Definitely Yes." Responses are recorded; outcome is total number of targets correct and subscores for each type of material. False-positive responses are considered in the interpretation of the test results. For the designs, a second recognition task is administered, in which all nine designs are shown simultaneously, and the patient is asked to "Select the three that you think you might have seen earlier during the test." To assess emotional change during the IAT, behavioral observations are made regarding affective changes following injection. All patients are interviewed by the attending neuropsychologist after the procedure to elicit any subjective reactions. Interpretation of IAT data includes conclusions regarding language laterality based on the comprehensive language assessment. Memory performance is compared for each injection following adjustment for false-positive responses. Any atypical features of the examination (e.g., cortical crossflow, obtundation) also are noted.

Replacement of the IAT with Functional Neuroimaging

Given the limitations of the IAT, suggestions for alternative technologies for gathering presurgical data regarding brain regions supporting cognitive functions have included event-related potentials[39] and transcranial magnetic stimulation.[40] Functional MRI[20,23,41,42] and ^{15}O-water positron emission tomography (PET)[43,44] have been proposed as alternatives to the IAT to localize language and memory cortex more precisely. Disadvantages of ^{15}O-water PET include invasiveness, lower availability and repeatability than fMRI, and lower spatial resolution. In this chapter, fMRI studies of memory and language functioning as related to the IAT will be the focus, although aspects of relevant PET studies will be addressed where appropriate.

The IAT demonstrates functional lateralization through unilateral hemispheric suppression of neuronal activity by anesthetization of the anterior and middle cerebral arterial distribution, followed by assessment of the cognitive functions of interest. In contrast, as described elsewhere in this volume, fMRI detects blood oxygen level-dependent (BOLD) signal during cognitive processing in an unsedated patient. This BOLD signal serves as an endogenous contrast agent and as a marker of task-related neuronal activity. As with the IAT, fMRI paradigms designed to assess language and memory functioning vary considerably. Although some language tasks (e.g., verbal fluency paradigms) have been more widely used, specific task and scan parameters are rarely consistent across studies, making direct comparison of fMRI activation patterns difficult. Despite this concern, some broad conclusions regarding the status of fMRI assessment of language and memory can be made.

fMRI Language Paradigms and the IAT

Significant progress has been made in the past decade with regard to the development of language-based fMRI paradigms. Although different tasks have been used to elicit language-related activation, including word generation, naming, and reading paradigms, most studies have found near-perfect agreement between lateralization based on fMRI activation patterns and that based on IAT. In the few studies where discrepancies between fMRI and IAT have been noted, these more typically reflect a nondiagnostic study in one modality, or bilateral language participation in one study, but not in the other, rather than frank disagreement regarding hemispheric language dominance (see Table 9.1 for summary of studies comparing language lateralization using fMRI and IAT).

While replicating IAT language results would require only establishing hemispheric dominance for language, most groups designing fMRI language paradigms to replace the IAT are interested in achieving activation of the broad neural networks subserving various language functions in order not only to lateralize language at the hemispheric level, but to localize specific aspects of language functioning to more focal brain regions. Some groups have used auditory paradigms to activate temporal lobe receptive language cortex in healthy controls and in epilepsy patients.[20,45–49] These tasks often activate primary auditory cortex bilaterally and may show additional activation in posterior superior temporal gyrus.[50–52] As bilateral primary auditory cortex activation is of less utility in assessing hemispheric language dominance, some tasks use auditory control conditions to allow for subtraction of primary auditory cortex activation. However, such strategies may also remove from analysis activation of brain regions important in language processing,[20,45–48] potentially resulting in a reduction of the laterality index many studies have used as a measure of language dominance, thus making dominance appear less marked.[46,53] Reading-based tasks[28–30,53,54] offer an alternative for localization of middle and superior temporal lobe receptive language areas involved in reading decoding and comprehension, as well as frontal regions involved in grammatical language processing or verbal

Table 9.1. Summary of Concordance between IAT and fMRI Language Lateralization Results and Regions of fMRI Activation[a]

Authors	Sample (Age range, years)[b]	IAT language tasks	fMRI language tasks	IAT/fMRI concordance	fMRI language regions activated
Desmond et al., 1995[61]	$n = 7$ (20–53)	Presence of speech arrest, paraphasic errors, and errors in naming, repetition, reading, and aural comp	Visually presented words 1. Semantic encoding: Abstract vs. Concrete 2. Perceptual encoding: Upper vs. Lower case	100%	Frontal
Binder et al., 1996[20]	$n = 22$ (17–64)	Numerical rating of speech arrest, ability to follow commands, paraphasic errors, naming, repetition, reading, and comp	Aurally presented noun-categorization task	100%	Frontal, temporal, temporo-parieto-occipital junction
Bahn et al., 1997[63]	$n = 7$ (mean = 29)	Assessment of naming, reading, and recall	Covert word generation to a target letter and to rhyme with a target word (aural stimuli-au)	100%	Frontal, temporal
Hertz-Pannier et al., 1997[23]	$n = 6$ (10–18)	Not reported	Covert and overt word generation to a target letter and to a target semantic category (au)	100%	Frontal, temporal
Worthington et al, 1997[64]	$n = 12$ (12–56)	Assessment of naming, repetition, reading, and comp	Covert word generation to a target letter	42%[c]	Not reported
Berbadis et al., 1998[62] (subset of patients from Binder et al., 1996)[20]	$n = 21$ (17–64)	Numerical rating of speech arrest, ability to follow commands, paraphasic errors, naming, repetition, reading, and comp	Aurally presented noun-categorization task	71–100%[d]	Frontal, temporal, temporo-parieto-occipital junction
Yetkin et al., 1998[65]	$n = 13$ (22–43)	Numerical rating of speech arrest, ability to follow commands, paraphasic errors, naming, repetition, reading, and comp	Covert word generation to a target letter (aural stimuli)	100%	Frontal
Benson et al, 1999[66]	$n = 12$ (19–70)	Assessment of speech arrest, paraphasic errors, naming, reading and comp	Visually presented verb-generation task	92%[e]	Not reported[f]

(continued)

Table 9.1. (continued)

Authors	Sample (Age range, years)[b]	IAT language tasks	fMRI language tasks	IAT/fMRI concordance	fMRI language regions activated
Lehéricy et al., 2000[46]	$n = 10$ (18–55)	Assessment of serial speech, naming, reading, spelling, and ability to follow commands	Covert word generation and sentence repetition, story listening (all aural stimuli)	100%[g]	Frontal, temporal
Carpentier et al., 2001[67]	$n = 10$ (24–51)	Assessment of speech arrest, paraphasic errors, comp, repetition, and naming	Identification of syntactic and semantic errors in sentences (aural and visual stimuli)	80–90%[h]	Frontal, temporal
Baciu et al., 2001[68]	$n = 10$ (20–48)	Presence/absence of speech arrest followed by transient aphasia	Visually presented rhyming/visual task	80–100%[i]	Frontal, temporal
Gaillard et al., 2002[29]	$n = 20$ (8–56)	Not reported	Covert naming in response to reading	75%[j]	Frontal, temporal
Rutten et al., 2002[100]	$n = 18$ (20–54)	Assessment of naming, expressive language, and paraphasic errors	Visually presented verb-generation, verbal-fluency, picture-naming, and sentence-comp task	83%[k]	Frontal, temporoparietal

[a] Adapted from Baxendale S. The role of functional MRI in the presurgical investigation of temporal lobe epilepsy patients: A clinical perspective and review. *J Clin Exp Neuropsychol* 2002;24(5):664-676. Adapted with permission from Psychology Press Ltd., *http://www.psypress.co.uk/journals.asp*.

[b] excluding healthy control subjects and epilepsy patients who did not receive IAT.

[c] Five patients demonstrated identical language laterality on IAT and fMRI. Three patients had disagreement between IAT and fMRL one patient had bilateral IAT but lateralized fMRL and three patients had a nondiagnostic fMRI study.

[d] 71% agreement was found between fMRI lateralization and IAT lateralization based solely on speech arrest; 100% concordance was found when IAT lateralization incorporated comprehensive language assessment.

[e] Eleven patients demonstrated identical language laterality on IAT and fMRI. One patient had equivocal findings on IAT and lateralized fMRI.

[f] While images are presented highlighting activation patterns in selected subjects, discussion of specific language regions activated is not included.

[g] Nine patients demonstrated left hemisphere dominance on both IAT and fMRI language measures, although strength of lateralization varied. One patient showed bilateral IAT, with strong right hemisphere fMRI lateralization of frontal language regions, but weak left lateralization of temporal areas.

[h] IAT and fMRI findings were concordant in eight patients when the whole brain was considered in fMRI analysis, and in nine patients when Brodmann's area 41/42 was excluded from analysis.

[I] Functional fMRI and IAT were entirely consistent in eight patients with conclusive IAT studies. Two patients had inconclusive IAT studies. In one of these, VEEG findings confirmed fMRI language lateralization. In the other, no other data was conclusive with regard to language lateralization.

[j] Five patients demonstrated identical language laterality on IAT and fMRI. One patient had a nondiagnostic IAT study, and another had a nondiagnostic fMRI study. One patient with left hemisphere language dominance on IAT showed bilateral language representation on fMRI and two patients with bilateral language functioning on IAT showed left hemisphere dominance on fMRI. In no case was there frank disagreement between IAT and fMRI.

[k] Of the three patients in whom fMRI and IAT were discordant, one was left dominant on fMRL but mixed dominant on IAT; one was mixed dominant on fMRL but left dominant on IAT; and one was right dominant on fMRI but left dominant on IAT.

working memory.[55–57] Semantic retrieval aspects of these tasks are thought to engage anterior language regions.[19,23,28,43,58–60]

Desmond and colleagues[61] were the first researchers to publish the results of a group of patients in whom language dominance was studied with both IAT and fMRI. In their series of seven epilepsy patients, 100% concordance was observed between the two methods with regard to language lateralization. In addition, they provided data on intrahemispheric localization, namely activation of frontal lobe language regions (Brodmann's areas 45, 46, and 47) when patients were asked to make semantic as compared to perceptual judgments about visually presented words. While seminal, the use of a reading task prohibited more general conclusions about localization of speech and speech comprehension, which are important for surgical planning. In a series of 22 consecutive epilepsy surgery patients, Binder and colleagues[20] likewise found complete agreement between IAT and fMRI language lateralization and a high concordance ($r = 0.96$) between IAT and fMRI language lateralization indices. These authors also were able to demonstrate intrahemispheric activation of lateral frontal and heteromodal temporo-parieto-occipital cortex during a single-word semantic decision-making task. The study employed a baseline tone discrimination task to control for activation of auditory and attentional systems; this task design permitted elegant localization of areas involved in speech comprehension, but, it could be argued, prohibited examination of language as a multidimensional ability intimately related to both hearing and attention. In a later study, Benbadis and colleagues[62] reanalyzed fMRI and IAT data from the Binder[20] sample to determine whether IAT speech arrest alone constitutes sufficient criteria for determination of language dominance, in comparison to the comprehensive language evaluation cited in Binder and colleagues.[20] They found that a laterality index calculated solely based on speech arrest did not correlate significantly with either the comprehensive IAT laterality index or with fMRI language lateralization. Categorical classification of language dominance as right, left, or bilateral was likewise discordant in several cases when using the speech arrest index, as compared to the complete agreement between IAT and fMRI reported by Binder and colleagues[20] when IAT lateralization was based on comprehensive speech assessment. Therefore, Benbadis and colleagues[62] concluded that IAT speech arrest alone is not a valid indicator of language lateralization, highlighting the importance of the consideration of assessment techniques in the evaluation of IAT and fMRI concordance, as an inappropriate strategy (e.g., a nonspecific measure such as speech arrest) in either modality may lead to spurious conclusions regarding concordance.

Bahn and colleagues[63] reported a series of seven epilepsy patients who received both IAT and fMRI assessment of language functioning. These authors utilized aurally presented covert word generation paradigms in which subjects were asked either to think of words beginning with a certain letter or to think of words that rhymed with a target word. Functional MRI laterality was judged by comparing the number of voxels activated above threshold in language regions (specifically Broca's and Wernicke's areas) of each hemisphere. Intracarotid amobarbital test language laterality was judged using assessment of object naming, reading, and object recall, with dysnomia as a principal measure of language integrity. Intracarotid amobarbital test and fMRI lateralization agreed in all cases, including two right-handed participants with atypical right hemisphere dominance.

No disagreement was found in lateralization of fMRI activation patterns between the two language tasks in any case, nor were there any instances of discordant lateralization of frontal and temporal language regions. Overall, however, asymmetric activation of Broca's area was visualized more reliably than activation of posterior language regions, including Wernicke's area. The rhyming task tended to demonstrate more robust activation and clearer hemispheric asymmetry than the naming to letter task, although a potential confound of task order was noted. While these findings were generally consistent with those of previous studies[20,61] demonstrating agreement between IAT and fMRI assessment of language dominance, the authors noted that fMRI conventions for classification of mixed or codominance of language were not well established, requiring further experience with this technique.

In the first extension of this type of research to pediatric populations, Hertz-Pannier and colleagues[23] used fMRI to assess language dominance in 11 children and adolescents with complex partial seizures (CPS) using word generation tasks. In all seven cases where either IAT, electrostimulation mapping, or surgical outcome results were available for comparison, findings regarding language dominance were concordant with fMRI asymmetry indices. All subjects demonstrated highest activation in the vicinity of Broca's area (inferior frontal gyrus), as well as in the middle and superior frontal gyri, and cingulate gyrus activation was observed in all but two subjects. With regard to the technical difficulties inherent in studying children using fMRI, these authors noted that second studies were successful in four children whose initial studies were uninterpretable due to noncompliance or motion artifact. Studies also were repeated in two other children to assess reproducibility of the fMRI findings; language lateralization and spatial extent of activation were comparable across studies. These findings offered promising preliminary evidence that fMRI is a feasible technique for assessing language dominance in pediatric epilepsy surgery candidates without the potential risks of IAT or ESM.

In one of the very few studies demonstrating poor concordance between fMRI and IAT language lateralization, Worthington and colleagues[64] studied frontal and temporal brain regions using an fMRI verbal fluency task in 12 adolescents and adults who had completed IAT. The method used for determining hemispheric laterality appeared to involve counting the number of significantly activated voxels in each hemisphere. Language dominance was concordant in five of 12 patients who completed both IAT and fMRI. Three cases apparently demonstrated overt disagreement between IAT and fMRI lateralization, while one case demonstrated bilateral representation of language on IAT, but lateralized findings on fMRI. Three fMRI studies were nondiagnostic due to motion artifact or unclear activation. While these authors concluded that their findings suggest that fMRI lacks the sensitivity and specificity to be of clinical utility in presurgical evaluation of language dominance, several shortcomings in their study may explain their findings. The task used for some subjects included the requirement that subjects count the number of words generated as a method of monitoring task performance. Such a working memory component is uncommon in fMRI word generation tasks and may have led to atypically broad brain activation patterns, which may have obscured laterality. In addition, it is unclear if data analysis accounted for the different tasks used between subjects. Furthermore, 25% of fMRI data collected in this study was reportedly unusable. The authors do not discuss whether additional motion correction strategies were attempted, if alteration of a statistical significance threshold improved interpretability, or if second fMRI studies were attempted to obtain adequate data. Overall, while the unusually low concordance between fMRI and IAT language lateralization reported in this study should not be dismissed, several technical and methodological issues raise important questions regarding the validity of these findings and suggest that they should not be weighted heavily in general consideration of the research findings in this area.

Yetkin and colleagues[65] also used a word-generation task to compare fMRI and IAT language lateralization in 13 CPS patients. In all subjects, frontal lobe language regions (predominantly inferior frontal gyrus and precentral gyrus) demonstrated activation during fMRI word generation. Functional MRI language lateralization was 100% concordant with IAT results, offering a further contribution to the now-growing evidence that fMRI language lateralization paradigms are a reliable and feasible option for replacement of the IAT. In an attempt to broaden the scope of fMRI language lateralization techniques, Benson and colleagues[66] developed and validated an fMRI language paradigm to determine hemispheric dominance for a group of subjects with potentially resectable brain lesions near language cortex in addition to epilepsy. Using whole-brain fMRI, only a verb generation task (versus object naming and single word reading measures) reliably lateralized language in 19 control subjects. The clinical applications of this task were evaluated in a group of 23 patients who had IAT and/or ESM results available for comparison with fMRI laterality indices. Concordant findings with IAT/ESM were found in 96% of patients. In the sole patient with discordant findings, exclusion of a large tumor and its reflection in the opposite hemisphere from fMRI laterality analysis led to concordance.

Lehéricy and colleagues[46] utilized fMRI semantic verbal fluency, covert repetition, and story listening tasks to assess the reliability of fMRI frontal and temporal language systems activation in evaluating language dominance in ten TLE patients. Laterality indices were calculated for IAT and for several fMRI regions of interest (ROIs). For 90% of patients, language lateralization to the left hemisphere was concordant between IAT and fMRI frontal and temporal lobe activation, although the strength of lateralization varied, and fMRI activation in frontal regions tended to demonstrate a stronger relationship with IAT findings than more posterior brain activation. For the tenth patient, IAT suggested symmetric hemispheric support of language, while fMRI demonstrated strong right hemisphere lateralization for frontal regions and weak left hemisphere dominance for temporal regions. Lehéricy and colleagues concluded that fMRI demonstrated good sensitivity for detection of frontal language lateralization, but was less able to demonstrate lateralization in temporal lobe regions using these tasks. They also concluded, however, that use of multiple fMRI language tasks (i.e., story listening and repetition in addition to verbal fluency) might prove useful in demonstrating activation of posterior language regions in patients under consideration for surgical resection of brain lesions in these areas.

Carpentier and colleagues[67] utilized visual and aural language comprehension fMRI tasks to lateralize language functioning in ten epilepsy surgery candidates with left hemisphere seizure foci in or near presumed language cortex and ten healthy controls. Functional MRI tasks required subjects to make syntactic or semantic decisions regarding sentence accuracy.

While fMRI activation was observed in a wide neural network of brain regions involved in language comprehension, Broca's area was the most consistently activated region, demonstrating activation in all subjects for both tasks, with controls demonstrating more robust laterality indices than epilepsy patients. Using whole-brain analysis, 80% concordance was observed between IAT and fMRI language lateralization, which rose to 90% when Brodmann's area 41/42 was excluded from laterality scoring. Functional MRI language lateralization scores demonstrated greater agreement with IAT and neuropsychological testing for the visual versus the auditory task. Strongest agreement was found using an fMRI laterality index including only Brodmann's areas 44/45 and 22, and the conjunction analysis of both fMRI tasks. These authors concluded that application of fMRI to replace the IAT should consider both modality-specific and modality-nonspecific patterns of brain activation. They also noted that their finding of greater bilateral representation of language functioning in epilepsy patients relative to controls supported previous findings and may provide further evidence of language plasticity related to epilepsy.

Baciu and colleagues[68] used an fMRI rhyme-detection task to assess language dominance in 19 epilepsy patients and compared these findings with those obtained using IAT, intracranial EEG stimulation and recording (SEEG), and/or video EEG recording (VEEG). Concordant lateralization was observed in 16 of 17 patients in whom language lateralization could be conclusively determined by both fMRI and one of these alternate methods. In the remaining subject, VEEG suggested left hemisphere language dominance, while fMRI activation during the rhyming task suggested bilateral language participation. These authors noted that, despite low intellectual functioning in some subjects, all patients were able to complete the fMRI task appropriately, and fMRI activation was apparent in frontal and temporal language regions across subjects. Baciu and colleagues[68] concluded that their rhyming paradigm offers a useful method for fMRI lateralization of language functions, and note that, unlike in other language tasks (e.g., covert naming or word generation), subject performance accuracy can be directly assessed.

In a recent study, Gaillard and colleagues[29] assessed hemispheric language dominance in children and adults with partial epilepsy of presumed temporal or frontotemporal origin using a covert naming in response to reading fMRI paradigm, in which subjects silently named an object after reading a sentence describing the object. Functional MRI data analysis included visual inspection and ROI analysis using regional asymmetry indices (AIs) for ROIs in frontal, temporal, and parietal regions. Of 20 patients who had IAT language lateralization data, fMRI demonstrated agreement in 15 cases (75%). In the five cases with disagreement between IAT and fMRI, the discrepancy was that one measure predicted bilateral language participation, whereas the other suggested unilateral dominance. Clinical visual inspection was found to be comparable to statistical ROI analysis. This fMRI paradigm resulted in visualization of both frontal and temporal language regions in the majority of cases, which is a significant finding given that previous studies[17,20,22,23,41,42,66,69–71] reliably demonstrated frontal language activation, but could not typically show task-related activation in more posterior language regions (for exceptions, see Refs. 28, 30, 48, 54). Typically, group averaging has been necessary to demonstrate language-related temporal lobe activation, and reliable findings have been more difficult to achieve in individual subjects.[19,22,72,73]

Like Carpentier and colleagues,[67] Gaillard and colleagues[29] showed discrepancies in language lateralization between patients and controls, with all control subjects showing left hemisphere dominance, and greater right hemisphere language activation in patients, which seemed to be accounted for mainly by those with a left hemisphere seizure focus. These findings support previous research suggesting that early localization-related epilepsy can lead to intra- or interhemispheric alteration from normal language representation,[14,74] as well as the possibility that such activation also may reflect compensatory processes, such as atypical use of the intact right hemisphere to support the dysfunctional left hemisphere. Further analysis of this pattern of dominant and nondominant hemisphere language activation may help to identify individuals more likely to recover language functions after an acquired insult to dominant hemisphere language regions.[75–77]

Given the variability of language lateralization indices reported by prior studies, Rutten and colleagues[78] used four language tasks in combination to attempt to locate language cortex reliably in 18 TLE patients in an effort to provide a reliable distinction between patients with unilateral and bilateral language dominance, which they argued had thus far prevented the use of fMRI language assessment to replace the IAT. Through use of combined task analysis (CTA), these authors achieved more robust and reliable results than with any single task, and achieved concordance with IAT findings in 91% (10 out of 11) of patients who were left dominant by IAT, 75% (3 out of 4) of those with bilateral dominance by IAT, and 67% (2 out of 3) of those right dominant by IAT. Consistent with previous studies, verb generation was the most useful task in terms of providing language lateralization concordant with IAT, although it did not demonstrate similar effectiveness in bilateral hemispheric dominant patients. Of note, Rutten and colleagues[78] used a fixed user-independent approach to statistical analysis, which did not allow for individual variability in the threshold set for significant activation. As will be discussed below, this method may not be ideal for all subjects due to significant interindividual variability in the level of fMRI activation. Overall, however, they concluded that CTA offered a more effective means of differentiating typical (left) from atypical (right, bilateral) language dominance in the context of surgical planning than single-task fMRI assessment, and may in the future obviate the need for IAT language assessment in patients with clearly typical hemispheric dominance.

Overall, fMRI paradigms designed to lateralize and localize language functions typically have been successful in demonstrating activation patterns that are concordant with IAT results. Although a few studies have found surprisingly low concordance between IAT and fMRI language assessment, most have demonstrated perfect or near-perfect agreement. In studies with lower concordance rates, typical discrepancies involve technically inadequate or nondiagnostic IAT or fMRI studies, or bilateral representation in one study and unilateral hemispheric dominance in the other. In very few cases was there frank disagreement between fMRI and IAT. These infrequent instances in which IAT and fMRI language lateralization disagree highlight the importance of consideration of all available clinical data in presurgical epilepsy cases, including scalp and intracranial EEG recordings, seizure semiology, neuropsychological assessment, structural MRI, electrostimulation mapping, and other functional neuroimaging techniques such as PET and single photon emission computed tomography (SPECT).

While much remains to be learned regarding the most efficient method of precise fMRI localization of specific language skills, it appears that current fMRI paradigms can consistently lateralize language as effectively as the IAT, and can be used with confidence in place of the IAT in some circumstances. At DHMC, for example, fMRI verb generation tasks have been utilized effectively to determine language dominance and localization of Broca's area in presurgical tumor and arteriovenous malformation (AVM) patients, as well as in epilepsy patients who cannot undergo the IAT (e.g., due to vascular risk factors). In particular, use of fMRI language paradigms provides a potential alternative for language lateralization in epilepsy patients who would not necessarily be considered for IAT, including adults with medical contraindications and young children, who may be trained to tolerate the fMRI procedure, and thus have language laterality assessed without the potential morbidity risks of the IAT. Another potential advantage of fMRI in studying language functions in young patients is the potential to observe intrahemispheric reorganization in cases of early brain injury and recovery, which could not be visualized with the IAT.

While studies have noted technical issues that must be considered in the use of fMRI with children,[23,50,79–81] including tailoring of cognitive paradigms and adjustment of statistical thresholds, results from DHMC and other centers suggest that language can be lateralized successfully using fMRI in pediatric populations. At DHMC, we have achieved successful language lateralization using fMRI word generation paradigms in epilepsy patients as young as six years of age. Our experience has been that children can effectively perform such fMRI tasks following out-of-scanner preparation, including practicing the fMRI tasks and instruction regarding the importance of remaining motionless, and with minimal in-scanner head restraints (i.e., only foam padding and/or tape across the forehead). With modification of fMRI paradigms as appropriate for level of cognitive functioning and additional physical assistance in head stabilization, it seems likely that fMRI may come into wider use for lateralization of language in very young children, in whom the IAT often is considered unfeasible or its attendant medical risks too great.

As noted in a recent review of fMRI paradigms with potential to replace the IAT,[82] future directions for fMRI assessment of language skills in presurgical epilepsy patients should include not only consistent lateralization of language dominance, but also specific localization of regions subserving the cognitive functions most likely to be affected negatively by surgical resection in the dominant hemisphere. Previous research[83] has demonstrated postoperative declines in naming skills following dominant temporal lobe resection, and other complex language functions such as reading and semantic processing also may be disrupted. Therefore, while some of the language paradigms used in the studies discussed above may not provide maximal information regarding overall language lateralization, such tasks may be useful in demonstrating activation of extrafrontal language regions (e.g., temporoparietal association cortex), which may be helpful in assessing the likelihood of postsurgical cognitive impairment and the potential for recovery of function. As TLE patients are those most commonly considered for epilepsy surgery, the importance of delineating temporal lobe language regions, as well as memory circuitry, becomes evident. In addition, it is important to note that the specific fMRI language task used may not be critical to achieving adequate language lateralization. For example, Grandin and colleagues[22] found that the number of pixels activated in frontal and temporal language regions did not differ for semantic versus phonemic verbal fluency tasks. Similarly, both tasks lateralized language functioning to the dominant hemisphere, suggesting no particular advantage to one form of verbal fluency task over the other. This information is particularly useful in the study of children, who may not be able to accurately generate words beginning with a particular letter, but who often can generate words to a semantic category such as animals or foods.

The available literature suggests that functional neuroimaging techniques such as PET and fMRI can reliably identify language dominance in both adults and children, and typically produce findings that agree with results from IAT and electrocortical stimulation.[20,23,41,42,46,61,63,65,66,70,84,85] A small percentage of studies, however, have shown disagreement between IAT and PET,[43,44,46,63,65,66] or only partial agreement between IAT and fMRI in terms of language lateralization,[65,66] with surgery at times confirming the functional imaging findings.[43,44] These findings may reflect difficulties in sensitivity to functional reorganization in individuals with atypical dominance, or dissociation of receptive and expressive language,[86,87] at least for some methods. Therefore, a conservative approach would include IAT or cortical stimulation confirmation of fMRI results at present. In cases of dominant hemisphere resection or where language dominance is unclear, intraoperative language mapping often is essential.

Case Examples of fMRI Language Activation

At DHMC, patients referred for clinical fMRI language mapping most typically complete an aurally presented verb generation task similar to those described in the previous section. Patients are presented with blocks of nouns alternating with blocks of tones. For each noun presented, the patient is instructed to mentally generate as many verbs as possible that go with that noun (e.g., for "frog", the patient might think "leap", "croak", "hop", etc.). The patient is instructed not to say the words or make any mouth movements. During the control condition (tones), the patient is instructed to simply listen and clear his/her mind. As this task does not involve collection of objective performance data, successful completion of the task is assessed by postscanning debriefing and comparison with performance on similar measures during out-of-scanner neuropsychological testing. Analysis contrasts hemodynamic responses during the two task conditions. The typical pattern of brain activation for this task comprises dominant hemisphere frontal regions, with more posterior temporal lobe activation observed in some patients. Consistent with the literature, cingulate gyrus activation is also often noted. In Figure 9.1, data are presented from a 44-year-old, right-handed female epilepsy patient. This patient displayed a typical pattern of left frontal activation, with cingulate cortex and bilateral cerebellar activation also apparent.

We have observed similar activation patterns in children with epilepsy. Figures 11.2 and 11.3 demonstrate the variation that can be observed in individual patient activation for verb generation. In Figure 9.2, frontal language-related activation is observed bilaterally in a nine-year-old,

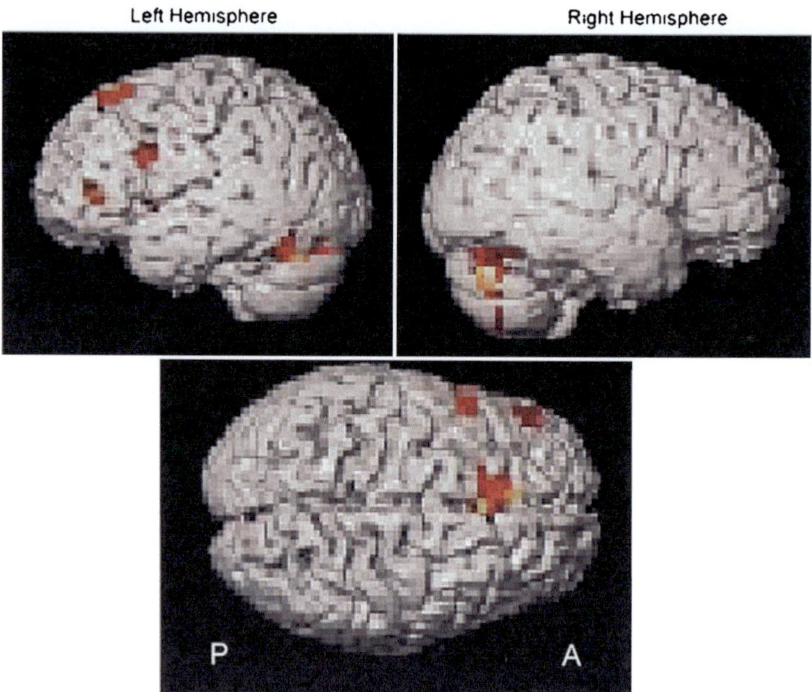

Figure 9.1. Functional MRI brain activation (p_{crit} = 0.01) during verb generation in a 44-year-old, right-handed female demonstrating strong left frontal fMRI brain activation. Bilateral cerebellar and medial cingulate gyrus activation also were noted. (Neurologic coordinates).

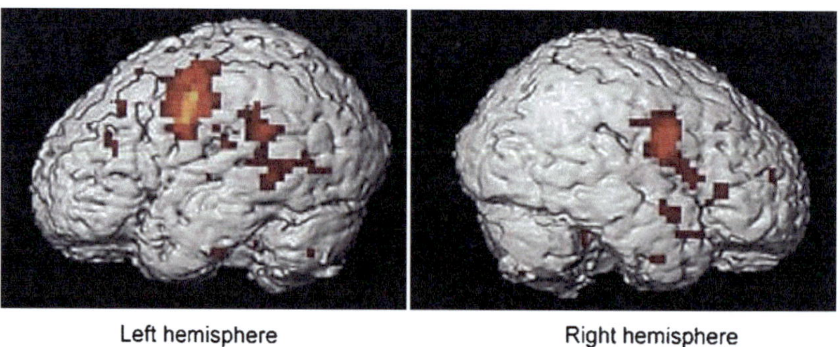

Figure 9.2. Functional MRI brain activation (p_{crit} = 0.0001) during verb generation in a 9-year-old, right-handed boy with an epileptogenic left orbitofrontal lesion. This patient displayed stronger left than right frontal activation in regions approximating Broca's area, suggesting left hemisphere dominance for language, with some right participation.

right-handed boy, in regions approximating Broca's area. Global peak activation is in the left frontal lobe, however, suggesting left hemisphere dominance for language. In addition, posterior temporal task-related activation is observed in the left, but not the right hemisphere. In contrast, in Figure 9.3, activation

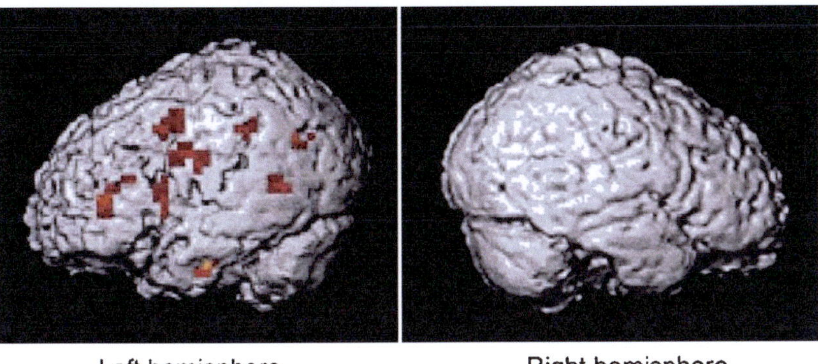

Figure 9.3. Functional MRI brain activation (p_{crit} = 0.01) during verb generation in an 11-year-old, right-handed girl with left TLE and left hippocampal sclerosis. This patient displayed clear left hemisphere dominance for language (confirmed by IAT), with activation of frontal and temporal language regions, including Broca's area.

maps from an 11-year-old, right-handed girl show only left hemisphere task-related activation, but in a more widely distributed network of frontal and temporal regions.

fMRI Memory Paradigms and the IAT

The development of fMRI memory paradigms to replace the IAT is in a state of relative infancy compared to the language lateralization literature. Whereas fMRI memory tasks cannot yet serve the critical IAT function of assessing unilateral support of memory functions on an individual basis, as neither hemisphere is anesthetized during stimulus presentation, research with fMRI and PET has examined episodic memory encoding and retrieval processes in healthy controls and TLE populations (see Table 9.2 for summary of studies assessing memory functioning in TLE using fMRI and IAT).

In TLE, Detre and colleagues[88] used a complex visual scene-encoding fMRI task, previously demonstrated to activate bilateral mesial temporal lobe structures in healthy controls,[89] to assess functional asymmetry in comparison with IAT memory lateralization in nine TLE patients. A tenth patient participated in fMRI, but IAT results were uninterpretable due to crossflow and subsequent obtundation. The fMRI paradigm involved memorization of novel complex scenes. In controls, comparison of activation during the task condition as compared to a visual control condition demonstrated bilateral posterior temporal and visual association cortex and right frontal activation, with a slight right hemisphere predominance overall in MTL ROIs. Epilepsy patients demonstrated markedly more asymmetric MTL activation. In nine out of ten patients, asymmetry ratios were greater than one standard deviation from the control mean; four out of ten patients showed asymmetry ratios greater than two standard deviations away from the control mean. In all patients, the direction of hemispheric asymmetry was concordant with IAT findings. As two patients demonstrated paradoxically greater fMRI activation and better IAT memory performance ipsilateral to the seizure focus,

Table 9.2. Summary of Studies Assessing Memory Performance in TLE Using fMRI

Authors	Sample (Age range, years)	IAT memory tasks	fMRI memory tasks	Findings
Detre et al., 1998[88]	Left TLE: $n = 6$ (17–48) Right TLE: $n = 3$ (18–37) Controls: $n = 8$ (18–40)	Assessment of free recall and recognition of common objects, low-imagery words, and abstract line drawings	Complex scene-encoding task	Controls demonstrated generally symmetric MTL activation. Patients showed asymmetric MTL activation, which agreed in all cases with memory asymmetry on IAT.
Bellgowan et al., 1998[90]	Left TLE: $n = 14$ (20–57) Right TLE: $n = 14$ (28–69)	Not described, although IAT memory lateralization data are presented	Semantic and tone decision task	Right TLE patients: similar activation in left MTL as previously observed in healthy controls in a separate study. Left TLE patients: decreased left MTL activation relative to right TLE patients, but similar whole-brain and left hemisphere activation and task performance.
Dupont et al., 2000[91]	Left TLE: $n = 7$ (18–53) Controls: $n = 10$ (23–30)	Not described, only IAT data presented are that all patients are left language dominant	Verbal episodic encoding and retrieval tasks	Bilateral parahippocampal gyms activation during retrieval in both groups, more so in controls, who had stronger task performance. Patients also activated left prefrontal regions during encoding and retrieval.
Dupont et al., 2001[92]	Left TLE: $n = 7$ (18–53) Controls: $n = 10$ (23–31)[a]	Not described, only IAT data presented are that all patients are left language dominant	Verbal retrieval task	Relative to the prior scan: Controls: decreased activation in parahippocampal, occipitotemporal, and ventrolateral frontal regions, but new activation in right posterior hippocampus and bilateral parietal cortex. Patients: slightly poorer task performance, absent MTL activation, and dramatic decrease in previously noted neocortical fMRI activation.
Jokeit et al., 2001[93]	Left TLE: $n = 16$ (13–55) Right TLE: $n = 14$ (14–54) Controls: $n = 17$ (7–63)	Assessment of free recall and recognition of 20 items (e.g., actual and drawn objects, words, abstract drawings)	Mental navigation and recall task	Both groups showed MTL activation; in controls, no significant asymmetry was evident. Patients: Hemispheric asymmetry in activation lateralized seizure onset in 90% (weaker activation on side of focus); left TLE patients showed correlation between left MTL activation and IAT memory performance using the left hemisphere.
Golby et al., 2002[94]	Left TLE: $n = 6$ (26–33) Right TLE: $n = 3$ (42–54)	Assessment of recognition memory for objects, words, and designs	Tasks requiring encoding and processing of words, faces, scenes, and patterns	Functional MRI and IAT memory lateralization concordant in 89% of subjects; in each group, greater encoding-related activation was observed in MTL structures contralateral to seizure focus; material-specific interaction between side of seizure focus and memory for verbal versus nonverbal stimuli.

[a] Same subjects as Dupont et al.,[91] rescanned 24 hours after scanning session reported in the previous study, and asked to recall words learned during the first scanning session.

this pattern was thought not entirely attributable to epilepsy-related structural abnormalities. This finding is clinically significant, as it demonstrates the potential utility of fMRI in demonstrating brain activation patterns that might by extension to the IAT predict memory deficits following temporal lobectomy, and thus inform risk–benefit discussions, or, in the extreme case, serve as a potential contraindication for surgery.

Bellgowan and colleagues[90] were able to discriminate left and right TLE patients based on their fMRI activation patterns on a semantic encoding task. Right TLE patients showed predominant left MTL activation involving the hippocampus, parahippocampal gyrus, and collateral sulcus, whereas those with a left hemisphere seizure focus demonstrated little activation in these regions. In contrast to the studies noted above, this task did not demonstrate bilateral activation of memory structures; neither right nor left TLE patients showed significant right hemisphere activation in MTL regions while completing the task. This is not unexpected, in that semantic tasks do not typically generate right hemisphere activation, and highlights a paradigm potentially useful for preferential activation of the left MTL in presurgical fMRI evaluation of epilepsy patients. The authors hypothesized that the lack of left MTL activation in left TLE patients in spite of relatively intact episodic memory functioning may indicate intra- or interhemispheric reorganization of memory functions in this group, which may be related to factors such as age at seizure onset. Bellgowan and colleagues[90] concluded that further demonstration of the reliability of similar techniques for evoking MTL activation in patients may in the future allow fMRI to replace the IAT for memory assessment.

In another study of fMRI memory patterns in TLE, Dupont and colleagues[91] utilized verbal episodic memory-encoding and retrieval tasks to demonstrate memory functioning in ten healthy control subjects and seven left TLE patients with left hippocampal sclerosis in an attempt to illustrate reallocation of verbal memory functions in left TLE. During fMRI scanning, subjects were asked to encode a supraspan list of 17 words over repeated presentations, then to covertly recall the words. In addition to activation across broader neural networks, both patients and controls demonstrated bilateral parahippocampal gyrus activation (right greater than left) during retrieval, although this effect was more marked in controls. Patients also recruited left prefrontal regions for encoding and retrieval, which were not activated in controls. Controls demonstrated significantly stronger memory for the word list on postscanner testing. Given the performance deficit noted in patients, Dupont and colleagues[91] hypothesized that this frontal cortex recruitment reflects ineffective reallocation of memory functions (i.e., cortical dysfunction rather than efficient reorganization) in the patient group due either to hippocampal dysfunction or epileptogenesis. In a later study,[92] this group analyzed differences in brain activation in the same subjects for 24-hour delayed retrieval of the verbal material. At the follow-up fMRI session, subjects were asked only to retrieve the words memorized the day before (i.e., the word list was not presented again). Memory was tested again through free recall following the scanner session. For controls, retrieval was similar to prior performance, whereas patient performance was slightly poorer. Analysis of changes in fMRI brain activation patterns in controls revealed decreases in parahippocampal, occipitotemporal, and ventrolateral frontal activation, and emergence of a new focus of activation in the right posterior hippocampus and bilateral parietal cortex. In the epilepsy patients, no MTL activation was apparent, and activation in neocortical brain regions observed at the previous session was dramatically decreased. The authors concluded that these findings support the assertion that MTL structures play a critical role in the neural networks involved in episodic verbal memory, including retrieval of stored information, and that dysfunction of these regions in TLE patients likely underlies the memory deficits and alterations in fMRI activation they observed in patients relative to controls.

Jokeit and colleagues[93] utilized fMRI to lateralize declarative memory functioning in a group of 30 TLE (16 left TLE, 14 right TLE) patients and 17 healthy control subjects using a mental navigation task involving mental recall and navigation of the subject's hometown, contrasted with a covert counting baseline condition. Both controls and patients (including children, older subjects, and some subjects with lower intellectual functioning) reliably activated MTL structures. Hemispheric asymmetry in MTL activation lateralized seizure onset in 90% of TLE patients, with diminished activation observed on the side of seizure focus. Controls did not demonstrate significant fMRI MTL activation asymmetry. The authors concluded that these activation patterns were related specifically to memory rather than to visuospatial abilities based on correlations between out-of-scanner neuropsychological testing of memory functions and fMRI MTL activation. Examination of fMRI activation patterns and IAT results demonstrated a significant correlation between number of activated voxels in the left MTL and left hemisphere IAT performance. Unfortunately, too few right TLE subjects were available for the authors to correlate hemispheric asymmetry indices from fMRI and IAT across TLE groups.

In another study attempting to lateralize memory functions in TLE patients, Golby and colleagues[94] evaluated hemispheric asymmetry of MTL activation in nine TLE patients during novel stimuli encoding. Subjects were asked to remember four types of stimuli: patterns, faces, scenes, and words. They were also asked to perform stimulus-related tasks. Performance accuracy was assessed by a recognition paradigm following the encoding phase. In 89% of subjects, fMRI lateralization of memory was concordant with IAT. Overall, right TLE patients demonstrated greater left than right MTL activation across encoding conditions, whereas the reverse was true for left TLE patients. In addition, group analysis demonstrated an interaction between side of seizure focus and material specificity for memory, such that left TLE patients showed right MTL activation for encoding of verbal material, whereas right TLE subjects showed left MTL activation for nonverbal information. The authors concluded that their data demonstrated functional reorganization of memory circuitry due to TLE, and noted that their findings, if replicated in larger samples, might provide an fMRI memory paradigm suitable for assessment of memory lateralization in individual patients, and thus possibly lead to eventual replacement of the IAT. Future directions in the study of fMRI memory lateralization and localization in TLE should likewise include assessment of memory across multiple stimulus modalities in order to capitalize upon the potential material specificity of hemispheric MTL functioning in memory encoding.

Case Examples of fMRI Memory Activation

At DHMC, fMRI probes have been used to elicit activation of memory systems in epilepsy patients before and after resective surgery.[95,96] Currently, the primary fMRI memory activation task used at DHMC is an event-related continuous performance recognition memory task. This task was patterned after the paradigm used by Swick and Knight[97] in their ERP studies of working memory versus delayed recognition, where reaction time and pattern of evoked responses differentiated between patients with focal frontal and hippocampal lesions. This task consists of a list of words or low-verbalizability line drawings[98] with a pseudo-random jittered interstimulus interval of five to eight seconds. Each stimulus is presented twice; the second occurrence may be immediately following the first (0 to 2 intervening stimuli), or may be nine to eighteen items later in the list. The subject responds by button press to indicate whether a stimulus is being presented for the first or second time. Analysis is performed by dividing items into three event types; first presentations ("new" items, encoding condition), second presentations with a short delay ("working memory" items, up to two stimuli between presentations), and second presentations with a long delay ("long delay" items, from nine to eighteen items between presentations). Contrasts then are made to compare hemodynamic responses between these three types of events. We have observed MTL activation across subjects during encoding on both the verbal and nonverbal (designs) analogs of this task. Functional MRI memory paradigms might prove to be a powerful tool for studying epilepsy-related brain functional reorganization. In Figure 9.4, data is presented from a 25-year-old, right-handed male patient with left TLE who underwent fMRI pre- and postsurgery. Presurgery, no hippocampal activation was evident in the right (nonepileptogenic) hemisphere. Postsurgery, however, right hippocampal activation was observed during learning of new words. These findings suggest a possible functional release from the irritative seizure focus following surgery.[95] In Figure 9.5, data are presented from two right-handed female patients with right TLE who were studied following temporal lobe resection. In both subjects, left hippocampal activation was apparent during encoding of new words, demonstrating functional activity in the nonepileptic MTL.[95]

Methodological Issues in Creating fMRI Paradigms to Replace the IAT

Technical Concerns

A critical issue highlighted by review of the current literature in fMRI language and memory paradigms is that of imaging methodology. Whereas some researchers choose only to image specific ROIs (e.g., scanning only frontal and temporal regions), others conduct whole-brain imaging. Within groups that obtain images of the whole brain, some analyze only activation within discrete ROIs, whereas others assess alterations in activation patterns throughout the brain. Choices made with regard to which brain regions to image or analyze obviously may have a pivotal effect on statistical power and the results and conclusions that can be drawn regarding the nature

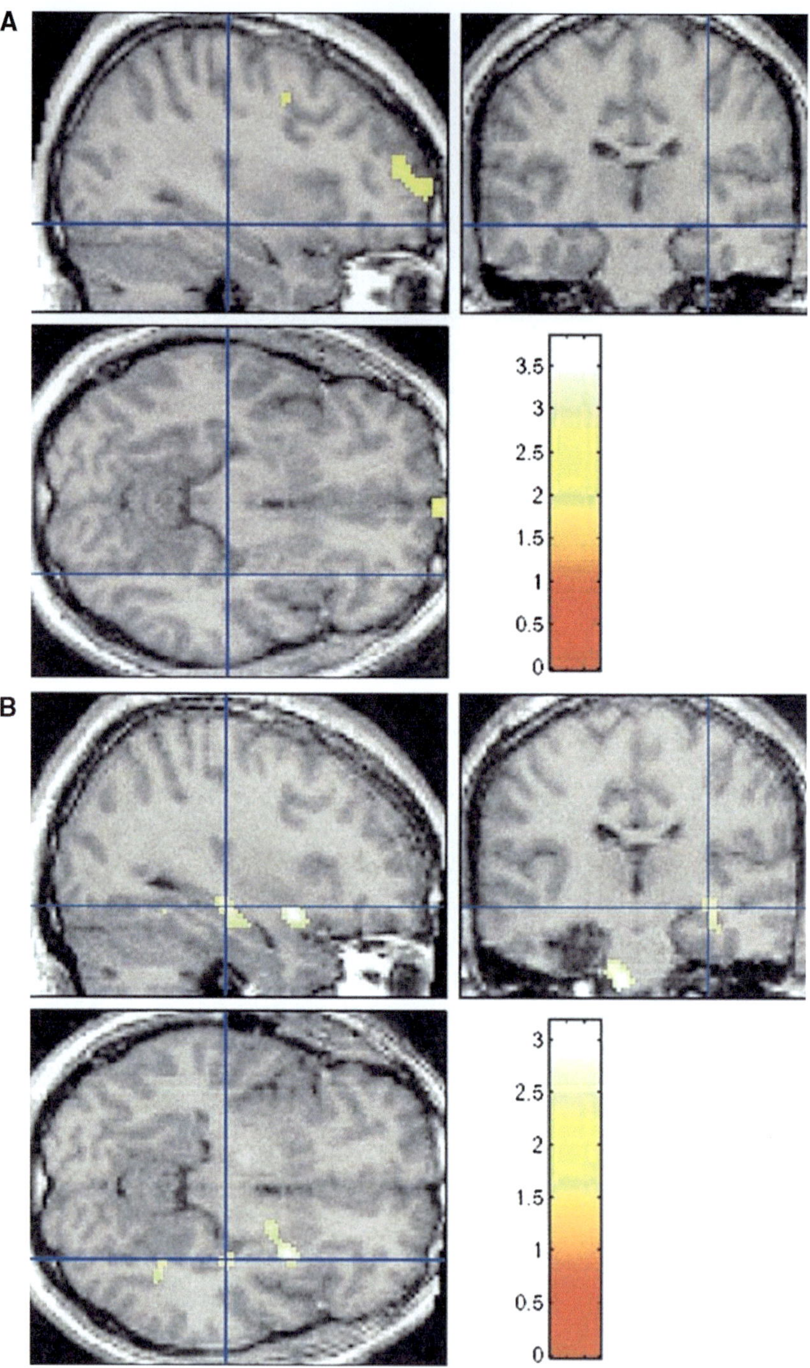

Figure 9.4. Right hippocampal activation ($p_{crit} = 0.01$) in a 25-year-old, right-handed male during verbal encoding before (A) and after (B) left selective amygdalohippocampectomy. Right MTL activation observed after, but not before, surgery in the nonepileptic hippocampus suggests a possible functional release from the irritative seizure focus (see McDonald and colleagues[95]). (Neurologic coordinates).

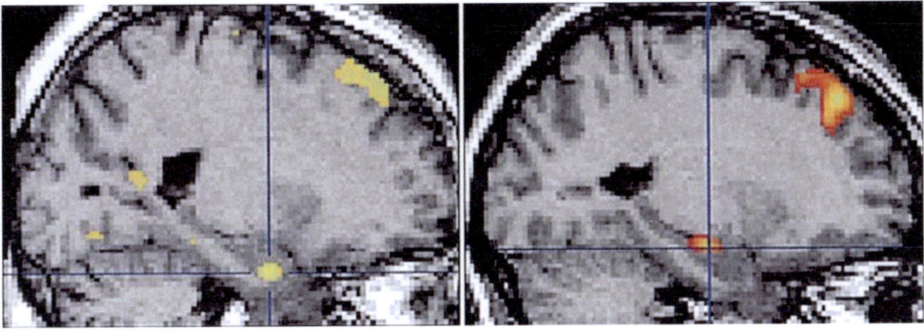

Figure 9.5. Left medial temporal lobe activation (p_{crit} = 0.05) in two female right temporal lobe resection patients (both right-handed and left hemisphere dominant for language on IAT), during encoding of novel words showing contralateral memory functioning after surgery (fMRI conducted 2.8 and 4.8 years after surgery, see McDonald and colleagues[95]).

and extent of the neural circuits subserving various cognitive functions. For example, those studies that obtain images only of the frontal lobes cannot, by definition, detect functional lateralization or localization of extrafrontal language or memory regions. The choice of imaging plane and slice thickness and positioning (axial, coronal, sagittal, or oblique) also may differentially affect the visualizability of brain regions. The problems of signal dropout and other susceptibility artifacts in memory-related structures (e.g., medial temporal lobes, frontal poles) also need to be addressed. The effect of various epileptogenic brain abnormalities (e.g., AVM and related flow disruption, tumor, cortical dysplasia) on brain anatomy, function, and activation patterns is also of critical importance in evaluation of the effectiveness of fMRI activation tasks in lateralizing and localizing cognitive functions. The statistical significance threshold chosen for a given study also can alter the conclusions drawn from fMRI data in ways that are particularly salient for surgical cases. As noted above,[23,29] lowering statistical thresholds for significant activation can lead to increased observed activation and assist in language lateralization. In some cases, however, lowering the significance threshold can lead to a spurious increase in regionally nonspecific activation and loss of a significant AI. The need to lower the threshold for significant activation may be greater in younger subjects due to developmental differences in overall levels of observed activation, although such a technique in these subjects could likewise lower the AI due to increased spurious activation or activation in homologous regions in the contralateral hemisphere.

The question of whether or not fMRI measures of cognition produce reproducible results is also of direct relevance whenever surgical intervention is under consideration. In a sophisticated statistical approach to analyzing the reproducibility of fMRI activation patterns, Fernandez and colleagues[99] examined the reliability of fMRI lateralization of language functions within and between individual subjects, and within and between scanning sessions. They administered a semantic judgment task to 34 epilepsy patients on one occasion and to 12 other patients at two separate scanning sessions on the same day using alternate task forms. Results demonstrated good within-test and test–retest reliability of task-related activation patterns.

For test–retest patients, a significant amount of overlap was noted between the first and second evaluations on a voxel-by-voxel basis, with higher significance levels for activation in frontal (e.g., Broca's area, premotor region) than more posterior regions (temporoparietal cortex). This method provided similarly reliable activation patterns for patients with right or mixed hemisphere dominance for language as those with left hemisphere dominance. The authors concluded that fMRI holds great promise for replacing the IAT in terms of language lateralization for lateralizing frontal language regions. They pointed out, however, that fMRI may activate some, but not necessarily all, brain regions participating in a given function; consequently, they recommend caution in replacing deactivation procedures (e.g., cortical stimulation mapping) entirely for planning surgical resection margins. Furthermore, they noted that their data cannot speak to the definition of such surgical margins, as the normalization paradigm required for group statistical analysis introduces spatial distortion of individual activation data. It should be noted, however, that such spatial normalization is not required for fMRI, and analyses can be performed in native brain space, as is typically done at DHMC for individual presurgical cases. With regard to setting the surgical margin, the statistical threshold chosen will necessarily affect degree and extent of activation observed. As the overall level of observed fMRI brain activation varies between individuals, it generally is not considered appropriate or feasible to set the same a priori threshold for all subjects. Rutten and colleagues[100] examined fMRI activation patterns in the temporal lobes in nonnormalized scans as compared to cortical stimulation mapping. Their study demonstrated a specificity of 61% of subjects, and false-positive activation in 51%, suggesting that fMRI cannot yet be used for direct delineation of the surgical resection margin. Fernandez and colleagues[99] suggest that one method to alleviate this difficulty would be to create individualized normalization of language regions in relation to brain regions with known, quantifiable relationships between fMRI task stimulation and activation response (e.g., primary visual cortex, where a linear relationship has been demonstrated between changes in neural activity and fMRI signal[101]).

Clinical Concerns

Future fMRI studies of cognition in epilepsy patients attempting to replace the IAT also will need to address issues related to neurodevelopmental abnormalities in cognition due to factors unique to epilepsy patients. For example, previous research[83,102–104] has demonstrated an interaction between factors such as age at seizure onset and age at first risk factor for epilepsy (e.g., febrile convulsions, traumatic brain injury, meningitis, encephalitis) and cognitive outcomes following temporal lobectomy. In a study of eight TLE patients, Killgore and colleagues[105] reported that presurgical fMRI memory lateralization predicted postsurgical seizure freedom as effectively as IAT, with asymmetry of fMRI MTL activation favoring the nonepileptogenic hemisphere, demonstrating an association with seizure freedom one year postsurgery. Similarly, Sabsevitz and colleagues[106,107] demonstrated that presurgical activation during an fMRI semantic decision-making task in a group of left TLE patients showed a significant relationship with performance on an out-of-scanner naming task postsurgery, suggesting that fMRI might be a useful tool in predicting postsurgical cognitive outcome. Another study from this group[108] showed that earlier age of seizure onset is associated with greater atypical language lateralization, and that subjects with a left hemisphere seizure focus whose language skills appear to have undergone reorganization demonstrated poorer naming skills. These findings point to the need for further investigation of the relationship of early risk factors for epilepsy and related abnormalities in neurodevelopment to later brain organization of cognitive functions such as language and memory. Functional MRI may be an ideal tool to study the reorganization suggested by earlier neuropsychological[83,109] and IAT studies.[110]

To date, fMRI studies of cognition in epilepsy generally have not explicitly addressed the potential contribution of antiepileptic drugs (AEDs) to observed activation patterns. Antiepileptic drugs have known or presumed effects on cerebral blood flow and metabolism[111–116], although, at present, these effects remain unelucidated or poorly understood for many AEDs. Direct or indirect effects on cortical blood flow may differentially affect the observed BOLD response in epilepsy patients in comparison to healthy medication-free control subjects. There are differences between AEDs in the nature and extent of influence on neural activity, cortical blood flow, and metabolism, and the role these mechanisms play in the BOLD response requires systematic investigation. This potential confound has not been addressed directly in fMRI studies of epilepsy patients. Sex differences in brain language organization also merit consideration when using presurgical IAT results to assess feasibility of surgery or predict postsurgical risk for cognitive deficits.[117,118] Baxter and colleagues[119] have utilized fMRI to examine brain activation during a semantic processing task in healthy adult subjects to assess the applicability of models of intra- versus interhemispheric sex differences in language organization. The results of this study offered some support for both models of language organization; females showed greater bilateral representation of language functions than did males, while males demonstrated more diffuse activation within the left hemisphere than did females. These findings are consistent with previous studies demonstrating sex differences in language lateralization, which may affect predictions regarding cognitive outcome following epilepsy surgery and warrant consideration in presurgical evaluation.

As noted previously, it can be difficult to directly compare fMRI and IAT results, as different aspects of language and memory functioning typically are measured in these paradigms. In addition, given the current state of fMRI technology, observed activation patterns may reflect not only activation of regions critical for the function under examination, but also activation of areas related to other functions tapped by a particular fMRI task; for example, some language tasks may reflect brain activation related to attention and planning functions rather than language per se.[84] Therefore, it may be possible to include some activated areas within the resection margin to increase the likelihood of obtaining seizure control without leading to impairment in language and/or memory (though such resection may affect other cognitive functions). Furthermore, brain regions important for a given function may fail to activate during a particular task, suggesting that appropriate caution must be used when interpreting fMRI findings as they relate to surgical intervention.

Conclusions and Future Directions: Can We Replace the IAT with fMRI?

At present, the potential for replacement of the IAT with fMRI is quite different for language versus memory. Using the simple standard of language lateralization, it appears that fMRI paradigms are poised to replace the IAT, and that they can reliably lateralize language in children and adults, even in subjects with atypical (right or mixed) dominance. Functional MRI also has the advantage of providing information beyond that of the IAT in terms of intrahemispheric localization of language regions, although it does not yet have the proven reliability and validity required to replace current techniques used for setting the surgical margin, including electrostimulation mapping. For memory, while the few available fMRI studies provide promising data that suggest that IAT might eventually be able to be replaced, further investigation is necessary to ascertain the functional utility of these data with regard to surgical planning and outcome, as well as to extend the applicability to pediatric populations. Evidence-based standards for the recommendation of new diagnostic tests and treatments have been articulated by relevant professional organizations,[120] with the highest (Class I) standard being prospective, randomized controlled clinical trials (RCTs), with masked outcome assessment. Clearly, none of the fMRI research discussed above meets these stringent standards, but instead falls at the Class IV level (reports of case series). The IAT has likewise never undergone Class I trials, but has become the de facto clinical standard due to its long history and the lack of available alternatives. As with fMRI, a few case studies (e.g., Ref. 121) are available demonstrating reproducibility of IAT results and offering evidence towards reliability and validity. Based on the currently available data, it seems unlikely that the field will reach consensus in terms of the acceptability of replacing the IAT with fMRI, particularly for memory. The early results are promising, however, and much more systematic research is needed, including RCTs. A true gold standard for language and memory localization will only be ascertained through systematic assessment of postsurgical outcome data in relation to presurgical localization data, a task that has not yet been adequately completed for the IAT or for fMRI.

Overall, it seems certain that fMRI prardigms designed to replace the IAT will include multiple language and memory tasks in order to elicit activation of broad neural networks, including frontal and temporal language and memory circuitry. Future directions in the development of an fMRI paradigm to replace the IAT may be similar to work recently conducted by Deblaere and colleagues.[122] In a study unique in its attempt to include fMRI measures for both language and memory functioning, these authors utilized a group of activation paradigms, including complex scene encoding, picture naming, reading, word generation, and semantic decision-making tasks. While this study included only healthy control subjects, its findings are promising for future research, as these investigators were able to demonstrate bilateral MTL activation consistent with prior studies[88,89] during memory encoding, as well as robust language lateralization. While IAT results are obviously not available for comparison, the authors noted their intention to utilize this group of fMRI tasks with epilepsy patients to attempt to determine its feasibility in replicating, and eventually replacing, the IAT.

The next decade of clinical research is likely to establish fMRI firmly as a valuable tool for preoperative assessment of language and memory, as well as other eloquent cortical functions, in various neurosurgical contexts. Functional MRI is expected to be seen combined with structural imaging and other advanced diagnostic modalities. Further technical advances in field strength, gradient and radiofrequency coils, software, and cognitive paradigms will improve the sensitivity and specificity of fMRI. In the not too distant future, accurate results of preoperative fMRI mapping will be registered in the neurosurgeon's computer and microscope and routinely used to guide surgery.

Acknowledgments: The authors thank Barbara C. Jobst, MD, Jennifer D. Schoenfeld, PhD, the Department of Diagnostic Radiology, and the Epilepsy and Epilepsy Surgery Programs at Dartmouth-Hitchcock Medical Center for their contributions to the data presented in this chapter.

References

1. Medina LS, Aguirre E, Bernal B, Altman NR. Functional MR imaging versus Wada test for evaluation of language lateralization: Cost analysis. *Radiology.* 2004;230(1):49–54.
2. Loring DW, Meador KJ, Lee GP, King DW. *Amobarbital Effects and Lateralized Brain Function: The Wada Test.* New York: Springer-Verlag; 1992.
3. van Emde Boas W, Juhn A. Wada and the sodium amytal test in the first (and last?) 50 years. *J Hist Neurosci.* 1999;8(3):286–292.
4. Gardner WJ. Injection of procaine into the brain to locate speech area in left-handed persons. *Arch Neurol Psychiatry.* 1941;46:1035–1038.
5. Wada J, Rasmussen T. Intracarotid injection of sodium amytal for the lateralization of cerebral speech dominance. *J Neurosurgery.* 1960;17:266–282.
6. Milner B, Branch C, Rasmussen T. Study of short-term memory after intracarotid injection of sodium amytal. *Trans Am Neurol Assoc.* 1962;87:224–226.
7. Sperling MR, Saykin AJ, Glosser G, Moran M, French JA, Brooks M, et al. Predictors of outcome after anterior temporal lobectomy: The intracarotid amobarbital test. *Neurology.* 1994;44(12):2325–2330.
8. Rausch R. Role of the neuropsychological evaluation and the intracarotid sodium amobarbital procedure in the surgical treatment for epilepsy. *Epilepsy Res Suppl.* 1992;5:77–86.
9. Tatum WO, IV, Benbadis SR, Vale FL. The neurosurgical treatment of epilepsy. *Arch Fam Med.* 2000;9(10):1142–1147.
10. Assessment: Neuropsychological testing of adults. Considerations for neurologists. Report of the Therapeutics and Technology Assessment Subcommittee of the American Academy of Neurology. *Neurology.* 1996;47(2):592–599.
11. Surgery for epilepsy. NIH Consensus Statement Online 1990;8(2):1–20.
12. Devinsky O, Perrine K, Llinas R, Luciano DJ, Dogali M. Anterior temporal language areas in patients with early onset of temporal lobe epilepsy. *Ann Neurol.* 1993;34(5):727–732.
13. Mizrahi EM, Kellaway P, Grossman RG, Rutecki PA, Armstrong D, Rettig G, et al. Anterior temporal lobectomy and medically refractory temporal lobe epilepsy of childhood. *Epilepsia.* 1990;31(3):302–312.
14. Rasmussen T, Milner B. The role of early left-brain injury in determining lateralization of cerebral speech functions. *Ann N Y Acad Sci.* 1977;299:355–369.

15. Satz P, Strauss E, Wada J, Orsini DL. Some correlates of intra- and interhemispheric speech organization after left focal brain injury. *Neuropsychologia.* 1988;26(2): 345–350.
16. Woods RP, Dodrill CB, Ojemann GA. Brain injury, handedness, and speech lateralization in a series of amobarbital studies. *Ann Neurol.* 1988;23(5):510–518.
17. Pujol J, Deus J, Losilla JM, Capdevila A. Cerebral lateralization of language in normal left-handed people studied by functional MRI. *Neurology.* 1999;52(5): 1038–1043.
18. Szaflarski JP, Binder JR, Possing ET, McKiernan KA, Ward BD, Hammeke TA. Language lateralization in left-handed and ambidextrous people: fMRI data. *Neurology.* 2002;59(2):238–244.
19. Binder JR, Rao SM, Hammeke TA, Frost JA, Bandettini PA, Jesmanowicz A, et al. Lateralized human brain language systems demonstrated by task subtraction functional magnetic resonance imaging. *Arch Neurol.* 1995;52(6):593–601.
20. Binder JR, Swanson SJ, Hammeke TA, Morris GL, Mueller WM, Fischer M, et al. Determination of language dominance using functional MRI: A comparison with the Wada test. *Neurology.* 1996;46(4):978–984.
21. Gaillard WD, Hertz-Pannier L, Mott SH, Barnett AS, LeBihan D, Theodore WH. Functional anatomy of cognitive development: fMRI of verbal fluency in children and adults. *Neurology.* 2000;54(1):180–185.
22. Grandin CB, Gaillard WD, Hunter KE, Petrella JR, Braniecki SH, Whitnah JR, et al. Comparison of phonemic and semantic verbal fluency tasks: An fMRI study. *Neuroimage.* 1998;7:S133.
23. Hertz-Pannier L, Gaillard WD, Mott SH, Cuenod CA, Bookheimer SY, Weinstein S, et al.Noninvasive assessment of language dominance in children and adolescents with functional MRI: A preliminary study. *Neurology.* 1997;48(4): 1003–1012.
24. Beauregard M, Chertkow H, Bub D, Murtha S, Dixon R, Evans A. The neural substrate for concrete, abstract, and emotional word lexica: A positron emission tomography study. *J Cogn Neurosci.* 1997;9(4):441–461.
25. Beeman M. Semantic processing in the right hemisphere may contribute to drawing inferences from discourse. *Brain Lang.* 1993;44(1):80–120.
26. Beeman M, Friedman RB, Grafman J, Perez E, Diamond S, Lindsay MB. Summation priming and coarse coding in the right hemisphere. *J Cogn Neurosci.* 1994;6:26–45.
27. Fletcher PC, Happe F, Frith U, Baker SC, Dolan RJ, Frackowiak RS, et al. Other minds in the brain: A functional imaging study of "theory of mind" in story comprehension. *Cognition.* 1995;57(2):109–128.
28. Gaillard WD, Pugliese M, Grandin CB, Braniecki SH, Kondapaneni P, Hunter K, et al. Cortical localization of reading in normal children: An fMRI language study. *Neurology.* 2001;57(1):47–54.
29. Gaillard WD, Balsamo L, Xu B, Grandin CB, Braniecki SH, Papero PH, et al. Language dominance in partial epilepsy patients identified with an fMRI reading task. *Neurology.* 2002;59(2):256–265.
30. Just MA, Carpenter PA, Keller TA, Eddy WF, Thulborn KR. Brain activation modulated by sentence comprehension. *Science.* 1996;274:114–116.
31. Ross ED, Mesulam MM. Dominant language functions of the right hemisphere? Prosody and emotional gesturing. *Arch Neurol.* 1979;36(3):144–148.
32. Scoville W, Milner B. Loss of recent memory after bilateral hippocampal lesions. *J Neurol Neurosurg Psychiatry.* 1957;20:11–21.
33. Loddenkemper T, Morris HH, 3rd, Perl J, 2nd. Carotid artery dissection after the intracarotid amobarbital test. *Neurology.* 2002;59(11):1797–1798.
34. Morris P. *Practical Neuroangiography.* Baltimore: Williams & Wilkins; 1997.
35. Rausch R, Silfvenius H, Wieser H-G, Dodrill CB, Meador KJ, Jones-Gotman M. Intraarterial amobarbital procedures. In: Engel J Jr, ed. *Surgical Treatment of the Epilepsies.* 2nd ed. New York: Raven Press, Ltd.; 1993:341–357.

36. Saykin AJ, Sussman NM, Gur RC. Neuropsychological methods in temporal lobectomy: Comparison of traditional batteries and specialized procedures. *J Clin Exp Neuropsychol.* 1987;9(1):33–34.

37. Kimura D. Right temporal damage. *Arch Neurol.* 1963;8:264–271.

38. Green D, Swets J. *Signal Detection Theory and Psychophysics.* New York: Krieger: 1974.

39. Gerschlager W, Lalouschek W, Lehrner J, Baumgartner C, Lindinger G, Lang W. Language-related hemispheric asymmetry in healthy subjects and patients with temporal lobe epilepsy as studied by event-related brain potentials and intracarotid amobarbital test. *Electroencephalog Clin Neurophysiol.* 1998;108(3): 274–282.

40. Epstein CM, Woodard JL, Stringer AY, Bakay RA, Henry TR, Pennell PB, et al. Repetitive transcranial magnetic stimulation does not replicate the Wada test. *Neurology.* 2000;55(7):1025–1027.

41. Fitzgerald DB, Cosgrove GR, Ronner S, Jiang H, Buchbinder BR, Belliveau JW, et al. Location of language in the cortex: A comparison between functional MR imaging and electrocortical stimulation. *AJNR Am J Neuroradiol.* 1997;18(8): 1529–1539.

42. Stapleton SR, Kiriakopoulos E, Mikulis D, Drake JM, Hoffman HJ,Humphreys R, et al.Combined utility of functional MRI, cortical mapping, and frameless stereotaxy in the resection of lesions in eloquent areas of brain in children. *Pediatr Neurosurg.* 1997;26(2):68–82.

43. Hunter KE, Blaxton TA, Bookheimer SY, Figlozzi C, Gaillard WD, Grandin C, et al. (15)O water positron emission tomography in language localization: A study comparing positron emission tomography visual and computerized region of interest analysis with the Wada test. *Ann Neurol.* 1999;45(5):662–665.

44. Pardo JV, Fox PT. Preoperative assessment of the cerebral hemispheric dominance for language with CBF PET. *Hum Brain Mapp.* 1993;1:57–68.

45. Dehaene S, Dupoux E, Mehler J, Cohen L, Paulesu E, Perani D, et al. Anatomical variability in the cortical representation of first and second language. *Neuroreport.* 1997;8(17):3809–3815.

46. Lehéricy S, Cohen L, Bazin B, Samson S, Giacomini E, Rougetet R, et al. Functional MR evaluation of temporal and frontal language dominance compared with the Wada test. *Neurology.* 2000;54(8):1625–1633.

47. Mazoyer BM, Tzourio N, Frak V, Syrota A, Murayama N, Levrier O, et al. The cortical representation of speech. *J Cogn Neurosci.* 1993;5(4):467–479.

48. Schlosser MJ, Aoyagi N, Fulbright RK, Gore JC, McCarthy G. Functional MRI studies of auditory comprehension. *Hum Brain Mapp.* 1998;6(1):1–13.

49. Schlosser MJ, Luby M, Spencer DD, Awad IA, McCarthy G. Comparative localization of auditory comprehension by using functional magnetic resonance imaging and cortical stimulation. *J Neurosurg.* 1999;91(4):626–635.

50. Bookheimer SY, Dapretto M, Karmarkar U. Functional MRI in children with epilepsy. *Dev Neurosci.* 1999;21(3–5):191–199.

51. Booth JR, Macwhinney B, Thulborn KR, Sacco K, Voyvodic J, Feldman HM. Functional organization of activation patterns in children: Whole brain fMRI imaging during three different cognitive tasks. *Prog Neuropsychopharmacol Biol Psychiatry.* 1999;23:669–682.

52. Howard D, Patterson K, Wise R, Brown WD, Friston K, Weiller C, et al. The cortical localization of the lexicons. Positron emission tomography evidence. *Brain.* 1992;115:1769–1782.

53. Gaillard WD, Xu B, Balsamo LM, Grandin CB, Papero PH, Weinstein S, et al. fMRI identification of language dominance in patients with complex partial epilepsy using an auditory based language comprehension task. *Epilepsia.* 2000;41 (Suppl 7):83.

54. Bavelier D, Corina D, Jezzard P, Padmanabhan S, Clark VP, Karni A, et al. Sentence reading: A functional MRI study at 4 Tesla. *J Cogn Neurosci.* 1997;9(5):664–686.

55. Dapretto M, Bookheimer SY. Form and content: Dissociating syntax and semantics in sentence comprehension. *Neuron.* 1999;24(2):427–432.

56. Embick D, Marantz A, Miyashita Y, O'Neil W, Sakai KL. A syntactic specialization for Broca's area. *Proc Nat Acad Sci U S A.* 2000;97(11):6150–6154.

57. Gabrieli JD, Poldrack RA, Desmond JE. The role of left prefrontal cortex in language and memory. *Proc Nat Acad Sci U S A.* 1998;95(3):906–913.

58. Bookheimer SY, Zeffiro TA, Blaxton TA, Gaillard WD, Malow B, Theodore WH. Regional cerebral blood flow during auditory responsive naming: Evidence for cross-modality neural activation. *Neuroreport.* 1998;9(10):2409–2413.

59. Demb JB, Desmond JE, Wagner AD, Vaidya CJ, Glover GH, Gabrieli JD. Semantic encoding and retrieval in the left inferior prefrontal cortex: A functional MRI study of task difficulty and process specificity. *J Neurosci.* 1995;15(9):5870–5878.

60. Poldrack RA, Wagner AD, Prull MW, Desmond JE, Glover GH, Gabrieli JD. Functional specialization for semantic and phonological processing in the left inferior prefrontal cortex. *Neuroimage.* 1999;10(1):15–35.

61. Desmond JE, Sum JM, Wagner AD, Demb JB, Shear PK, Glover GH, et al. Functional MRI measurement of language lateralization in Wada-tested patients. *Brain.* 1995;118(Pt 6):1411–1419.

62. Benbadis SR, Binder JR, Swanson SJ, Fischer M, Hammeke TA, Morris GL, et al. Is speech arrest during Wada testing a valid method for determining hemispheric representation of language? *Brain Lang.* 1998;65(3):441–446.

63. Bahn MM, Lin W, Silbergeld DL, Miller JW, Kuppusamy K, Cook RJ, et al. Localization of language cortices by functional MR imaging compared with intracarotid amobarbital hemispheric sedation. *AJR Am J Roentgenol.* 1997;169(2):575–579.

64. Worthington C, Vincent DJ, Bryant AE, Roberts DR, Vera CL, Ross DA, et al. Comparison of functional magnetic resonance imaging for language localization and intracarotid speech amytal testing in presurgical evaluation for intractable epilepsy. Preliminary results. *Stereotact Funct Neurosurg.* 1997;69(1–4 Pt 2):197–201.

65. Yetkin FZ, Swanson S, Fischer M, Akansel G, Morris G, Mueller W, et al. Functional MR of frontal lobe activation: Comparison with Wada language results. *AJNR Am J Neuroradiol.* 1998;19(6):1095–1098.

66. Benson RR, FitzGerald DB, LeSueur LL, Kennedy DN, Kwong KK, Buchbinder BR, et al. Language dominance determined by whole brain functional MRI in patients with brain lesions. *Neurology.* 1999;52(4):798–809.

67. Carpentier A, Pugh KR, Westerveld M, Studholme C, Skrinjar O, Thompson JL, et al. Functional MRI of language processing: Dependence on input modality and temporal lobe epilepsy. *Epilepsia.* 2001;42(10):1241–1254.

68. Baciu M, Kahane P, Minotti L, Charnallet A, David D, Le Bas JF, et al. Functional MRI assessment of the hemispheric predominance for language in epileptic patients using a simple rhyme detection task. *Epileptic Disord.* 2001;3(3):117–124.

69. Cuenod CA, Bookheimer SY, Hertz-Pannier L, Zeffiro TA, Theodore WH, Le Bihan D. Functional MRI during word generation, using conventional equipment: A potential tool for language localization in the clinical environment. *Neurology.* 1995;45(10):1821–1827.

70. Springer JA, Binder JR, Hammeke TA, Swanson SJ, Frost JA, Bellgowan PS, et al. Language dominance in neurologically normal and epilepsy subjects: A functional MRI study. *Brain.* 1999;122(Pt 11):2033–2046.

71. Yetkin FZ, Mueller WM, Morris GL, McAuliffe TL, Ulmer JL, Cox RW, et al. Functional MR activation correlated with intraoperative cortical mapping. *AJNR Am J Neuroradiol.* 1997;18(7):1311–1315.

72. Fiez JA, Petersen SE. Neuroimaging studies of word reading. *Proc Nat Acad Sci U S A.* 1998;95(3):914–921.

73. Price CJ, Moore CJ, Humphreys GW, Wise RJS. Segregating semantic from phonological processes during reading. *J Cogn Neurosci.* 1997;9(6):727–733.
74. Ojemann G, Ojemann J, Lettich E, Berger M. Cortical language localization in left, dominant hemisphere. An electrical stimulation mapping investigation in 117 patients. *J Neurosurg.* 1989;71(3):316–326.
75. Heiss WD, Kessler J, Thiel A, Ghaemi M, Karbe H. Differential capacity of left and right hemispheric areas for compensation of poststroke aphasia. *Ann Neurol.* 1999;45(4):430–438.
76. Warburton E, Wise RJ, Price CJ, Weiller C, Hadar U, Ramsay S, et al. Noun and verb retrieval by normal subjects. Studies with PET. *Brain.* 1996;119(Pt 1): 159–179.
77. Weiller C, Isensee C, Rijntjes M, Huber W, Muller S, Bier D, et al. Recovery from Wernicke's aphasia: A positron emission tomographic study. *Ann Neurol.* 1995;37(6):723–732.
78. Rutten GJ, Ramsey NF, van Rijen PC, Alpherts WC, van Veelen CW. fMRI-determined language lateralization in patients with unilateral or mixed language dominance according to the Wada test. *Neuroimage.* 2002;17(1):447–460.
79. Benson RR, Logan WJ, Cosgrove GR, Cole AJ, Jiang H, LeSueur LL, et al. Functional MRI localization of language in a 9-year-old child. *Can J Neurol Sci.* 1996;23(3):213–219.
80. Gaillard WD, Grandin CB, Xu B. Developmental aspects of pediatric fMRI: Considerations for image acquisition, analysis, and interpretation. *Neuroimage.* 2001;13(2):239–249.
81. Hertz-Pannier L, Chiron C, Vera P, Van de Morteele PF, Kaminska A, Bourgeois M, et al. Functional imaging in the work-up of childhood epilepsy. *Childs Nerv Syst.* 2001;17(4–5):223–228.
82. Baxendale S. The role of functional MRI in the presurgical investigation of temporal lobe epilepsy patients: A clinical perspective and review. *J Clin Exp Neuropsychol.* 2002;24(5):664–676.
83. Saykin AJ, Stafiniak P, Robinson LJ, Flannery KA, Gur RC, O'Connor MJ, et al. Language before and after temporal lobectomy: Specificity of acute changes and relation to early risk factors. *Epilepsia.* 1995;36(11):1071–1077.
84. Bookheimer SY, Zeffiro TA, Blaxton T, Malow BA, Gaillard WD, Sato S, et al. A direct comparison of PET activation and electrocortical stimulation mapping for language localization. *Neurology.* 1997;48(4):1056–1065.
85. Muller RA, Rothermel RD, Behen ME, Muzik O, Mangner TJ, Chugani HT. Differential patterns of language and motor reorganization following early left hemisphere lesion: A PET study. *Arch Neurol.* 1998;55(8):1113–1119.
86. Kurthen M, Helmstaedter C, Linke DB, Solymosi L, Elger CE, Schramm J. Interhemispheric dissociation of expressive and receptive language functions in patients with complex-partial seizures: An amobarbital study. *Brain Lang.* 1992;43(4):694–712.
87. Staudt M, Grodd W, Niemann G, Wildgruber D, Erb M, Krageloh-Mann I. Early left periventricular brain lesions induce right hemispheric organization of speech. *Neurology.* 2001;57(1):122–125.
88. Detre JA, Maccotta L, King D, Alsop DC, Glosser G, D'Esposito M, et al. Functional MRI lateralization of memory in temporal lobe epilepsy. *Neurology.* 1998;50(4):926–932.
89. Stern CE, Corkin S, Gonzalez RG, Guimaraes AR, Baker JR, Jennings PJet al.The hippocampal formation participates in novel picture encoding: Evidence from functional magnetic resonance imaging. *Proc Nat Acad Sci U S A.* 1996;93(16): 8660–8665.
90. Bellgowan PS, Binder JR, Swanson SJ, Hammeke TA, Springer JA, Frost JA, et al. Side of seizure focus predicts left medial temporal lobe activation during verbal encoding. *Neurology.* 1998;51(2):479–484.

91. Dupont S, Van de Moortele PF, Samson S, Hasboun D, Poline JB, Adam C, et al. Episodic memory in left temporal lobe epilepsy: A functional MRI study. *Brain.* 2000;123(Pt 8):1722–1732.

92. Dupont S, Samson Y, Van de Moortele PF, Samson S, Poline JB, Adam Cet al. Delayed verbal memory retrieval: A functional MRI study in epileptic patients with structural lesions of the left medial temporal lobe. *Neuroimage.* 2001;14(5): 995–1003.

93. Jokeit H, Okujava M, Woermann FG. Memory fMRI lateralizes temporal lobe epilepsy. *Neurology.* 2001;57(10):1786–1793.

94. Golby AJ, Poldrack RA, Illes J, Chen D, Desmond JE, Gabrieli JD. Memory lateralization in medial temporal lobe epilepsy assessed by functional MRI. *Epilepsia.* 2002;43(8):855–863.

95. McDonald BC, Saykin AJ, Jobst BC, Williamson PD, Roberts DW, Thadani VM, et al. Brain activation patterns in frontal and temporal memory circuitry following temporal lobe resection for intractable epilepsy: An fMRI study. *J Neuropsychiatry Clin Neurosci.* 2003;15(2):282.

96. Saykin AJ, Weaver JB, Burr RB, Riordan HJ, Roberts DW, Williamson PDet al. Functional magnetic resonance imaging in the evaluation of epilepsy surgery patients: A memory activation study. *Epilepsia.* 1994;35:86.

97. Swick D, Knight R. Contributions of prefrontal cortex to recognition memory: Electrophysiological and behavioral evidence. *Neuropsychology.* 1999;13(2): 155–170.

98. Martin A. Automatic activation of the medial temporal lobe during encoding: Lateralized influences of meaning and novelty. *Hippocampus.* 1999;9(1):62–70.

99. Fernandez G, Specht K, Weis S, Tendolkar I, Rueber M, Fell J, et al. Intra-subject reproducibility of presurgical language lateralization and mapping using fMRI. *Neurology.* 2003;60:969–975.

100. Rutten GJ, Ramsey NF, van Rijen PC, Noordmans HJ, van Veelen CW. Development of a functional magnetic resonance imaging protocol for intra-operative localization of critical temporoparietal language areas. *Ann Neurol.* 2002;51(3):350–360.

101. Boynton GM, Engel SA, Glover GH, Heeger DJ. Linear systems analysis of functional magnetic resonance imaging in human V1. *J Neurosci.* 1996;16(13): 4207–4221.

102. Saykin AJ, Gur RC, Sussman NM, O'Connor MJ, Gur RE. Memory deficits before and after temporal lobectomy:effect of laterality and age of onset. *Brain Cogn.* 1989;9:191–200.

103. Saykin AJ, Robinson LJ, Stafiniak P, Kester DB, Gur RC, O'Connor MJ, et al. Neuropsychological changes after anterior temporal lobectomy: Acute effects on memory, language, and music. In: Bennett TL, ed. *The Neuropsychology of Epilepsy.* New York: Plenum Press; 1992.

104. Stafiniak P, Saykin AJ, Sperling MR, Kester DB, Robinson LJ, O'Connor MJ, et al. Acute naming deficits following dominant temporal lobectomy: Prediction by age at 1st risk for seizures. *Neurology.* 1990;40(10):1509–1512.

105. Killgore WD, Glosser G, Casasanto DJ, French JA, Alsop DC, Detre JA. Functional MRI and the Wada test provide complementary information for predicting post-operative seizure control. *Seizure.* 1999;8(8):450–455.

106. Sabsevitz DS, Swanson SJ, Hammeke TA, Possing ET, Spanaki MV, Morris GL, et al. Predicting naming deficits following left anterior temporal lobectomy using fMRI. *J Int Neuropsychol Soc.* 2002;8(2):317.

107. Sabsevitz DS, Swanson SJ, Hammeke TA, Spanaki MV, Possing ET, Morris GL, 3rd, et al.Use of preoperative functional neuroimaging to predict language deficits from epilepsy surgery. *Neurology.* 2003;60(11):1788–1792.

108. Swanson SJ, Binder JR, Possing ET, Hammeke TA, Sabsevitz DS, Spanaki M, et al. fMRI language laterality during a semantic task: Age of onset and side of seizure focus effects. *J Int Neuropsychol Soc.* 2002;8(2):222.

109. Hermann BP, Seidenberg M, Haltiner A, Wyler AR. Relationship of age at onset, chronologic age, and adequacy of preoperative performance to verbal memory change after anterior temporal lobectomy. *Epilepsia.* 1995;36(2):137–145.

110. Glosser G, Saykin A, Deutsch G, Sperling M, O'Connor M. Patterns of reorganization of memory functions within and between cerebral hemispheres as assessed by the intracarotid amobarbital test. *Neuropsychology.* 1995;9(4): 449–456.

111. Ketter TA, Kimbrell TA, George MS, Willis MW, Benson BE, Danielson Aet al. Baseline cerebral hypermetabolism associated with carbamazepine response, and hypometabolism with nimodipine response in mood disorders. *Biol Psychiatry.* 1999;46(10):1364–1374.

112. Matheja P, Weckesser M, Debus O, Lottgen J, Schuierer G, Schober O, et al. Drug-induced changes in cerebral glucose consumption in bifrontal epilepsy. *Epilepsia.* 2000;41(5):588–593.

113. Roberts MA, Manshadi FF, Bushnell DL, Hines ME. Neurobehavioural dysfunction following mild traumatic brain injury in childhood: A case report with positive findings on positron emission tomography (PET). *Brain Inj.* 1995;9(5):427–436.

114. Theodore WH. Antiepileptic drugs and cerebral glucose metabolism. *Epilepsia.* 1988;29(Suppl 2):S48–S55.

115. Theodore WH, Bromfield E, Onorati L. The effect of carbamazepine on cerebral glucose metabolism. *Ann Neurol.* 1989;25(5):516–520.

116. Theodore WH. Therapeutics: Pharmacologic. In: Mazziotta JC, Toga AW, Frackowiak RSJ, eds. *Brain Mapping: The Disorders.* San Diego, CA: Academic Press; 2000:599–612.

117. Kimura D. Sex differences in cerebral organization for speech and praxic functions. *Can J Psychol.* 1983;38:19–35.

118. McGlone J. Sex differences in the cerebral organization of verbal functions in patients with unilateral brain lesions. *Brain.* 1977;100(4):775–793.

119. Baxter LC, Saykin AJ, Flashman LA, Johnson SC, Guerin SJ, Babcock DRet al. Sex differences in semantic language processing: A functional MRI study. *Brain Lang.* 2003;84(2):264–272.

120. American Academy of Neurology. *AAN Clinical Practice Handbook.* St. Paul, MN: American Academy of Neurology; 1995–2003.

121. Bramham J, Morris RG. Pre- and postoperative intracarotid amytal procedure: An assessment of validity. *Epilepsy Behav.* 2003;4(5):556–563.

122. Deblaere K, Backes WH, Hofman P, Vandemaele P, Boon PA, Vonck K, et al. Developing a comprehensive presurgical functional MRI protocol for patients with intractable temporal lobe epilepsy: A pilot study. *Neuroradiology.* 2002;44(8):667–673.

10

Cognitive Neuroscience Applications

Mark D'Esposito

Introduction

Cognitive neuroscience is a discipline that attempts to determine the neural mechanisms underlying cognitive processes. Specifically, cognitive neuroscientists test hypotheses about brain–behavior relationships organized along two conceptual domains: *functional specialization*—the idea that functional modules exist within the brain, that is, areas of the cerebral cortex that are specialized for a specific cognitive process, and *functional integration*—the idea that a cognitive process can be an emergent property of interactions among a network of brain regions that suggests that a brain region can play a different role across many functions.

Early studies of brain–behavior relationships consisted of careful observation of individuals with neurological injury resulting in focal brain damage. The idea of functional specialization evolved from hypotheses that damage to a particular brain region was responsible for a given behavioral syndrome that was characterized by a precise neurological examination; for instance, the association of nonfluent aphasia with right-sided limb weakness implicated the left hemisphere as the site of language abilities. Moreover, upon the death of a patient with a neurological disorder, clinico-pathological correlations provided confirmatory information about the site of damage causing a specific neurobehavioral syndrome such as aphasia; for example, in 1861, Paul Broca's observations of nonfluent aphasia in the setting of a damaged left inferior frontal gyrus cemented the belief that this brain region was critical for speech output.[1] The introduction of structural brain imaging more than 100 years after Broca's observations, first with computerized tomography and later with magnetic resonance imaging (MRI), paved the way for more precise anatomical localization in the living patient of the cognitive deficits that develop after brain injury. The superb spatial resolution of structural neuroimaging has reduced the reliance on the infrequently obtained autopsy for making brain–behavior correlations.

This chapter previously appeared in *Functional MRI: Basic Principles and Clinical Applications*, edited by S. Faro and F. Mohamed. New York: Springer Science+Business Media, LCC 2006.

From: *BOLD fMRI: A Guide to Functional Imaging for Neuroscientists*
Edited by: S.H. Faro and F.B. Mohamed, DOI 10.1007/978-1-4419-1329-6_10
© Springer Science+Business Media, LLC 2010

Functional neuroimaging, broadly defined as techniques that measure brain activity, has expanded our ability to study the neural basis of cognitive processes. One such method, functional MRI (fMRI) has emerged as an extremely powerful technique that affords excellent spatial and temporal resolution. Measuring regional brain activity in healthy subjects while they perform behavioral tasks links localized brain activity with specific behaviors; for example, functional neuroimaging studies have demonstrated that the left inferior frontal gyrus is consistently activated during the performance of speech-production tasks in healthy individuals.[2] Such findings from functional neuroimaging are complementary to findings derived from observations of patients with focal brain damage. This chapter focuses on the principles underlying fMRI as a cognitive neuroscience tool for exploring brain–behavior relationships.

Inference in Functional Neuroimaging Studies of Cognitive Processes

Insight regarding the link between brain and behavior can be gained through a variety of approaches. It is unlikely that any single neuroscience method is sufficient to investigate fully any particular question regarding the mechanism underlying cognitive function. From a methodological point of view, every method will offer different temporal and spatial resolution. From a conceptual point of view, every method will provide data that will support different types of inferences that can be drawn from it. Thus, data obtained addressing a single question but derived from multiple methods can provide more comprehensive and inferentially sound conclusions.

Functional neuroimaging studies support inferences about the association of a particular brain system with a cognitive process. However, it is difficult to prove in such a study that the observed activity is necessary for an isolated cognitive process because perfect control over a subject's cognitive processes during a functional neuroimaging experiment is never possible. Even if the task a subject performs is well designed, it is difficult to demonstrate conclusively that he/she is differentially engaging a single identified cognitive process. The subject may engage in unwanted cognitive processes that either have no overt measurable effects, or are perfectly confounded with the process of interest. Consequently, the neural activity measured by the functional neuroimaging technique may result from some confounding neural computation that is itself not necessary for executing the cognitive process seemingly under study. In other words, functional neuroimaging is an observational, correlative method.[3] It is important to note that the inferences that can be drawn from functional neuroimaging studies such as fMRI apply to all methods of physiological measurement [e.g., electroencephalogram (EEG) or magnetoencephalogram.]

The inference of necessity cannot be made without showing that inactivating a brain region disrupts the cognitive process in question. However, unlike precise surgical or neurotoxic lesions in animal models, lesions in patients are often extensive, damaging local neurons and fibers of passage; for example, damage to prominent white matter tracts can cause cognitive deficits similar to those produced by cortical lesions, such as the amnesia resulting from lesions of the fornix, the main white matter pathway projecting from the hippocampus.[4] In addition, connections from region A may support the continued metabolic function of region B, but region A may not be computationally involved in certain processes undertaken by region B. Thus, damage to region A could impair the function of region B via two possible mechanisms: (1) diaschisis[5] and (2) retrograde transsynaptic degeneration. Consequently, studies of patients with focal lesions cannot conclusively demonstrate that the neurons within a specific region are themselves critical to the computational support of an impaired cognitive process.

Empirical studies using lesion and electrophysiologic methods demonstrate these issues regarding the types of inferences that can logically be drawn from them. In monkeys, single-unit recording reveals neurons in the lateral prefrontal cortex that increase their firing during the delay between the presentation of information to be remembered and a few seconds later when that information must be recalled.[6,7] These studies are taken as evidence that persistent neural activity in the prefrontal cortex is involved in temporary storage of information, a cognitive process known as working memory. The necessity of prefrontal cortex for working memory was demonstrated in other monkey studies showing that prefrontal lesions impair performance on working memory tasks, but not on tasks that do not require temporarily holding information in memory.[8] Persistent neural activity during working memory tasks are also found in the hippocampus.[9,10] Hippocampal lesions, however, do not impair performance on most working memory tasks,[11] which suggests that the hippocampus is involved in maintaining information over short periods of time, but is not necessary for this cognitive operation. Observations in humans support this notion. For example, the well-studied patient H.M., with complete bilateral hippocampal damage and the severe inability to learn new information, could nevertheless perform normally on working memory tasks such as digit span.[12] The hippocampus is implicated in long-term memory, especially when relations between multiple items or multiple features of a complex novel item must be retained. Thus, the hippocampus may only be engaged during working memory tasks that requires someone to subsequently remember novel information.[13]

When the results from lesion and functional neuroimaging studies are combined, a stronger level of inference emerges. As in the examples of Broca's aphasia or working memory, a lesion of a specific brain region causes impairment of a given cognitive process, and when engaged by an intact individual, that cognitive process evokes neural activity in the same brain region. In this type of finding, the inference that this brain region is computationally necessary for the cognitive process is stronger than data derived from each study performed in isolation. Thus, lesion and functional neuroimaging studies are complementary, each providing inferential support that the other lacks.

Other types of inferential failure can occur in the interpretation of functional neuroimaging studies when other common assumptions do not hold true. First, it is assumed that if a cognitive process activates a particular brain region (evoked by a particular task), the neural activity in that brain region must depend on engaging that particular cognitive process; for example, a brain region showing greater activation during the presentation of faces than to other types of stimuli, such as photographs of cars or buildings, is considered to engage face perception processes. However, this region also may support other higher-level cognitive processes such as memory processes, in addition to lower-level perceptual processes.[14] Second, it is assumed that if a particular brain region is activated during the performance of a cognitive task, the subject must have engaged the cognitive process supported by that region during the task; for example, observing activation of the frontal lobes during a mental rotation task, it was proposed that subjects engaged working memory processes to recall the identity of the rotated target.[15] (They derived this assumption from other imaging studies showing activation of the frontal lobes during working memory tasks.) However, in this example, because some other cognitive process supported by the frontal lobes could have activated this region,[16] one cannot be sure that working memory was engaged leading to the activation of the frontal lobes.

In summary, interpretation of the results of functional neuroimaging studies attempting to link brain and behavior rests on numerous assumptions. Familiarity with the types of inferences that can and cannot be drawn from these studies should be helpful for assessing the validity of the findings reported by such studies.

Functional MRI as a Cognitive Neuroscience Tool

Functional MRI has become the predominant functional neuroimaging method for studying the neural basis of cognitive processes in humans. Compared to its predecessor, positron emission tomography (PET) scanning, fMRI offers many advantages; for example, MRI scanners are much more widely available, and imaging costs are less expensive because MRI does not require a cyclotron to produce radioisotopes. Magnetic resonance imaging is also a noninvasive procedure because there is no requirement for injection of a radioisotope into the bloodstream. In addition, given the half-life of available radioisotopes, PET scanning is unable to provide comparable temporal resolution to that of fMRI, which can provide images of behavioral events occurring on the order of seconds rather than the summation of many behavioral events over tens of seconds.

In selected circumstances, however, PET can provide an advantage over fMRI for studying certain questions concerning the neural basis of cognition; for example, at present, fMRI does not adequately image the regions within the orbitofrontal cortex and the anterior or inferior temporal lobe because of the susceptibility artifact near the interface of the brain and sinuses. These artifacts worsen at higher magnetic fields (i.e., 3 or 4 Tesla), and such scanners are becoming commonly available and increasingly utilized by cognitive neuroscientists. Improvements in pulse sequences for acquiring fMRI data and development of algorithms for distortion correction of images should eventually eliminate or reduce these artifacts.[17–19] Currently, however, such sequences and methods are not widely available and implemented. Position emission tomography scanning may remain desirable or necessary when studying certain populations of individuals; for example, amnesic patients resulting from cerebral anoxia often have implanted cardiac pacemakers precluding them from having an MRI scan due to the magnetic field. However, PET scanning is unacceptable for studies of children due to the radiation exposure.

The MRI scanner, compared to a behavioral testing room, is less than ideal for performing most cognitive neuroscience experiments. Experiments are performed in the awkward position of lying on one's back, often requiring subjects to visualize the presentation of stimuli through a mirror in an acoustically noisy environment. Moreover, most individuals develop some degree of claustrophobia due to the small bore of the MRI scanner and find it difficult to remain completely motionless for a long duration of time that is required for most experiments (e.g., usually 60 to 90 minutes). These constraints of the MRI scanner make it especially difficult to scan children, which has resulted in many fewer fMRI studies involving children than adults.[20,21] In addition, it has been a technical challenge to develop equipment within the MRI environment that successfully presents different types of stimuli to the individual (e.g., olfactory, tactile), as well as to collect ancillary response or physiological data necessary for a particular experiment.

All sensory systems have been investigated with fMRI, including the visual, auditory, somatosensory, olfactory, and gustatory systems. Each system requires different technologies for successful presentation of relevant stimuli within an MRI environment. At the time of this writing, very few off-the-shelf commercial products exist that are MRI compatible, and most in use today have been engineered locally by individual laboratories. Most published fMRI studies have utilized visual stimuli, although great strides have been made to allow the presentation of other types of stimuli. Details regarding the issues related to presenting visual and auditory stimuli in the MRI environment can be reviewed furthered in a comprehensive chapter on the topic by Savoy and colleagues.[22] In brief, the most common means of presenting visual stimuli is via a LCD projector system, with the sophistication of the system depending on the quality of image resolution required for the experiment. Several options exist for auditory stimuli, such as piezoelectric or electrostatic headphones. However, the biggest challenge is the acoustically noisy scanner environment. The pulsing of the fMRI gradient coils is the source of such noise, making the study of auditory processes challenging;[23,24] for example, during echoplanar imaging within a 4 Tesla magnet using a high-performance head gradient set, sound levels can reach 130 decibels. As a reference point, Food and Drug Administration (FDA) safety regulations require no greater than an average of 105 decibels for one hour. With placement of absorbing materials within the scanner and on the walls of the room, as well as a fiberglass bore liner surrounding the gradient set, we have been able to reduce sound levels by about 25 decibels. For further discussion concerning sound reduction techniques, refer to the chapter on Auditing MRI. One of the biggest technical challenges within an MRI scanner has been the ability to present olfactory stimuli. However, sophisticated MR-compatible olfactometers have been designed and utilized successfully. Such methods use a nasal-mask in which the change from odorant to no-odorant conditions occurs within a few milliseconds.[25,26]

Acquiring ancillary electrophysiological data such as electromyographic recordings to measure muscle contraction or electrodermal responses to measure autonomic activity enhances many cognitive neuroscience experiments. Devices have been developed that are MR compatible for these types of measurements, as well other physiological measures such as heart rate, electrocardiography, oxygen saturation, and respiratory rate. The recording of eye movements is becoming commonplace in MRI scanners, predominantly with the use of an infrared video camera equipped with long-range optics.[27,28] Video images of the pupil–corneal reflection can be sampled at 60/120/240 hertz, allowing for the accurate (less than one degree) localization of gaze within 50 horizontal and 40 vertical degrees of visual angle. Although most behavioral tasks used in cognitive neuroscience experiments rely on collecting manual responses, the ability to reliably collect verbal responses without significant artifact being introduced into the data has been demonstrated by several laboratories.[29–31]

Electroencephalogram recordings also have been performed successfully during MRI scanning.[32,33] However, the recording of event-related potentials, a signal that is much smaller in amplitude than the signal in EEG, can be more difficult in a magnetic field due to artifacts induced by gradient pulsing and head movement from cardiac pulsation. New monitoring devices and algorithms to remove artifact are being developed, allowing for reliable measurements of event-related potentials during MRI scanning.[34,35]

In summary, most initial challenges facing performing cognitive and behavioral experiments within the MRI environment have been overcome, creating an environment that is comparable to standard psychophysical testing labs outside of a scanner. Although individual laboratories have achieved most of these advancements, MRI scanners originally designed for clinical use by manufacturers are now being designed with consideration of many of these research-related issues.

Temporal Resolution

Two types of temporal resolution need to be considered for cognitive neuroscience experiments. First, what is the briefest neural event that can be detected as an fMRI signal? Second, how close together can two neural events occur and be resolved as separable fMRI signals?

The time scale on which neural changes occur are quite rapid; for example, neural activity in the lateral intraparietal area of monkeys increases within 100 milliseconds of the visual presentation of a saccade target.[36] In contrast, the fMRI signal gradually increases to its peak magnitude within four to six seconds after an experimentally induced brief (less than one second) change in neural activity, and then decays back to baseline after several more seconds.[37–39] This slow time course of fMRI signal change in response to such a brief increase in neural activity is informally referred to as the BOLD fMRI hemodynamic response, or simply, the hemodynamic response (see Figure 10.1). Thus, neural dynamics and neurally evoked hemodynamics, as measured with fMRI, are on quite different time scales.

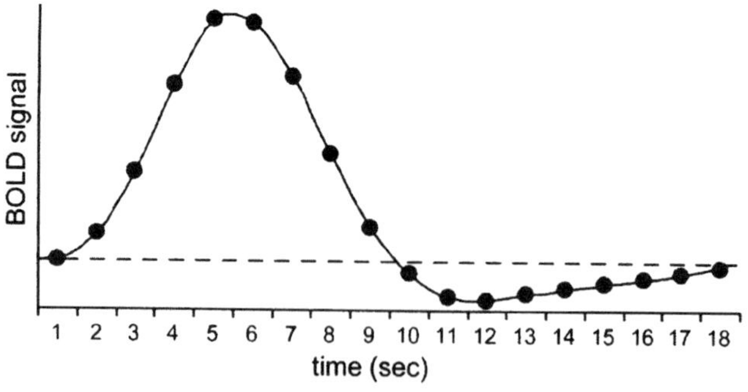

Figure 10.1. A typical hemodynamic response (i.e., fMRI signal change in response to a brief increase of neural activity) from the primary sensorimotor cortex. The fMRI signal peaked approximately five seconds after the onset of the motor response (at time zero).

The sluggishness of the hemodynamic response limits the temporal resolution of the fMRI signal to hundreds of milliseconds to seconds as opposed to the millisecond temporal resolution of electrophysiological recordings of neural activity, such as from single-unit recording in monkeys and EEG or magnetoencephalogram in humans. However, it has been clearly demonstrated that brief changes in neural activity can be detected with reasonable statistical power using fMRI; for example, appreciable fMRI signal can be observed in sensorimotor cortex in association with single finger movements[40] and in visual cortex during very briefly presented (34 milliseconds) visual stimuli.[41] In contrast, the temporal resolution of fMRI limits the detection of sequential changes in neural activity that occurs rapidly with respect to the hemodynamic response. That is, the ability to resolve the changes in the fMRI signal associated with two neural events, often requires the separation of those events by a relatively long period of time compared with the width of the hemodynamic response. This is because two neural events closely spaced in time will produce a hemodynamic response that reflects the accumulation from both neural events, making it difficult to estimate the contribution of each individual neural event. In general, evoked fMRI responses to discrete neural events separated by at least four seconds appear to be within the range of resolution.[42] However, provided that the stimuli are presented randomly, studies have shown significant differential functional responses between two events (e.g., flashing visual stimuli) spaced as closely as 500 milliseconds apart.[43–45] The effect at fixed and randomized intertrial intervals on the BOLD signal is illustrated in Figure 10.2.

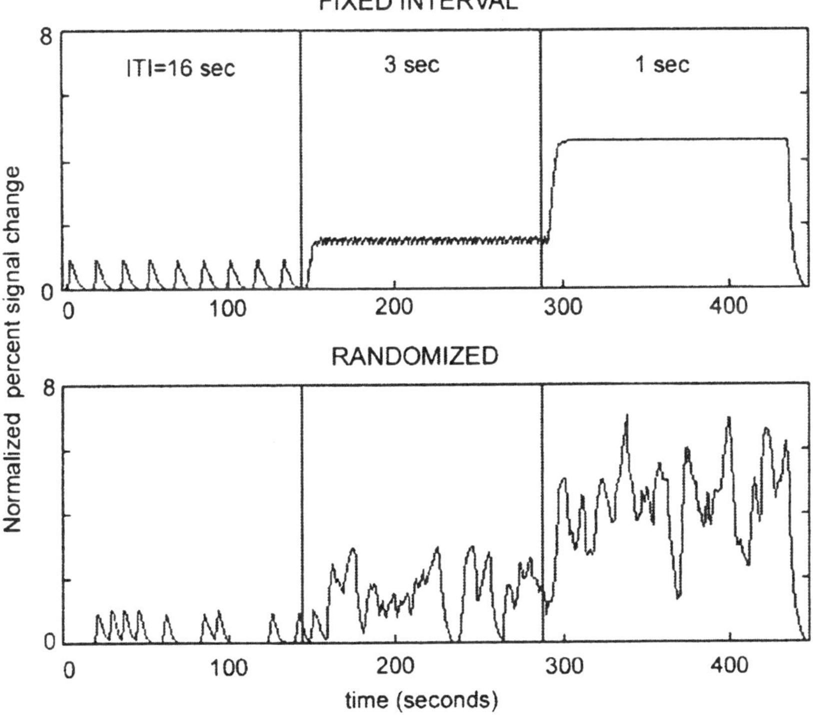

Figure 10.2. Effect of fixed versus randomized intertrial intervals on the BOLD fMRI signal. Adapted from Burock MA, Buckner RL, Woldorff MG, Rosen BR, Dale AM. Randomized event related experimental designs allow for extremely rapid presentation rates using functional MRI. *Neuroreport*. 1998;9:3735–3739.

In some tasks, the order of individual trial events cannot be randomized; for example, in certain types of working memory tasks, the presentation of the information to be remembered during the delay period, and the period when the subject must recall the information, are individual trial events whose order cannot be randomized. In these types of tasks, short time scales (less than four seconds) cannot be temporally resolved. These temporal resolution issues in fMRI have been extensively considered regarding their impact on experimental design.[46,47]

Spatial Resolution

It has yet to be determined how precisely the measured BOLD fMRI signal, which arises from the vasculature, reflects adjacent neural activity. Thus, the ultimate spatial resolution of BOLD fMRI is unknown. Functional MRI studies in both monkey and man at high field (4 to 4.7 Tesla) have demonstrated that BOLD signal can be obtained with high spatial resolution— approximately $0.75 \times 0.75mm^2$ in-plane resolution.[48,49] In monkeys, with novel approaches such as using a small, tissue-compatible, intraosteally implanted radiofrequency coil, ultra high spatial resolution of $125 \times 125mm^2$ has been obtained.[50] Using this method, Logothetis and colleagues[50] demonstrated cortical lamina-specific activation in a task that compared responses to moving stimuli with those elicited by flickering stimuli. This contrast elicited BOLD signal mostly in the granular layers of the striate cortex of the monkey, which are known to have a high concentration of directionally selective cells. Advances in such methods would allow for imaging of hundreds of neurons per voxel as opposed to hundreds of thousands of neurons per voxel, which is more typical for a human cognitive neuroscience fMRI experiment.

Virtually all fMRI studies model the large BOLD signal increase, which is due to a local low-deoxyhemoglobin state (see Figure 10.1), in order to detect changes correlating with a behavioral task. However, optical imaging studies have demonstrated that preceding this large positive response is an initial negative response reflecting a localized increase in oxygen consumption, causing a high-deoxyhemoglobin state.[51] This early hemodynamic response is called the initial dip and is thought to be more tightly coupled to the actual site of neural activity evoking the BOLD signal as compared to the later positive portion of the BOLD response; for example, Kim and colleagues,[52] scanning cats in a high field scanner, demonstrated that the early negative BOLD response (e.g., initial dip) produced activation maps that were consistent with orientation columns within visual cortex. This finding is quite remarkable given that the average spacing between two adjacent orientation columns in cortex is approximately one millimeter. In contrast, the activation maps produced by the delayed positive BOLD response appeared more diffuse, and cortical columnar organization could not be identified.[52] Thus, empirical evidence suggests that deriving activation maps by correlating behavioral responses with the initial dip may markedly improve spatial resolution. However, it is important to note that observation of the initial dip of the BOLD signal has been inconsistently observed in humans across laboratories for reasons that are still unclear. Several groups, however, were able to detect columnar architecture (in this case, ocular dominance columns) by modeling the positive BOLD response in humans scanning at 4 Tesla.[49,53] These investigators attributed their success to optimized radiofrequency coils, limiting head motion, optimizing slice orientation, and the enhanced signal-to-noise ratio (SNR) provided by a high magnetic field.

Another unique method for improving spatial resolution has been called functional magnetic resonance–adaptation (fMR-A), which could provide a means for identifying and assessing the functional attributes of sharply defined neuronal populations within a given region of the brain.[54] Even if the spatial resolution of fMRI evolves to the point of being able to resolve a population of a few hundred neurons within a voxel, it is still likely that this small population will contain neurons with very different functional properties that will be averaged together. The adaptation method is based on several basic principles. First, repeated presentation of the same type of stimuli (i.e., a picture of the one object) causes neurons to adapt to those stimuli (i.e., neuronal firing is reduced). Second, if these neurons are then exposed to a different type of stimulus (i.e., a picture of another object) or a change in some property of the stimulus (i.e., the same object in a different orientation), recovery from adaptation can be assessed (i.e., whether or not the BOLD signal returns to its original state). If the signal remains adapted, it implies that the neurons are invariant to the attribute that was changed. If the signal recovers from the adapted state, it would imply that the neurons are sensitive to that attribute; for example, Grill-Spector and colleagues demonstrated that an area of lateral occipital cortex thought to be important for object recognition was less sensitive to changes in object size and position as compared to changes in illumination and viewpoint.[55] Thus, with this method, it is possible to investigate the functional properties of neuronal populations with a level of spatial resolution that is beyond that obtained from conventional fMRI data analysis methods.

Considering all the neuroscientific methods available today for studying human brain–behavior relationships, fMRI provides an excellent balance of temporal and spatial resolution (see Figure 10.3). Improvements on both fronts will clearly add to the increasing popularity of this method.

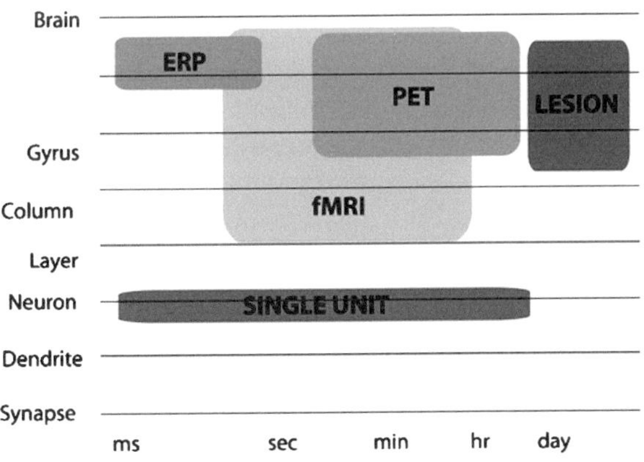

Figure 10.3. Temporal and spatial resolution of different neuroscience methods[114]. Adapted from Churchland PS, Sejnowski TJ. Perspectives on cognitive neuroscience. *Science.* 1988;242:741–745. Copyright © 1988 AAAS.

Issues in Functional MRI Experimental Design

Numerous options exist for designing experiments using fMRI (see Chapter 3 by Aguirre for more in-depth discussion of experimental design). The prototypical fMRI experimental design consists of two behavioral tasks presented in blocks of trials alternating over the course of a scanning session, and the fMRI signal between the two tasks is compared. This is known as a blocked design; for example, a given block might present a series of faces to be viewed passively, which evokes a particular cognitive process, such as face perception. The experimental block alternates with a control block, which is designed to evoke all of the cognitive processes present in the experimental block except for the cognitive process of interest. In this experiment, the control block may comprise a series of objects. In this way, the stimuli used in experimental and control tasks have similar visual attributes, but differ in the attribute of interest (i.e., faces). The inferential framework of cognitive subtraction[56] attributes differences in neural activity between the two tasks to the specific cognitive process (i.e., face perception). Cognitive subtraction was originally conceived by Donders[57] in the late 1800s for studying the chronometric substrates of cognitive processes (see Sternberg[58]) and was a major innovation in imaging.[56,59] The assumptions required for cognitive subtraction may not always hold and could produce erroneous interpretation of functional neuroimaging data.[42] Cognitive subtraction relies on two assumptions: pure insertion and linearity. Pure insertion implies that a cognitive process can be added to a preexisting set of cognitive processes without affecting them. This assumption is difficult to prove because one needs an independent measure of the preexisting processes in the absence and presence of the new process.[58] If pure insertion fails as an assumption, a difference in the neuroimaging signal between the two tasks might be observed, not because a specific cognitive process was engaged in one task and not the other, but because the added cognitive process and the preexisting cognitive processes interact.

An example of this point is illustrated in working memory studies using delayed-response tasks.[60] These tasks (for an example, see Jonides and colleagues[61]) typically present information that the subject must remember (engaging an encoding process), followed by a delay period during which the subject must hold the information in memory over a short period of time (engaging a memory process), followed by a probe that requires the subject to make a decision based on the stored information (engaging a retrieval process). The brain regions engaged by evoking the memory process theoretically are revealed by subtracting the BOLD signal measured by fMRI during a block of trials that the subject performs that do not have a delay period (only engaging the encoding and retrieval processes) from a block of trials with a delay period (engaging the encoding, memory, and retrieval processes). In this example, if the addition or insertion of a delay period between the encoding and retrieval processes affects these other behavioral processes in the task, the result is failure to meet the assumptions of cognitive subtraction. That is, these non-memory processes may differ in delay trials and no-delay trials, resulting in a failure to cancel each other out in the two types of trials that are being compared.

Empirical evidence of such failure exists.[62] For example, Figure 10.4 demonstrates BOLD signal derived from the prefrontal cortex from a subject

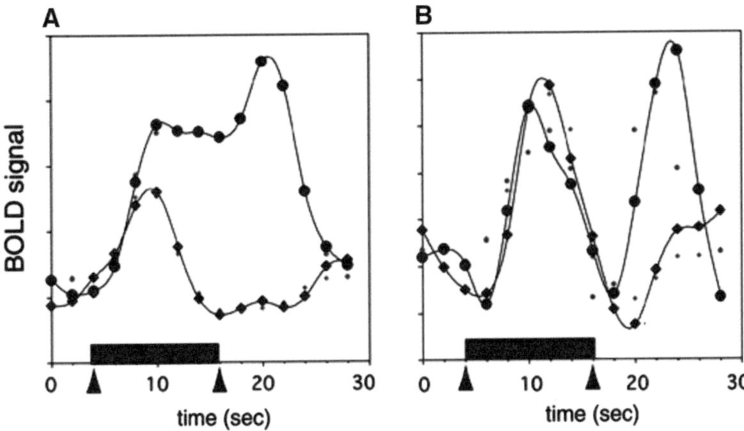

Figure 10.4. Data derived from the performance of a normal subject on a spatial delayed-response task. This task comprised both delay trials (circles), as well as trials without a delay period (no-delay trials; diamonds). (A) Trial-averaged fMRI signal from prefrontal cortex that displayed delay-correlated activity. The gray bar along the x-axis denotes the 12-second delay period during delay trials. The delay trials display a level of fMRI signal greater than baseline throughout the period of time corresponding to the retention delay (taking into account the delay and dispersion of the fMRI signal). The peaks seen in the signal correspond to the encoding and retrieval periods. (B) Trial-averaged fMRI signal from a region in prefrontal cortex that did not display the characteristics of delay-correlated activity. This region displays a significant functional change associated with the no-delay trials, and a significant functional change associated with the encoding and retrieval periods of the delay trials, but not one associated with the retention delay of delay trials. Adapted from Zarahn E, Aguirre GK, D'Esposito M. Temporal isolation of the neural correlates of spatial mnemonic processing with fMRI. *Cogn Brain Res.* 1999;7:255–268.

performing a delayed response task similar to the tasks described above. The left side of the figure illustrates BOLD signal consistent with delay period activity, whereas the right side of the figure illustrates BOLD signal from another region of prefrontal cortex that did not display sustained activity during the delay, yet showed greater activity in the delay trials as compared to the trials without a delay. In any blocked functional neuroimaging study that compares delay versus no-delay trials with subtraction, such a region would be detected and likely assumed to be a memory region. Thus, this result provides empirical grounds for adopting a healthy doubt regarding the inferences drawn from imaging studies that rely exclusively on cognitive subtraction.

In functional neuroimaging, the transform between the neural signal and the hemodynamic response (measured by fMRI) must also be linear for the cognitive subtractive method to yield valid results. In other words, it is assumed that the BOLD signal being measured is approximately proportional to the local neural activity that evokes it. Surprisingly, although thousands of empirical studies using fMRI to study brain–behavior relationships have been published, only a handful exist that have explored the neurophysiological basis of the BOLD signal (for reviews, see Attwell and Iadecola[63] and Heeger and Ress[64]). In several studies, linearity did not strictly hold for the BOLD fMRI system, but the linear transform model was reasonably consistent with the data; for example, Boynton and colleagues tested whether

BOLD signal in response to long duration stimuli can be predicted by summing the responses to shorter duration stimuli.[39] Using pulses of flickering checkerboard patterns and measuring within human primary visual cortex, these investigators found that the BOLD signal response to various durations of stimulus presentation (6, 12, or 24 seconds) could be predicted from the responses they obtained from shorter stimulus presentations; for example, the BOLD signal response to a six-second pulse could be predicted from the summation of the BOLD signal response to the three-second pulse with a copy of the same response delayed by three seconds. However, temporal summation did not always hold, and there are clearly nonlinear effects in the transform of neural activity to a hemodynamic response that must be considered.[65–68] If these nonlinearities lead to saturation of the BOLD effect at a certain stimulus intensity, erroneous interpretation of particular results of fMRI experiments may occur.

Another class of experimental designs, called event-related fMRI, attempt to detect changes associated with individual trials, as opposed to the larger unit of time comprising a block of trials.[69,70] Each individual trial may be composed of one behavioral event, such as the presentation of a single stimulus (e.g., a face or object to be perceived), or several behavioral events, such as in the delayed-response task described above, (e.g., an item to be remembered, a delay period, and a motor response in a delayed-response task); for example, with an event-related design, activity within the prefrontal cortex has consistently been shown to correlate with the delay period,[62] supporting the role of the PFC in temporarily maintaining information. This finding is consistent with single-neuron recording studies in the PFC of monkeys.[7] Event-related designs offer numerous advantages; for example, it allows for stimulus or trial randomization, avoiding the behavioral confounds of blocked trials. It also permits the separate analysis of functional responses, which are identified only in retrospect (i.e., trials on which the subject made a correct or incorrect response). Of course, an experiment does not have to be limited to either a block or event-related designs—a mixed-type (both event-related and blocked) design, where particular trial types are randomized within a block, is perfectly feasible. In this type of design, both item-related processes (e.g., transient responses to stimuli), as well as state-related processes (processes sustained throughout a block of trials or a task)[71,72] are perfectly feasible. Overall, much flexibility exists in the type of experimental design that can be utilized in an fMRI experiment, and continued innovation in this area will greatly expand the types of neuroscientific questions that can be addressed.

Issues in Interpretation of fMRI Data

Statistics

Many statistical techniques are used for analyzing fMRI data, but no single method has emerged as the ideal or gold standard (see Chapter 3 by Aguirre for more in-depth discussion of statistical analysis of fMRI data). The analysis of any fMRI experiment designed to contradict the null hypothesis (i.e., there is no difference between experimental conditions) requires inferential statistics. If the difference between two experimental conditions is too large to reasonably be due to chance, then the null hypothesis is rejected in favor of the alternative hypothesis, which typically is the experimenter's hypothesis (e.g., the fusiform gyrus is activated to a greater extent by viewing faces than objects). Unfortunately, because errors can occur in any statistical test, experimenters will never know when an error is committed, and they can only try to minimize them.[73] Knowledge of several basic statistical issues provides a solid foundation for the correct interpretation of the data derived from functional neuroimaging studies.

Two types of statistical errors can occur. A Type I error is committed when the null hypothesis is falsely rejected when it is true, that is, a difference between experimental conditions is found but a difference does not truly exist. This type of error is also called a false-positive error. In a functional neuroimaging study, a false-positive error would be finding a brain region activated during a cognitive task, when actually it is not. A Type II error is committed when the null hypothesis is accepted when it is false, that is, no difference between experimental conditions exists when a difference does exist. This type of error is called a false-negative error. A false-negative error in a functional neuroimaging study would be failing to find a brain region activated during the performance of a cognitive task when actually it is.

In fMRI experiments, like all experiments, a tolerable probability for Type I error, typically less than five percent, is chosen for adequate control of specificity, that is, control of false-positive rates. Two features of imaging data can cause unacceptable false-positive rates, even with traditional parametric statistical tests. First, there is the problem of multiple comparisons. For the typical resolution of images acquired during fMRI scans, the full extent of single slice (matrix-128^2, slice-5mm) of the human brain could comprise 15000 voxels. Thus, with any given statistical comparison of two experimental conditions, there are actually 15000 statistical comparisons being performed. With such a large number of statistical tests, the probability of finding a false-positive activation, that is, committing a Type I error, somewhere in the brain increases. Several methods exist to deal with this problem. One method, a Bonferroni correction, assumes that each statistical test is independent and calculates the probability of Type I error by dividing the chosen probability ($p = 0.05$) by the number of statistical tests performed. Another method is based on Gaussian field theory,[74] and calculates the probability of Type I error when imaging data are spatially smoothed. Many other methods for determining thresholds of statistical maps are proposed and utilized,[75,76] but unfortunately, no single method has been universally accepted. Nevertheless, all fMRI studies must apply some type of correction for multiple comparisons to control the false-positive rate.

The second feature that might increase the false-positive rate is the noise in fMRI data. Data from BOLD fMRI are temporally autocorrelated, with more noise at some frequencies than at others. The shape of this noise distribution is characterized by a 1/frequency function, with increasing noise at lower frequencies.[77] Traditional parametric and nonparametric statistical tests assume that the noise is not temporally autocorrelated, that is, each observation is independent. Therefore, any statistical test used in fMRI studies must account for the noise structure of fMRI data. If not, the false-positive rates will inflate.[77,78]

Type II error is rarely considered in functional neuroimaging studies. When a brain map from an fMRI experiment is presented, several areas of activation are typically attributed to some experimental manipulation.

The focus of most imaging studies is on brain activation, whereas it is often implicitly assumed that all of the other areas (typically, most of the brain) were not activated during the experiment. Power as a statistical concept refers to the probability of correctly rejecting the null hypothesis.[73] As the power of a fMRI study to detect changes in brain activity increases, the false-negative rate decreases. Unfortunately, power calculations for particular fMRI experiments are rarely performed, although this methodology is evolving.[79–81] Reports that specific brain areas were not active during an experimental manipulation should provide an estimate of the power required for detection of a change in the region. All experiments should be designed to maximize power. Relatively simple strategies can increase power in an fMRI experiment in certain circumstances, such as increasing the amount of imaging data collected or increasing the number of subjects studied. It is also important to note that task designs can affect sensitivity;[82] for example, because BOLD fMRI data are temporally autocorrelated, experiments with fundamental frequencies in the lower range (e.g., a box-car design with 60-second epochs) will have reduced sensitivity due to the presence of greater noise at these lower frequencies. Finally, in a study that simultaneously measured neural signal via intracortical recording and BOLD signal in a monkey, it was observed that the SNR of the neural signal was, on average, at least one order of magnitude higher than that of the BOLD signal. The investigators of this study concluded that "the statistical and thresholding methods applied to the hemodynamic responses probably underestimate a great deal of actual neural activity related to a stimulus or task."[83] Thus, the magnitude of Type II error in BOLD fMRI may currently be underestimated and warrants further consideration in the interpretation of almost any cognitive neuroscience experiment.

Altered Hemodynamic Response

When comparing changes in BOLD signal levels within the brain of an individual subject across different cognitive tasks and making conclusions regarding changes in neural activity and the pattern of activity, numerous assumptions are made regarding the steps comprising neurovascular coupling (stimulus → neural activity → hemodynamic response → BOLD signal) and the regional variability of the metabolic and vascular parameters influencing the BOLD signal. It should be obvious that fMRI studies of cognition and behavior of individuals with local vascular compromise or diffuse vascular disease (e.g., patients with strokes or normal elderly) are potentially problematic; for example, many fMRI studies have sought to identify age-related changes in the neural substrates of cognitive processes. These studies that directly compare changes in BOLD signal intensity across age groups rely upon the assumption of age-equivalent coupling of neural activity to BOLD signal. However, there is empirical evidence that suggests that this general assumption may not hold true. Extensive research on the aging neurovascular system has revealed that it undergoes significant changes in multiple domains in a continuum throughout the human lifespan, probably as early as the fourth decade (for a review, see Farkas and Luiten[84]). These changes affect the vascular ultrastructure,[85] the resting cerebral blood flow (CBF),[86,87] the vascular responsiveness of the vessels,[88] and the cerebral metabolic rate of oxygen consumption.[89,90] Aging is also frequently associated with co-morbidities such as diabetes, hypertension, and hyperlipidemia, all of which may affect the BOLD signal by affecting CBF and neurovascular coupling.[91] Any one of these age-related differences in the vascular system could conceivably produce age-related differences in BOLD fMRI signal responsiveness, greatly affecting the interpretation of results from such studies.

Our laboratory compared the hemodynamic response function (HRF) characteristics in the sensorimotor cortex of young and older subjects in response to a simple motor reaction-time task.[92] The provisional assumption was made that there was identical neural activity between the two populations based on physiological findings of equivalent movement-related electrical potentials in subjects under similar conditions.[93] Thus, it was presumed that any changes that were observed in BOLD fMRI signal between young and older individuals in motor cortex would be due to vascular, and not neural, activity changes in normal aging. Several important similarities and differences were observed between age groups. Although there was no significant difference in the shape of the hemodynamic response curve or peak amplitude of the signal, a significantly decreased SNR in the BOLD signal was found in older individuals as compared to young individuals. This was attributed to a greater level of noise in the older individuals. A decrease in the spatial extent of the BOLD signal was also observed in older individuals compared to younger individuals in sensorimotor cortex (i.e., the median number of suprathreshold voxels). Similar results have been replicated by two other laboratories.[94,95] These findings suggest that there is some property of the coupling between neural activity and BOLD signal that changes with age.

The notion that vascular differences among individuals may affect BOLD signal is especially a concern when considering studies of patient populations with known vascular changes such as stroke. A recent fMRI study addressed the issue of the influence of vascular factors on the BOLD signal in a symptomatic stroke population.[96] They analyzed the time course of the BOLD HRF in the sensorimotor cortex of patients with an isolated subcortical lacunar stroke compared to a group of age-matched controls. They found a decrease in the rate of rise and the maximal BOLD HRF to a finger- or hand-tapping task in both the sensorimotor cortex of the hemisphere affected by the stroke and the unaffected hemisphere. These investigators proposed that, given the widespread changes of these BOLD signal differences, the change was unlikely a direct consequence of the subcortical lacunar stroke, but rather a manifestation of preexisting diffuse vascular pathology.

In summary, comparing BOLD signal in two different groups of individuals that may differ in their vascular system should be done with caution; for example, in one scenario, a comparison of activation of young and elderly individuals during a cognitive task may show less activation by elderly (as compared to young subjects) in some brain regions, but greater activation in other regions (e.g., see Rypma and colleagues[97]). In this scenario, it is unlikely that regional variations in the hemodynamic coupling of neural activity to imaging signal would account for such age-related differences in patterns of activation. In another scenario, a comparison of young and elderly subjects may show less activation by elderly (as compared to young subjects) in some brain regions, but no evidence of greater activation in any other region. In this case, it is possible that the observed age-related differences are not due to differences in intensity of neural activity, but rather to other non-neuronal contributions to the imaging signal, that is, neurovascular coupling. Several statistical approaches towards the imaging data are being developed that will attempt to address these potential confounds.[72,98,99]

Types of Hypotheses Tested Using fMRI

Functional neuroimaging experiments test hypotheses regarding the anatomical specificity for cognitive processes (functional specialization), basic mechanisms of cognition (cognitive theory), and direct or indirect interactions among brain regions (functional integration). The experimental design and statistical analyses chosen will determine the types of questions that can be addressed. Ultimately, the most powerful approach for the testing of theories on brain–behavior relationships is the analysis of converging data from multiple methods.

Functional Specialization

The major focus of fMRI studies of cognition is testing theories on functional specialization. The concept of functional specialization is based on the premise that functional modules exist within the brain, that is, areas of the cerebral cortex are specialized for a specific cognitive process; for example, facial recognition is a critical primary function likely served by a functional module. Prosopagnosia is the selective inability to recognize faces. Patients with prosopagnosia, however, can recognize familiar faces, such as those of relatives, by other means, such as the voice, dress, or body shape. Other types of visual recognition, such as identifying common objects, are normal. Prosopagnosia arises from lesions of the inferomedial temporo-occipital lobe, which usually are due to a stroke within the posterior cerebral artery circulation. No lesion studies have precisely localized the area crucial for facial perception. However, they provide strong evidence that a brain area is specialized for processing faces. Functional imaging studies have provided anatomical specificity for such a module; for example, Kanwisher and colleagues[100] used fMRI to test a group of healthy individuals and found that the fusiform gyrus was significantly more active when the subjects viewed faces than when they viewed assorted common objects. The specificity of a fusiform face area was further demonstrated by the finding that this area also responded significantly more strongly to passive viewing of faces than to scrambled two-tone faces, front-view photographs of houses, and photographs of human hands. These elegant experiments allowed the investigators to reject alternative functions of the face area, such as visual attention, subordinate-level classification, or general processing of any animate or human forms, demonstrating that this region selectively perceives faces.

Cognitive Theory

An exciting new direction for studies using functional neuroimaging are those that test theories of the underlying mechanisms of cognition; for example, an fMRI study[101] attempted to answer the question, "To what extent does perception depend on attention?" One hypothesis is that unattended stimuli in the environment receive very little processing,[102] but another hypothesis is that the processing load in a relevant task determines the extent to which irrelevant stimuli are processed.[103] These alternative hypotheses were tested by asking normal individuals to perform linguistic tasks of low or high load while ignoring irrelevant visual motion in the periphery of a display. Visual motion was used as the distracting stimulus because it activates a distinct region of the brain (cortical area MT or V5, another functional module in the visual system). Activation of area MT would indicate that irrelevant visual motion was processed. Although task and irrelevant stimuli were unrelated, fMRI of motion-related activity in MT showed a reduction in motion processing during the high-processing load condition in the linguistic task. These findings support the hypothesis that perception of irrelevant environmental information depends on the information processing load that is currently relevant and being attended to. Thus, by the finding that perception depends on attention, this fMRI experiment provides insight regarding underlying cognitive mechanism.

Functional Integration

Functional neuroimaging experiments can also test hypotheses about interactions between brain regions by focusing on covariances of activation levels between regions.[104,105] These covariances reflect functional connectivity, a concept that was originally developed in reference to temporal interactions among individual neurons.[106] Newer approaches, often using a statistical test called structural equation modeling, attempt to determine whether covariances among brain regions result from direct or indirect interactions, a concept called effective connectivity. Using this method, McIntosh and colleagues[105] found shifting prefrontal and limbic interactions in a working memory task for faces as the retention delay increased (see Figure 10.5). The different interactions between brain regions at short and long delays

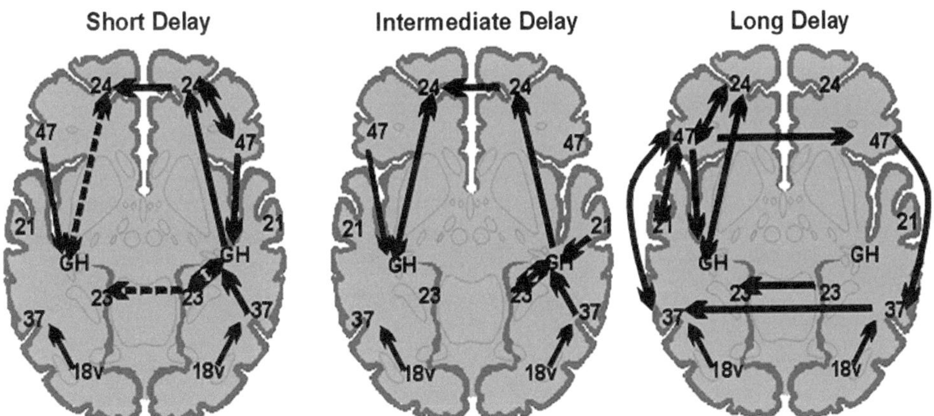

Figure 10.5. Network analysis of fMRI data during performance of a working memory task cross three different delay periods.[105] Areas of correlated increases in activation (*solid lines*) and areas of correlated decreases in activation (*dotted lines*) are shown. Note the different pattern of interactions among brain regions at short and long delays. Adapted from McIntosh AR, Grady CL, Haxby JV, Ungerleider LG, Horwitz B. Changes in limbic and prefrontal functional interactions in working memory task for faces. *Cereb Cortex.* 1996;6:571–584.

were interpreted as a functional change; for example, strong corticolimbic interactions were found at short delays, but at longer delays, when the image of the face was more difficult to maintain, strong fronto-cingulate-occipital interactions were found. The investigators postulated that the former finding was due to maintaining an iconic facial representation, and that the latter finding was due to an expanded encoding strategy, resulting in more resilient memory. By characterizing changes in regional activity and the interactions between regions over time, the network analysis in this study added to the original analysis, that of only assessed regional changes in mean activity.

Integration of Multiple Methods

The most powerful approach toward understanding brain–behavior relationships comes from analyzing converging data from multiple methods. There are several ways in which different methods can provide complementary data; for example, one method can provide superior spatial resolution (e.g., fMRI), whereas the other can provide superior temporal resolution (e.g., event-related potetials). In addition, the data from one method may allow for different conclusions to be drawn from it, such as whether a particular brain region is necessary to implement a cognitive process (i.e., lesion methods) or whether it is only involved during its implementation (i.e., physiological methods). The following sections describe examples of such approaches.

Combined fMRI/Lesion Studies

The combined use of functional neuroimaging and lesions studies can be illustrated with studies of the neural basis of semantic memory, the cognitive system that represents our knowledge of the world. Early studies of patients with focal lesions supported the notion that the temporal lobes mediate the retrieval of semantic knowledge;[107] for example, patients with temporal lobe lesions may show a disproportionate impairment in the knowledge of living things (e.g., animals) compared with nonliving things. Other patients have a disproportionate deficit in knowledge of nonliving things.[108] These observations led to the notion that the semantic memory system is subdivided into different sensorimotor modalities, that is, living things, compared with nonliving things, are represented by their visual and other sensory attributes (e.g., a banana is yellow), whereas nonliving things are represented by their function (e.g., a hammer is a tool but comes in many different visual forms). The small number of patients with these deficits, and often large lesions, limits precise anatomical–behavioral relationships. However, functional neuroimaging studies in normal subjects can provide spatial resolution that the lesion method lacks.[109]

These original observations regarding the neural basis of semantic memory conflicted with functional neuroimaging studies consistently showing activation of the left inferior frontal gyrus (IFG) during the retrieval of semantic knowledge; for example, an early cognitive activation PET study revealed IFG activation during a verb-generation task compared with a simple word-repetition task.[59] A subsequent fMRI study[110] offered a fundamentally different interpretation of the apparent conflict between lesion and functional neuroimaging studies of semantic knowledge: left IFG activity is associated with the need to select some relevant feature of semantic knowledge from competing alternatives, not retrieval of semantic knowledge per se. This interpretation was supported by an fMRI experiment in normal individuals in which selection, but not retrieval, demands were varied across three semantic tasks. In a verb-generation task, in a high-selection condition, subjects generated verbs to nouns with many appropriate associated responses without any clearly dominant response (e.g., wheel), but in a low-selection condition, nouns with few associated responses or with a clear dominant response (e.g., scissors) were used. In this way, all tasks required semantic retrieval, and differed only in the amount of selection required. The fMRI signal within the left IFG increased as the selection demands increased (see Figure 10.6). When the degree of semantic processing varied independently of selection demands, there was no difference in left IFG activity, suggesting that selection, not retrieval, of semantic knowledge drives activity in the left IFG.

To determine if left IFG activity was correlated with, but not necessary for, selecting information from semantic memory, the same task used during the fMRI study was used to examine the ability of patients with focal frontal lesions to generate verbs.[111] Supporting the earlier claim regarding left IFG function derived from an fMRI study,[110] the overlap of the lesions

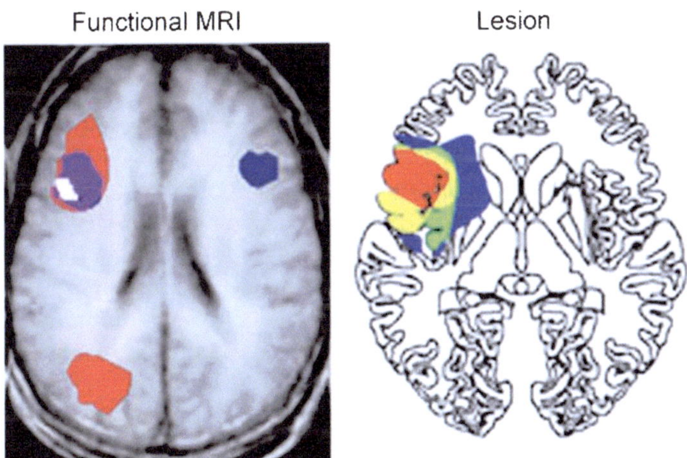

Figure 10.6. Regions of overlap of fMRI activity in healthy human subjects (left side of figure) during the performance of three semantic memory tasks, with the convergence of activity within the left inferior frontal gyrus (white region). Adapted from Thompson-Schill SL, D'Esposito M, Aguirre GK, Farah MJ. Role of left inferior prefrontal cortex in retrieval of semantic knowledge: a reevaluation. *Proc Natl Acad Sci USA.* 1997;94:14792–14797. Copyright © 1997 National Academy of Sciences, U.S.A. Regions of overlap of lesion location in patients with selection-related deficits on a verb-generation task (right side of figure) with maximal overlap within the left inferior frontal gyrus (red region). Adapted from Thompson-Schill SL, Swick D, Farah MJ, D'Esposito M, Kan IP, Knight RT. Verb generation in patients with focal frontal lesions: a neurophysiological test of neuroimaging findings. *Proc Natl Acad Sci USA.* 1998;95:15855–15960. Copyright © 1998 National Academy of Sciences, U.S.A. (Neurologic coordinates).

in patients with deficits on this task corresponded to the site of maximum fMRI activation in healthy young subjects during the verb-generation task (see Figure 10.6). In this example, the approach of using converging evidence from lesion and fMRI studies differs in a subtle but important way from the study described earlier that isolated the face-processing module. Patients with left IFG lesions do not present with an identifiable neurobehavioral syndrome reflecting the nature of the processing in this region. Guided by the fMRI results from healthy young subjects, the investigators studied patients with left IFG lesions to test a hypothesis regarding the necessity of this region in a specific cognitive process. Coupled with the well-established finding that lesions of the left temporal lobe impair semantic knowledge, these studies further our understanding of the neural network mediating semantic memory.

Combined fMRI/Transcranial Magnetic Stimulation Studies Transcranial magnetic stimulation (TMS) is a noninvasive method that can induce a reversible virtual lesion of the cerebral cortex in a normal human subject.[112] Using both fMRI and TMS provides another means of combining brain activation data with data derived from the lesion method. There are several advantages for using TMS as a lesion method. First, brain injury likely results in brain reorganization after the injury, and studies of patients with lesions assume that the non-lesioned brain areas have not been affected, whereas, in TMS, it is performed on the normal brain. Another advantage for using TMS is that it has excellent spatial resolution and can target specific locations in the brain, whereas lesions in patients with brain injury are markedly variable in location and size across individuals. Such an approach can be illustrated in a recent investigation of the role of the medial frontal cortex in task-switching.[113] In this study, subjects first performed an fMRI study that identified the regions that were active when they stayed on the current task versus when they switched to a new task. It was found that medial frontal cortex is activated when switching between tasks. In order to determine if the medial frontal cortex was necessary for the processes involved in task-switching, the same paradigm was utilized during inactivation of the medial frontal cortex with TMS. Guided by the locations of activation observed in the fMRI study, and using a MRI-guided frameless stereotaxic procedure, it was found that applying a TMS pulse over the medial frontal cortex disrupted performance only during trials during which the subject was required to switch between tasks. Transcranial magnetic stimulation over adjacent brain regions did not show this effect. Additionally, the excellent temporal resolution of TMS allowed the investigators to stimulate during precise periods of the task, determining that the observed effect was during the time when the subjects were presented a cue, indicating they must switch tasks prior to the actual performance of the new task. Thus, combining the results from both fMRI and TMS, it was concluded that medial prefrontal cortex was essential for allowing individuals to intentionally switch to a new task.

Combined fMRI/Event-Related Potential Studies

The strength of combining these two methods is coupling the superb spatial resolution of fMRI with the superb temporal resolution of event-related potential recording. An example of such a study was reported by Dehaene and colleagues, who asked the question "Does the human capacity for mathematical intuition depend on linguistic competence or on visuospatial representations?" In this study, subjects performed two addition tasks—one in which they were instructed to select the correct sum from two numerically close numbers (exact condition) and one in which there were instructed to estimate the result and select the closest number (approximate condition). During fMRI scanning, greater bilateral parietal lobe activation was observed in the approximation condition as compared to the exact condition. Because this activation was outside the perisylvian language zone, it was taken as support that visuospatial processes were engaged during the cognitive operations involved in approximate calculation. Greater left lateralized frontal lobe activation was observed to be greater in the exact condition as compared to the approximate condition, which was taken as evidence for language-dependent coding of exact addition facts. In order to consider an alternative explanation of the fMRI findings, the investigators also performed an ERP study. The alternative explanation was that in both the exact and approximate tasks, subjects would compute the exact result using the same representation for numbers, but later processing, when they had to make a decision as to the correct choice, was what led to the differences in brain activation. Because fMRI does not offer adequate temporal resolution to resolve these two behavioral events that occur on brief time scale, event-related potential was the appropriate method to test this hypothesis. In the event-related potential study, it was demonstrated that the evoked neural response during exact and approximate trials already differed significantly during the first 400 milliseconds of a trial before subjects had to make a decision.

Summary

Functional MRI is an extremely valuable tool for studying brain–behavior relationships, as it is widely available, noninvasive, and has superb temporal and spatial resolution. New approaches in fMRI experimental design and data analysis are appearing in the literature at an almost exponential rate, leading to numerous options for testing hypotheses on brain–behavior relationships. Combined with information from other complimentary methods, such as the study of patients with focal lesions, healthy individuals with transcranial magnetic stimulation, or event-related potentials, data from fMRI studies provide new insights regarding the organization of the cerebral cortex, as well as the neural mechanisms underlying cognition.

References

1. Broca P. Remarques sur le siege de la faculte du langage articule suivies d'une observation d'amphemie (perte de al parole). *Bull Mem Soc Anat Paris*. 1861;36.
2. Buckner RL, Raichle ME, Petersen SE. Dissociation of human prefrontal cortical areas across different speech production tasks and gender groups. *J Neurophysiol*. 1995;74:2163–2173.
3. Sarter M, Bernston G, Cacioppo J. Brain imaging and cognitive neuroscience: toward strong inference in attributing function to structure. *Am Psychol*. 1996;51:13–21.
4. Gaffan D, Gaffan EA. Amnesia in man following transection of the fornix: a review. *Brain*. 1991;114:2611–2618.

5. Feeney DM, Baron JC. Diaschisis. *Stroke.* 1986;17:817–830.
6. Fuster JM, Alexander GE. Neuron activity related to short-term memory. *Science.* 1971;173:652–654.
7. Funahashi S, Bruce CJ, Goldman-Rakic PS. Mnemonic coding of visual space in the monkey's dorsolateral prefrontal cortex. *J Neurophysiol.* 1989;61:331–349.
8. Funahashi S, Bruce CJ, Goldman-Rakic PS. Dorsolateral prefrontal lesions and oculomotor delayed-response performance: Evidence for mnemonic "scotomas". *J Neurosci.* 1993;13:1479–1497.
9. Watanabe T, Niki H. Hippocampal unit activity and delayed response in the monkey. *Brain Res.* 1985;325:241–254.
10. Cahusac PM, Miyashita Y, Rolls ET. Responses of hippocampal formation neurons in the monkey related to delayed spatial response and object-place memory tasks. *Behav Brain Res.* 1989;33:229–240.
11. Alvarez P, Zola-Morgan S, Squire LR. The animal model of human amnesia: long-term memory impaired and short-term memory intact. *Proc Natl Acad Sci U S A.* 1994;91:5637–5641.
12. Corkin S. Lasting consequences of bilateral medial temporal lobectomy: clinical course and experimental findings in H.M. *Sem Neurol.* 1984;4:249–259.
13. Ranganath C, D'Esposito M. Medial temporal lobe activity associated with active maintenance of novel information. *Neuron.* 2001;31:865–873.
14. Druzgal TJ, D'Esposito M. Activity in fusiform face area modulated as a function of working memory load. *Brain Res Cogn Brain Res.* 2001;10:355–364.
15. Cohen MS, Kosslyn SM, Breiter HC, et al. Changes in cortical activity during mental rotation: a mapping study using functional MRI. *Brain.* 1996;119:89–100.
16. D'Esposito M, Ballard D, Aguirre GK, Zarahn E. Human prefrontal cortex is not specific for working memory: a functional MRI study. *Neuroimage.* 1998;8:274–282.
17. Abduljalil AM, Robitaille PM. Macroscopic susceptibility in ultra high field MRI. *J Comput Assist Tomogr.* 1999;23:832–841.
18. Abduljalil AM, Kangarlu A, Yu Y, Robitaille PM. Macroscopic susceptibility in ultra high field MRI. II: acquisition of spin echo images from the human head. *J Comput Assist Tomogr.* 1999;23:842–844.
19. Zeng H, Constable RT. Image distortion correction in EPI: comparison of field mapping with point spread function mapping. *Magn Reson Med.* 2002;48:137–146.
20. Casey BJ, Thomas KM, Davidson MC, Kunz K, Franzen PL. Dissociating striatal and hippocampal function developmentally with a stimulus-response compatibility task. *J Neurosci.* 2002;22:8647–8652.
21. Schlaggar BL, Brown TT, Lugar HM, Visscher KM, Miezin FM, Petersen SE. Functional neuroanatomical differences between adults and school-age children in the processing of single words. *Science.* 2002;296:1476–1479.
22. Savoy RL, Ravicz ME, Gollub R. The psychophysiological laboratory in the magnet: stimulus delivery, response recording, and safety. In: Moonen CTW, Bandettini PA, eds. *Functional MRI.* Berlin: Springer; 1999:347–365.
23. Edminster WB, Talavage TM, Ledden PJ, Weisskoff RM. Improved auditory cortex imaging using clustered volume acquisitions. *Hum Brain Mapp.* 1999;7:88–97.
24. Belin P, Zatorre RJ, Hoge R, Evans AC, Pike B. Event-related fMRI of the auditory cortex. *Neuroimage.* 1999;10:417–429.
25. Sobel N, Prabhakaran V, Hartley CA, et al. Blind smell: brain activation induced by an undetected airborne chemical. *Brain.* 1999;122(Pt 2):209–217.
26. Sobel N, Prabhakaran V, Desmond JE, Glover GH, Sullivan EV, Gabrieli JD. A method for functional magnetic resonance imaging of olfaction. *J Neurosci Methods.* 1997;78:115–123.
27. Gitelman DR, Parrish TB, LaBar KS, Mesulam MM. Real-time monitoring of eye movements using infrared video-oculography during functional magnetic resonance imaging of the frontal eye fields. *Neuroimage.* 2000;11:58–65.

28. Kimmig H, Greenlee MW, Gondan M, Schira M, Kassubek J, Mergner T. Relationship between saccadic eye movements and cortical activity as measured by fMRI: quantitative and qualitative aspects. *Exp Brain Res.* 2001;141:184–194.

29. Palmer ED, Rosen HJ, Ojemann JG, Buckner RL, Kelley WM, Petersen SE. An event-related fMRI study of overt and covert word stem completion. *Neuroimage.* 2001;14:182–193.

30. Fu CH, Morgan K, Suckling J, et al. A functional magnetic resonance imaging study of overt letter verbal fluency using a clustered acquisition sequence: greater anterior cingulate activation with increased task demand. *Neuroimage.* 2002;17:871–879.

31. Barch DM, Sabb FW, Carter CS, Braver TS, Noll DC, Cohen JD. Overt verbal responding during fMRI scanning: empirical investigations of problems and potential solutions. *Neuroimage.* 1999;10:642–657.

32. Goldman RI, Stern JM, Engel J Jr., Cohen MS. Acquiring simultaneous EEG and functional MRI. *Clin Neurophysiol.* 2000;111:1974–1980.

33. Lazeyras F, Zimine I, Blanke O, Perrig SH, Seeck M. Functional MRI with simultaneous EEG recording: feasibility and application to motor and visual activation. *J Magn Reson Imaging.* 2001;13:943–948.

34. Kruggel F, Herrmann CS, Wiggins CJ, von Cramon DY. Hemodynamic and electroencephalographic responses to illusory figures: recording of the evoked potentials during functional MRI. *Neuroimage.* 2001;14:1327–1336.

35. Kruggel F, Wiggins CJ, Herrmann CS, von Cramon DY. Recording of the event-related potentials during functional MRI at 3.0 Tesla field strength. *Magn Reson Med.* 2000;44:277–282.

36. Gnadt JW, Andersen RA. Memory related motor planning activity in posterior parietal cortex of macaque. *Exp Brain Res.* 1988;70:216–220.

37. Aguirre GK, Zarahn E, D'Esposito M. The variability of human, BOLD hemodynamic responses. *Neuroimage.* 1998;8:360–369.

38. Bandettini PA, Wong EC, Hinks RS, Tikofsky RS, Hyde JS. Time course of EPI of human brain function during task activation. *Magn Reson Med.* 1992;25:390–397.

39. Boynton GM, Engel SA, Glover GH, Heeger DJ. Linear systems analysis of functional magnetic resonance imaging in human V1. *J Neurosci.* 1996;16:4207–4221.

40. Kim SG, Richter W, Ugurbil K. Limitations of temporal resolution in fMRI. *Magn Reson Med.* 1997;37:631–636.

41. Savoy RL, Bandettini PA, O'Craven KM, et al. Pushing the temporal resolution of fMRI: studies of very brief stimuli, onset of variability and asynchrony, and stimulu-correlated changes in noise. *Proc Soc Magn Reson Med.* 1995;3:450.

42. Zarahn E, Aguirre GK, D'Esposito M. A trial-based experimental design for functional MRI. *Neuroimage.* 1997;6:122–138.

43. Burock MA, Buckner RL, Woldorff MG, Rosen BR, Dale AM. Randomized event-related experimental designs allow for extremely rapid presentation rates using functional MRI. *Neuroreport.* 1998;9:3735–3739.

44. Clark VP, Maisog JM, Haxby JV. fMRI studies of visual perception and recognition using a random stimulus design. *Soc Neurosci Abstr.* 1997;23:301.

45. Dale AM, Buckner RL. Selective averaging of rapidly presented individual trials using fMRI. *Hum Brain Mapp.* 1997;5:1–12.

46. Miezin FM, Maccotta L, Ollinger JM, Petersen SE, Buckner RL. Characterizing the hemodynamic response: effects of presentation rate, sampling procedure, and the possibility of ordering brain activity based on relative timing. *Neuroimage.* 2000;11:735–759.

47. D'Esposito M, Zarahn E, Aguirre GK. Event-related functional MRI: implications for cognitive psychology. *Psychol Bull.* 1999;125:155–164.

48. Logothetis NK, Guggenberger H, Peled S, Pauls J. Functional imaging of the monkey brain. *Nat Neurosci.* 1999;2:555–562.

49. Cheng K, Waggoner RA, Tanaka K. Human ocular dominance columns as revealed by high-field functional magnetic resonance imaging. *Neuron.* 2001;32:359–374.

50. Logothetis N, Merkle H, Augath M, Trinath T, Ugurbil K. Ultra high-resolution fMRI in monkeys with implanted RF coils. *Neuron.* 2002;35:227–242.
51. Malonek D, Grinvald A. Interactions between electrical activity and cortical microcirculation revealed by imaging spectroscopy: implications for functional brain mapping. *Science.* 1996;272:551–554.
52. Kim SG, Duong TQ. Mapping cortical columnar structures using fMRI. *Physiol Behav.* 2002;77:641–644.
53. Menon RS, Ogawa S, Strupp JP, Ugurbil K. Ocular dominance in human V1 demonstrated by functional magnetic resonance imaging. *J Neurophysiol.* 1997;77:2780–2787.
54. Grill-Spector K, Malach R. fMR-adaptation: a tool for studying the functional properties of human cortical neurons. *Acta Psychol (Amst).* 2001;107:293–321.
55. Grill-Spector K, Kushnir T, Edelman S, Avidan G, Itzchak Y, Malach R. Differential processing of objects under various viewing conditions in the human lateral occipital complex. *Neuron.* 1999;24:187–203.
56. Posner MI, Petersen SE, Fox PT, Raichle ME. Localization of cognitive operations in the human brain. *Science.* 1988;240:1627–1631.
57. Donders FC. Over de snelheid van psychische processen. Onderzoekingen gedaan in het Physiologisch Laboratorium der Utrechtsche Hoogeschool. *Tweede Reeks.* 1868;II:92–120.
58. Sternberg S. The discovery of processing stages: extensions of Donders' method. *Acta Psychol.* 1969;30:276–315.
59. Petersen SE, Fox PT, Posner MI, Mintun M, Raichle ME. Positron emission tomographic studies of the cortical anatomy of single word processing. *Nature.* 1988;331:585–589.
60. Fuster J. *The Prefrontal Cortex: Anatomy, Physiology, and Neuropsychology of the Frontal Lobes.* Raven Press: New York; 1997.
61. Jonides J, Smith EE, Koeppe RA, Awh E, Minoshima S, Mintun MA. Spatial working memory in humans as revealed by PET. *Nature.* 1993;363:623–625.
62. Zarahn E, Aguirre GK, D'Esposito M. Temporal isolation of the neural correlates of spatial mnemonic processing with fMRI. *Cogn Brain Res.* 1999;7:255–268.
63. Attwell D, Iadecola C. The neural basis of functional brain imaging signals. *Trends Neurosci.* 2002;25:621–625.
64. Heeger DJ, Ress D. What does fMRI tell us about neuronal activity? *Nat Rev Neurosci.* 2002;3:142–151.
65. Friston KJ, Josephs O, Rees G, Turner R. Nonlinear event-related responses in fMRI. *Magn Reson Med.* 1998;39:41–52.
66. Glover GH. Deconvolution of impulse response in event-related BOLD fMRI. *Neuroimage.* 1999;9:416–429.
67. Miller KL, Luh WM, Liu TT, et al. Nonlinear temporal dynamics of the cerebral blood flow response. *Hum Brain Mapp.* 2001;13:1–12.
68. Vazquez AL, Noll DC. Nonlinear aspects of the BOLD response in functional MRI. *Neuroimage.* 1998;7:108–118.
69. D'Esposito M, Zarahn E, Aguirre GK. Event-related fMRI: implications for cognitive psychology. *Psychol Bull.* 1999;125:155–164.
70. Rosen BR, Buckner RL, Dale AM. Event-related functional MRI: past, present, and future. *Proc Natl Acad Sci U S A.* 1998;95:773–780.
71. Donaldson DI, Petersen SE, Ollinger JM, Buckner RL. Dissociating state and item components of recognition memory using fMRI. *Neuroimage.* 2001;13:129–142.
72. Mitchell KJ, Johnson MK, Raye CL, D'Esposito M. fMRI evidence of age-related hippocampal dysfunction in feature binding in working memory. *Brain Res Cogn Brain Res.* 2000;10:197–206.
73. Keppel G, Zedeck S. *Data Analysis for Research Design.* New York: W.H. Freeman & Company; 1989.
74. Worsley KJ, Friston KJ. Analysis of fMRI time-series revisited—again. *Neuroimage.* 1995;2:173–182.

75. Forman SD, Cohen JD, Fitzgerald M, Eddy WF, Mintun MA, Noll DC. Improved assessment of significant activation in functional magnetic resonance imaging (fMRI): use of a cluster-size threshold. *Magn Reson Med*. 1995;33: 636–647.

76. Everitt BS, Bullmore ET. Mixture model mapping of the brain activation in functional magnetic resonance images. *Hum Brain Mapp*. 1999;7:1–14.

77. Zarahn E, Aguirre GK, D'Esposito M. Empirical analyses of BOLD fMRI statistics. I. Spatially unsmoothed data collected under null-hypothesis conditions. *Neuroimage*. 1997;5:179–197.

78. Aguirre GK, Zarahn E, D'Esposito M. Empirical analyses of BOLD fMRI statistics. II. Spatially smoothed data collected under null-hypothesis and experimental conditions. *Neuroimage*. 1997;5:199–212.

79. D'Esposito M, Ballard D, Zarahn E, Aguirre GK. The role of prefrontal cortex in sensory memory and motor preparation: an event-related fMRI study [see comments]. *Neuroimage*. 2000;11:400–408.

80. Zarahn E, Slifstein M. A reference effect approach for power analysis in fMRI. *Neuroimage*. 2001;14:768–779.

81. Van Horn JD, Ellmore TM, Esposito G, Berman KF. Mapping voxel-based statistical power on parametric images. *Neuroimage*. 1998;7:97–107.

82. Aguirre GK, D'Esposito M. Experimental design for brain fMRI. In: Moonen CTW, Bandettini PA, eds. *Functional MRI*. Berlin: Springer Verlag; 1999:369–380.

83. Logothetis NK, Pauls J, Augath M, Trinath T, Oeltermann A. Neurophysiological investigation of the basis of the fMRI signal. *Nature*. 2001;412:150–157.

84. Farkas E, Luiten PG. Cerebral microvascular pathology in aging and Alzheimer's disease. *Prog Neurobiol*. 2001;64:575–611.

85. Fang HCH. Observations on aging characteristics of cerebral blood vessels, macroscopic and microscopic features. In: Gerson S, Terry RD, eds. *Neurobiology of Aging*. New York: Raven Press; 1976.

86. Bentourkia M, Bol A, Ivanoiu A, et al. Comparison of regional cerebral blood flow and glucose metabolism in the normal brain: effect of aging. *J Neurol Sci*. 2000;181:19–28.

87. Schultz SK, O'Leary DS, Boles Ponto LL, Watkins GL, Hichwa RD, Andreasen NC. Age-related changes in regional cerebral blood flow among young to mid-life adults. *Neuroreport*. 1999;10:2493–2496.

88. Yamamoto M, Meyer JS, Sakai F, Yamaguchi F. Aging and cerebral vasodilator responses to hypercarbia: responses in normal aging and in persons with risk factors for stroke. *Arch Neurol*. 1980;37:489–496.

89. Yamaguchi T, Kanno I, Uemura K, et al. Reduction in regional cerebral rate of oxygen during human aging. *Stroke*. 1986;17:1220–1228.

90. Takada H, Nagata K, Hirata Y, et al. Age-related decline of cerebral oxygen metabolism in normal population detected with positron emission tomography. *Neurol Res*. 1992;14:128–131.

91. Claus JJ, Breteler MM, Hasan D, et al. Regional cerebral blood flow and cerebrovascular risk factors in the elderly population. *Neurobiol Aging*. 1998;19:57–64.

92. D'Esposito M, Zarahn E, Aguirre GK, Rypma B. The effect of normal aging on the coupling of neural activity to the bold hemodynamic response. *Neuroimage*. 1999;10:6–14.

93. Cunnington R, Iansek R, Bradshaw JL, Phillips JG. Movement-related potentials in Parkinson's disease. Presence and predictability of temporal and spatial cues. *Brain*. 1995;118:935–950.

94. Buckner RL, Snyder AZ, Sanders AL, Raichle ME, Morris JC. Functional brain imaging of young, nondemented, and demented older adults. *J Cogn Neurosci*. 2000;12(Suppl 2):24–34.

95. Huettel SA, Singerman JD, McCarthy G. The Effects of Aging upon the Hemodynamic Response Measured by Functional MRI. *Neuroimage*. 2001,13: 161–175.

96. Pineiro R, Pendlebury S, Johansen-Berg H, Matthews PM. Altered hemodynamic responses in patients after subcortical stroke measured by functional MRI. *Stroke.* 2002;33:103–109.
97. Rypma B, Prabhakaran V, Desmond JE, Gabrieli JD. Age differences in prefrontal cortical activity in working memory. *Psychol Aging.* 2001;16:371–384.
98. Jonides J, Marshuetz C, Smith EE, Reuter-Lorenz PA, Koeppe RA, Hartley A. Age differences in behavior and PET activation reveal differences in interference resolution in verbal working memory. *J Cogn Neurosci.* 2000;12:188–196.
99. Rypma B, D'Esposito M. Isolating the neural mechanisms of age-related changes in human working memory. *Nat Neurosci.* 2000;3:509–515.
100. Kanwisher N, McDermott J, Chun MM. The fusiform face area: a module in huma extrastriate cortex specialized for face perception. *J Neurosci.* 1997;17:4302–4311.
101. Rees G, Frith CD, Lavie N. Modulating irrelevant motion perception by varying attentional load in an unrelated task. *Science.* 1997;278:1616–1619.
102. Treisman AM. Strategies and models of selective attention. *Psychol Rev.* 1969;76:282–299.
103. Lavie N, Tsal Y. Perceptual load as a major determinant of the locus of selection in visual attention. *Percept Psychophys.* 1994;56:183–197.
104. Buchel C, Coull JT, Friston KJ. The predictive value of changes in effective connectivity for human learning. *Science.* 1999;283:1538–1541.
105. McIntosh AR, Grady CL, Haxby JV, Ungerleider LG, Horwitz B. Changes in limbic and prefrontal functional interactions in a working memory task for faces. *Cereb Cortex.* 1996;6:571–584.
106. Gerstein GL, Perkel DH, Subramanian KN. Identification of functionally related neural assemblies. *Brain Res.* 1978;140:43–62.
107. McCarthy RA, Warrington EK. Disorders of semantic memory. *Philos Trans R Soc Lond B Biol Sci.* 1994;346:89–96.
108. Warrington EST. Category specific semantic impairments. *Brain.* 1984;107:829–854.
109. Thompson-Schill SL. Neuroimaging studies of semantic memory: inferring "how" from "where". *Neuropsychologia.* 2003;41:280–292.
110. Thompson-Schill SL, D'Esposito M, Aguirre GK, Farah MJ. Role of left inferior prefrontal cortex in retrieval of semantic knowledge: a reevaluation. *Proc Natl Acad Sci U S A.* 1997;94:14792–14797.
111. Thompson-Schill SL, Swick D, Farah MJ, D'Esposito M, Kan IP, Knight RT. Verb generation in patients with focal frontal lesions: a neuropsychological test of neuroimaging findings. *Proc Natl Acad Sci U S A.* 1998;95:15855–15860.
112. Pascual-Leone A, Tarazona F, Keenan J, Tormos JM, Hamilton R, Catala MD. Transcranial magnetic stimulation and neuroplasticity. *Neuropsychologia.* 1999;37:207–217.
113. Rushworth MF, Hadland KA, Paus T, Sipila PK. Role of the human medial frontal cortex in task switching: a combined fMRI and TMS study. *J Neurophysiol.* 2002;87:2577–2592.
114. Churchland PS, Sejnowski TJ. Perspectives on cognitive neuroscience. *Science.* 1988;242:741–745.

Part III

Neuroanatomical Atlas

11

Neuroanatomical Atlas

Feroze B. Mohamed and Scott H. Faro

In this chapter we have displayed several important areas of normal-functioning adult brain images generated using fMRI BOLD imaging. The fMRI shown here highlight areas of brain activation arising from simple motor tasks, visual functions, auditory and complex language, and listening paradigms. A somatotopic fMRI mapping of the human motor cortex was created for the foot, knee, trunk, shoulder, wrist, hand, face, tongue, and abdomen. The fMRI experiments in these conditions were carried out by simple box-car type block design experiments. These included a rest condition where no activity was performed, followed by an activation period where the subject was asked to perform a specific task. The representation of visual function, as well as language and auditory areas, were also obtained using a block design.

These pictures represent some of the most important and commonly studied areas of the brain and might serve as a reference or template for users of fMRI for brain mapping. The images shown here are represented in radiological co-ordinates and are presented in three different orientations (axial, coronal, and sagittal). The blue cross hair represents the area of interest, and the region was labeled based on the Talaraich atlas. The color map overlying the images are statistical maps and the graded change in color from yellow to orange represent varying statistical value from low to high statistical significance. A composite display showing the motor homunculus with corresponding fMRI activation maps is shown at the end of the chapter. The post-processing of the fMRI data was performed with SPM'99 software (Statistical Parametric Mapping, Wellcome Department of Cognitive Neurology, University College of London) running under the Matlab (The Mathworks, Inc.) environment. A Pentium-based PC was used to generate all the images shown in this section.

This chapter previously appeared in *Functional MRI: Basic Principles and Clinical Applications*, edited by S. Faro and F. Mohamed. New York: Springer Science+Business Media, LCC 2006.

From: *BOLD fMRI: A Guide to Functional Imaging for Neuroscientists*
Edited by: S.H. Faro and F.B. Mohamed, DOI 10.1007/978-1-4419-1329-6_11
© Springer Science+Business Media, LLC 2010

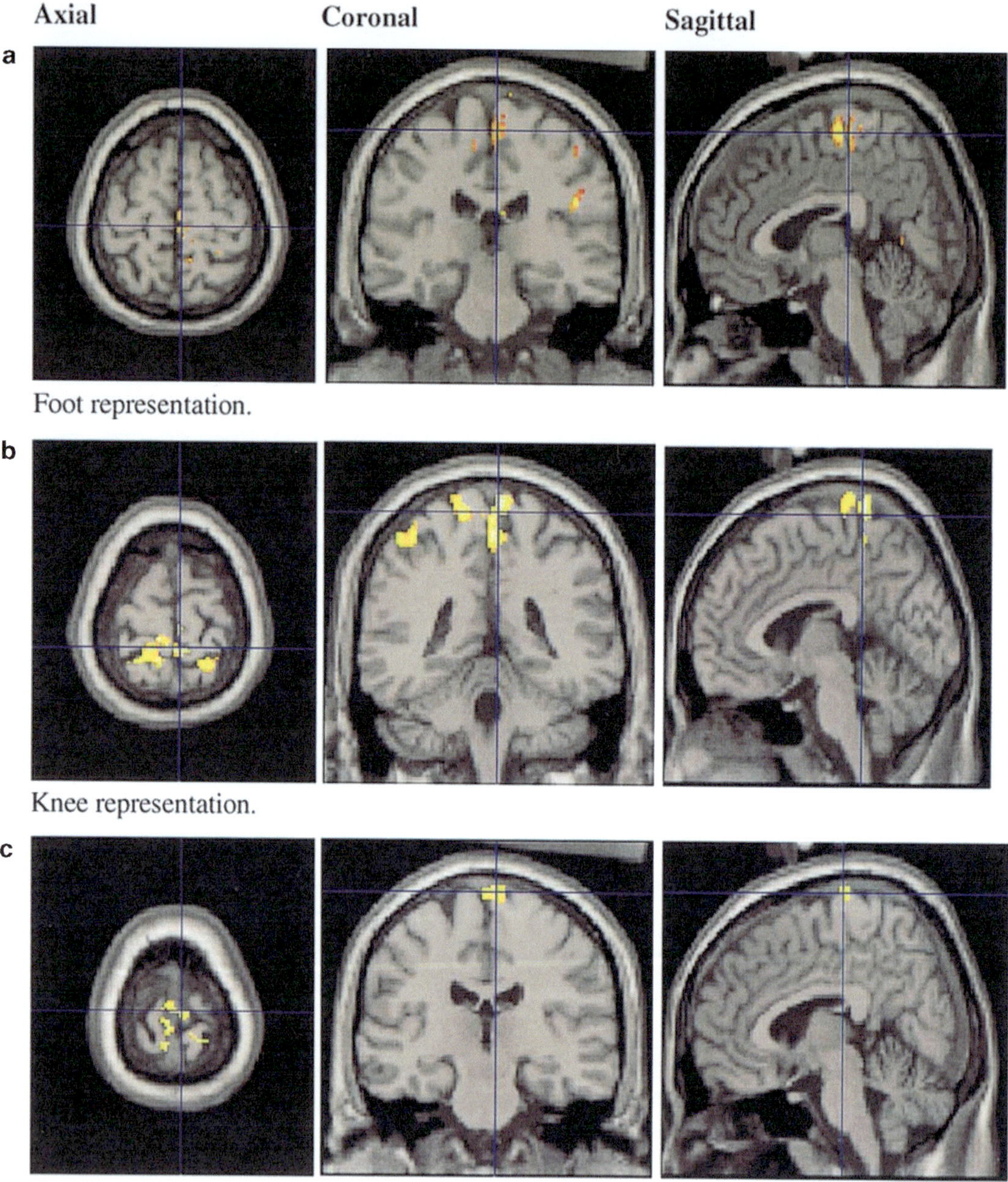

Axial
Coronal
Sagittal
a
Foot representation.
b
Knee representation.
c
Trunk representation.

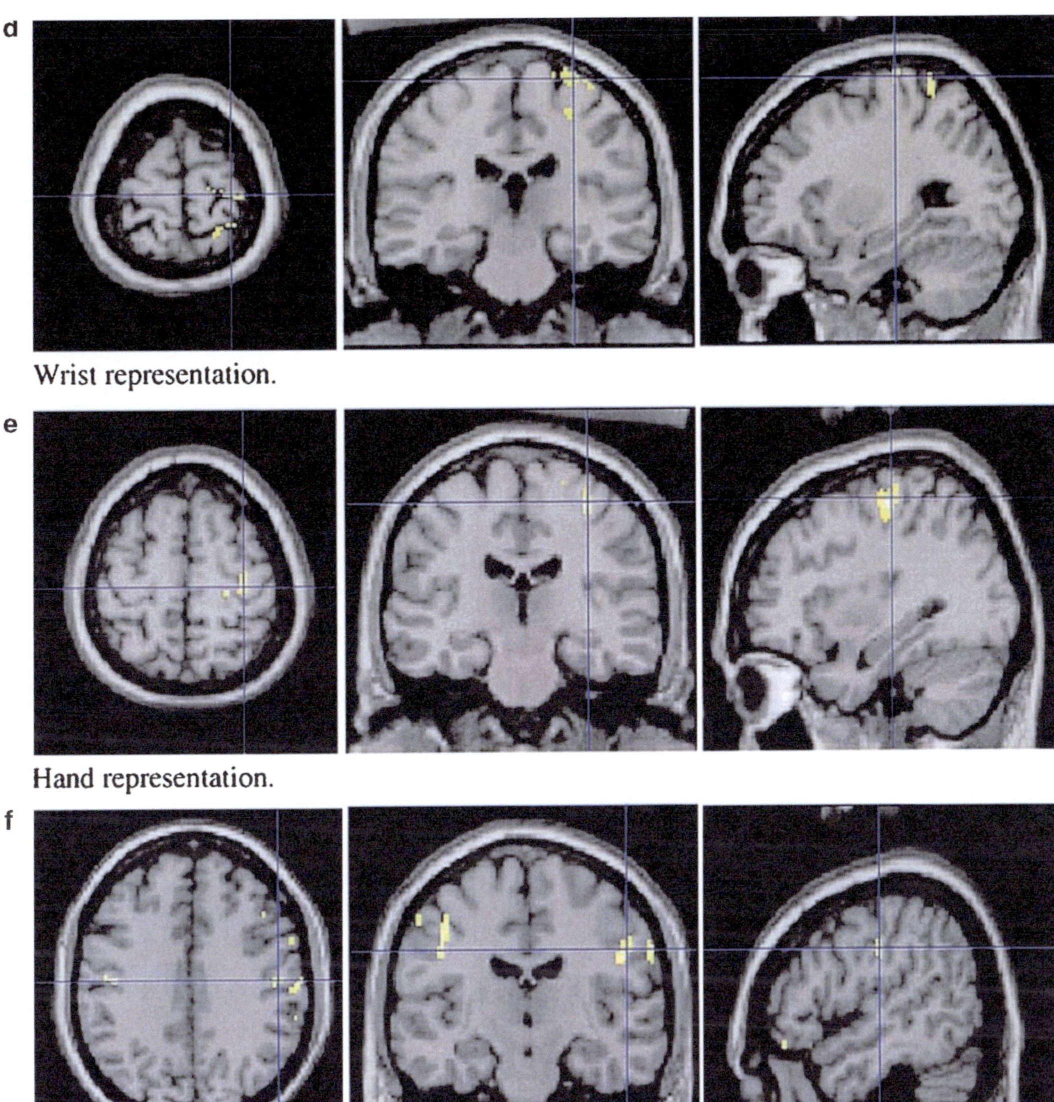

Wrist representation.

Hand representation.

Face representation.

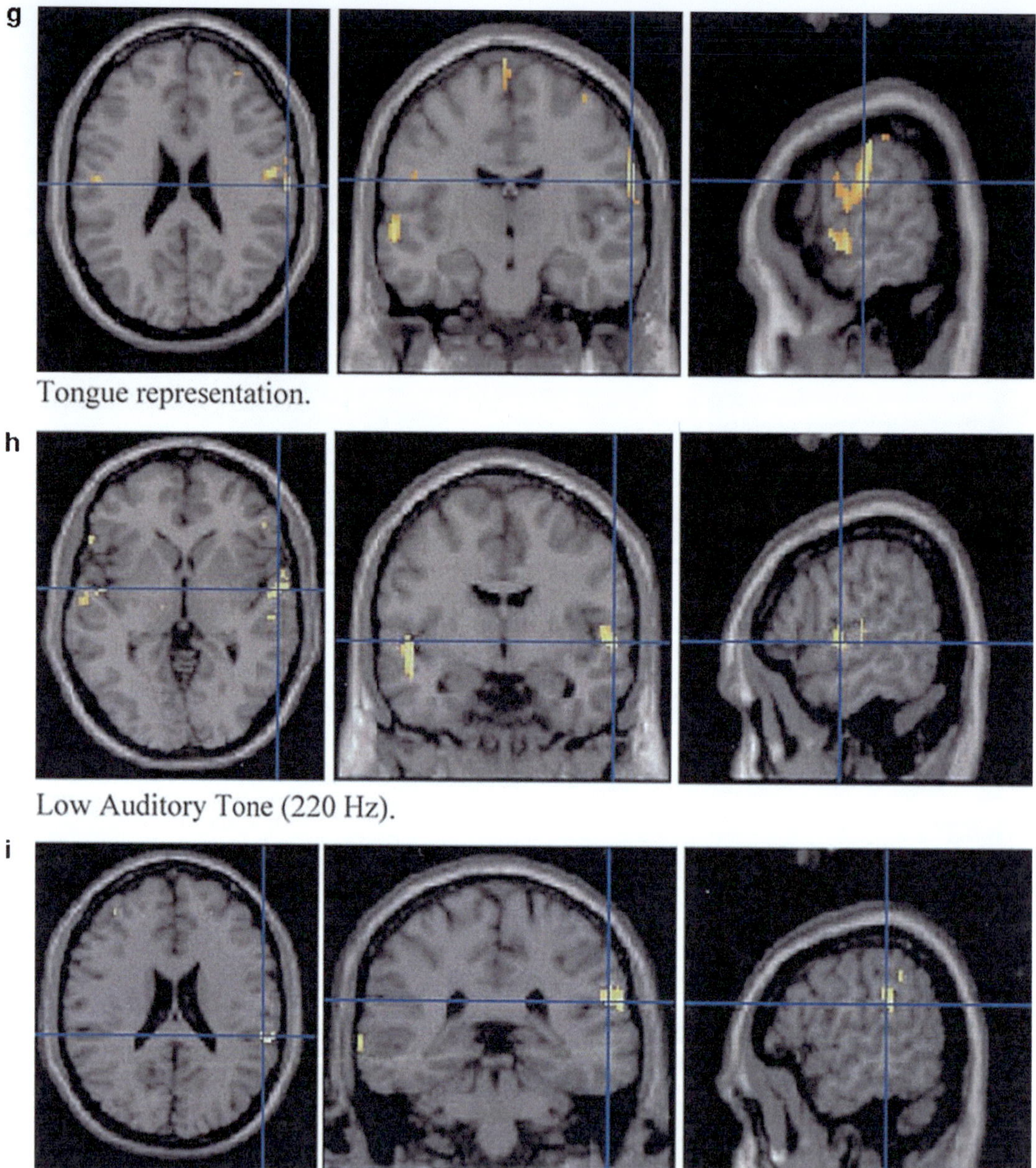

g Tongue representation.

h Low Auditory Tone (220 Hz).

i High Auditory Tone (1000 Hz).

j

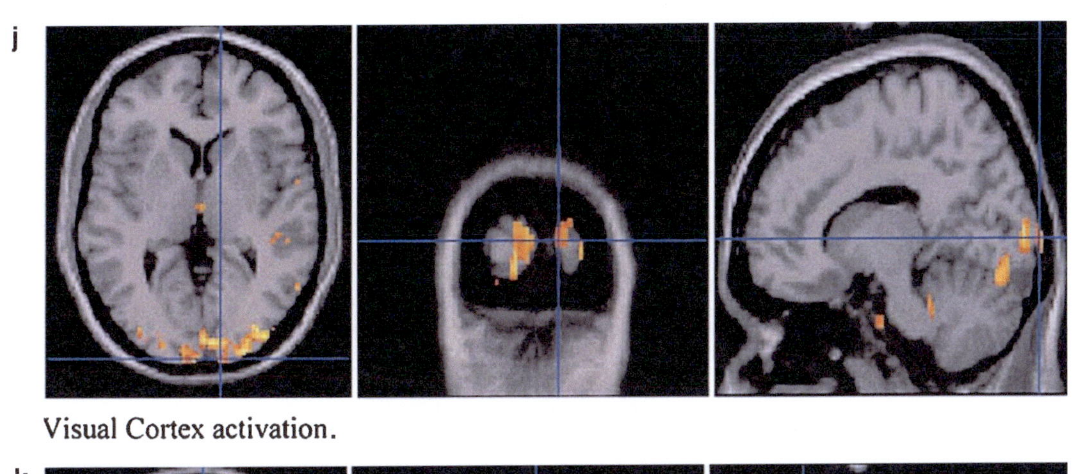

Visual Cortex activation.

k

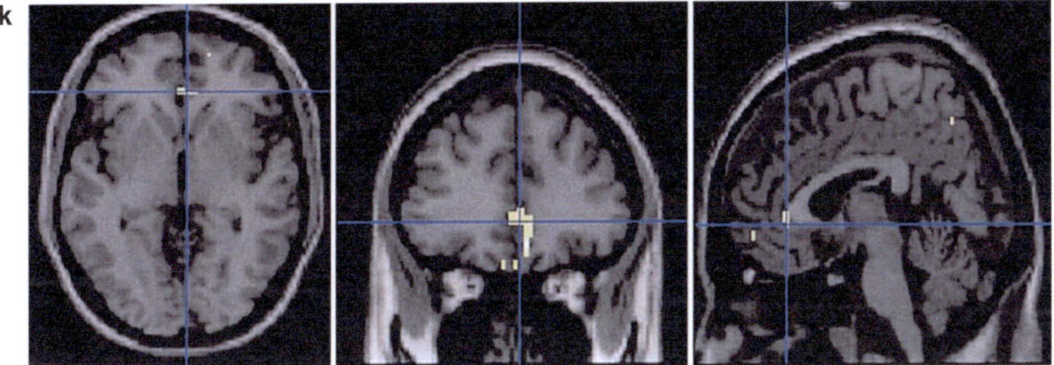

Limbic Lobe (Anterior Cingulate).

l

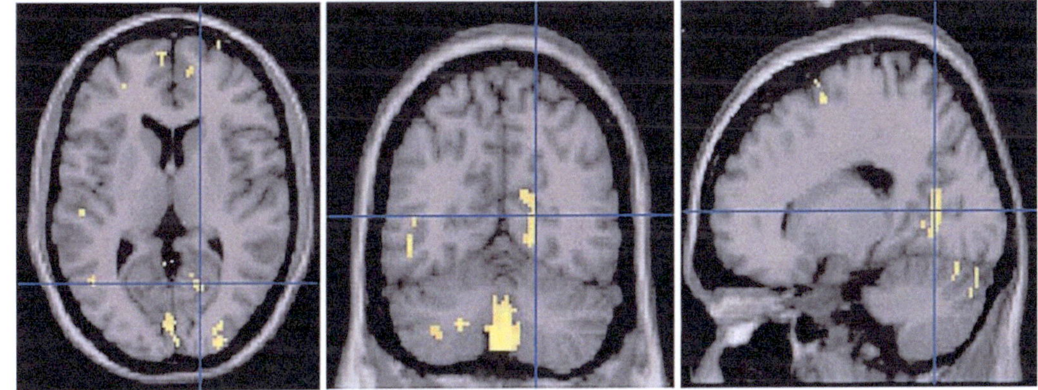

Limbic Lobe (Posterior Cingulate).

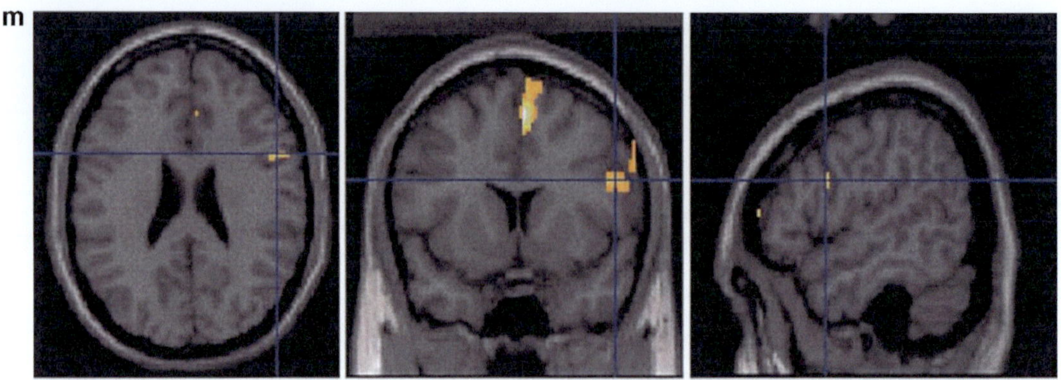

Frontal Lobe: Inferior Frontal Gyrus.

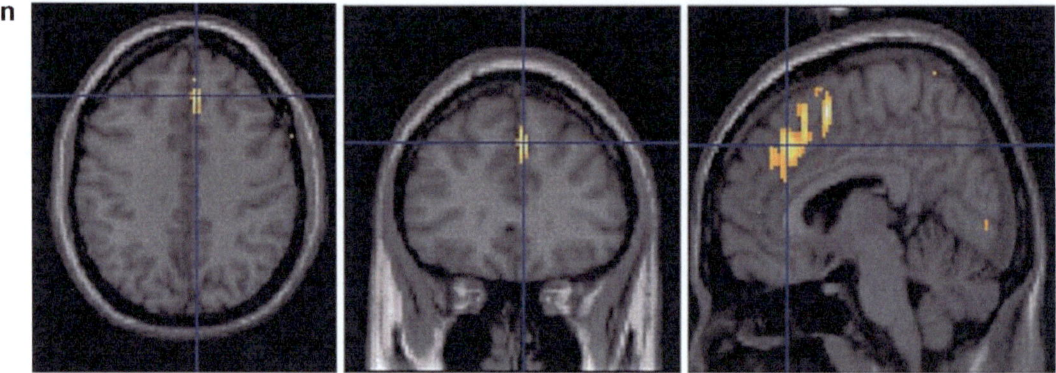

Frontal Lobe: Medial Frontal Gyrus.

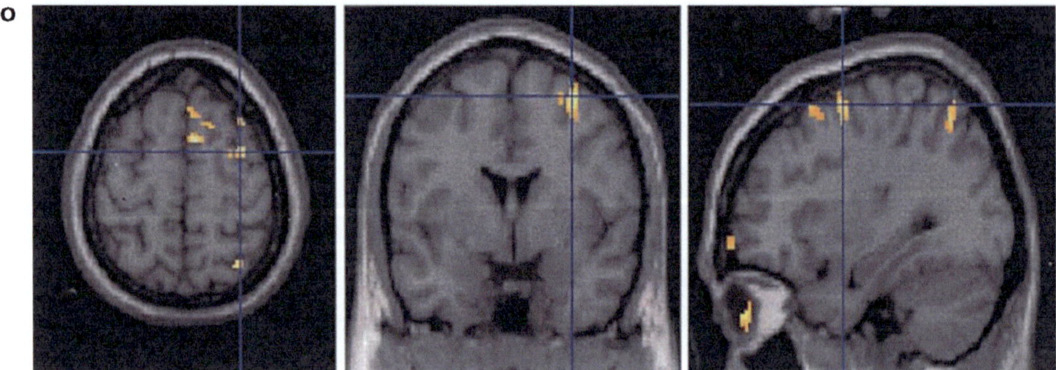

Frontal Lobe: Middle Frontal Gyrus.

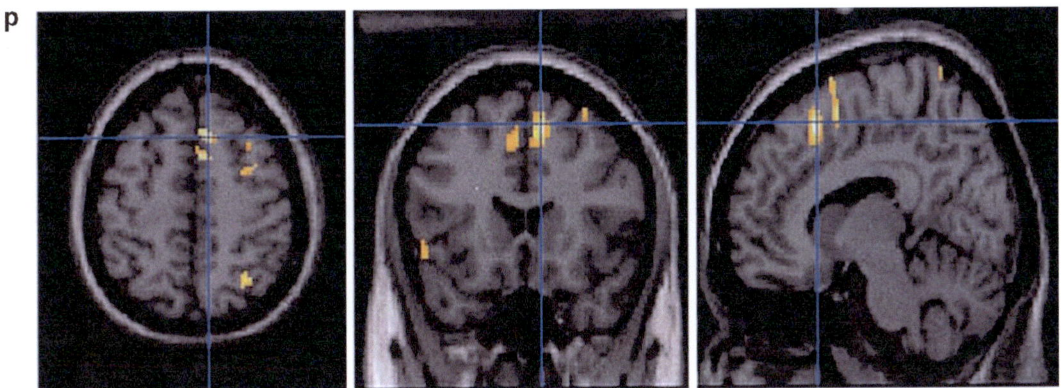

Frontal Lobe: Superior Frontal Gyrus.

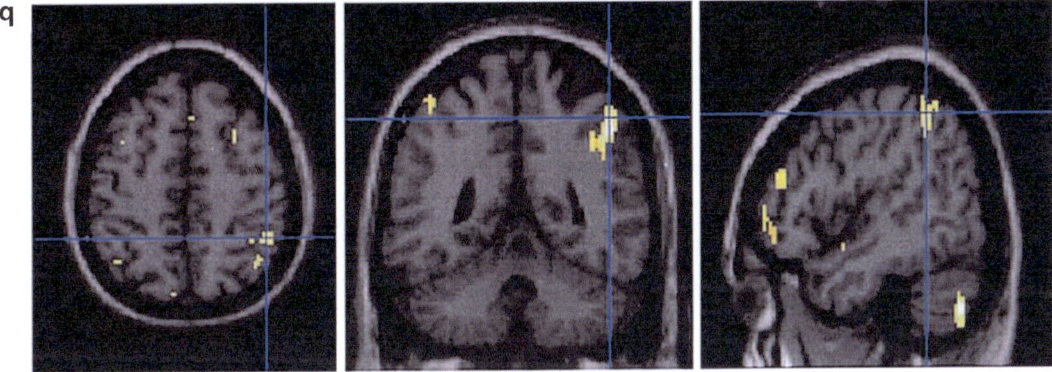

Parietal Lobe: Inferior Parietal Lobule.

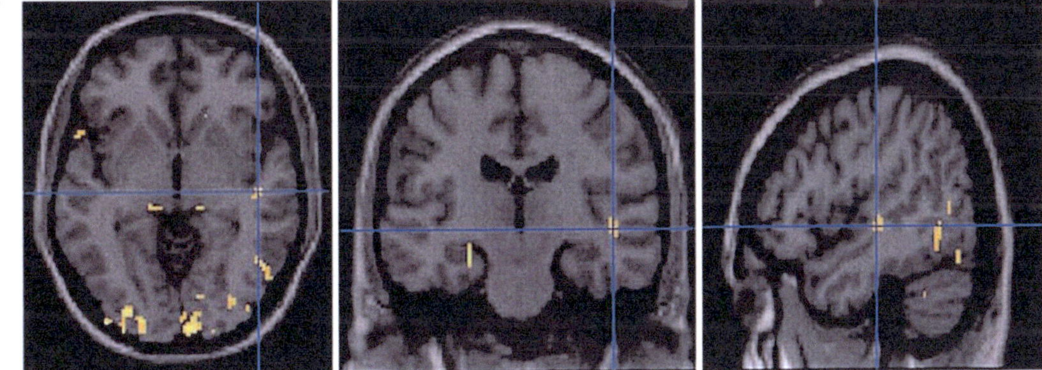

Temporal Lobe: Wernicke's Area.

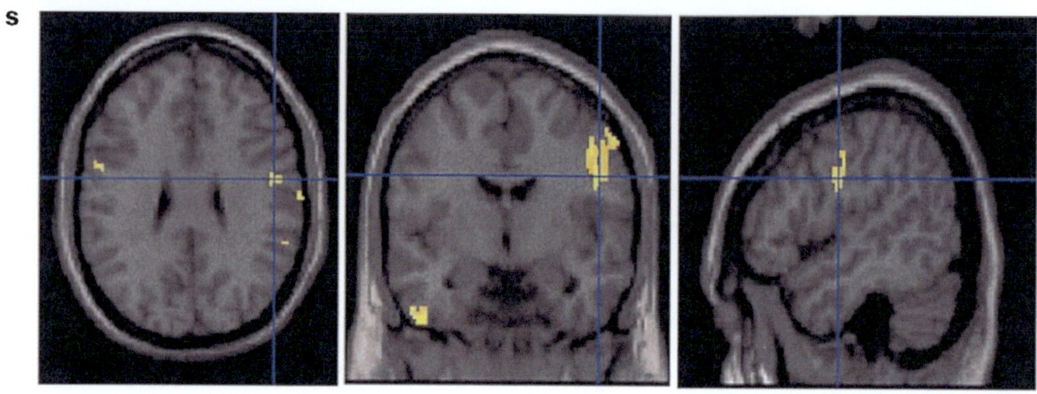

Broca's Motor Area.

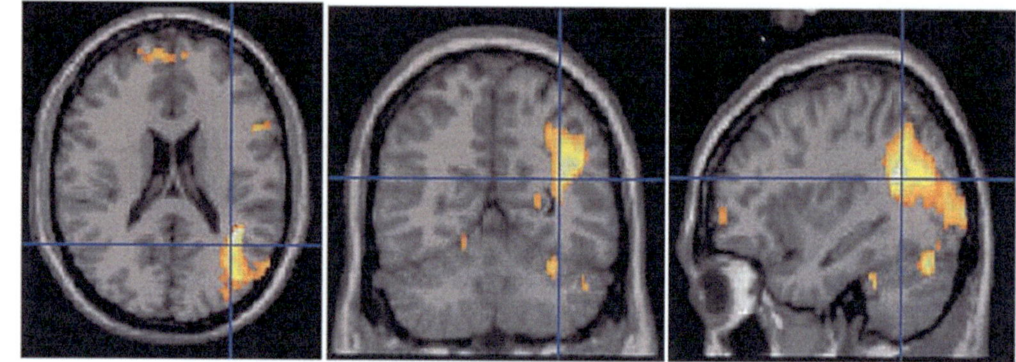

Parietal Occipital Lobe: Object Naming Task.

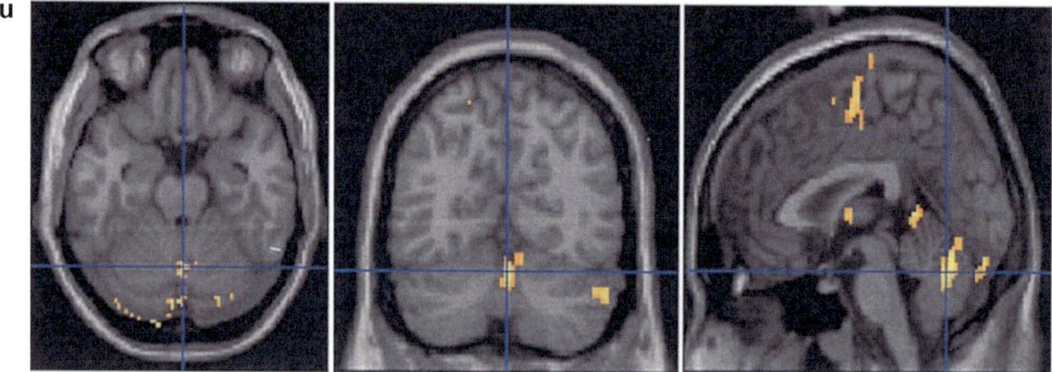

Cerebellum: Coordination Motor Task.

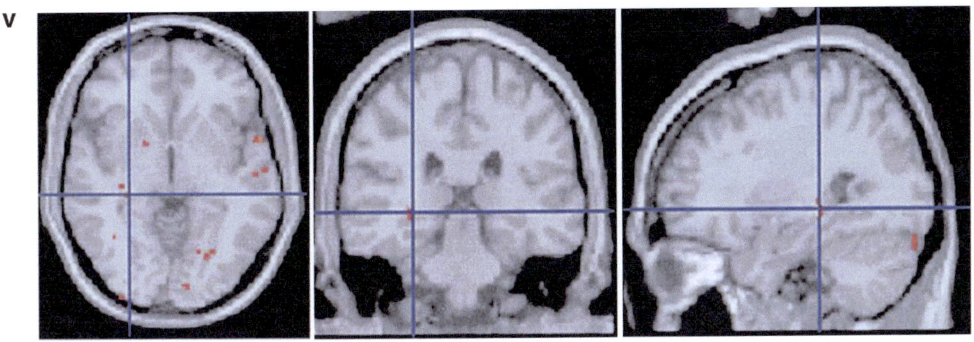

Temporal Lobe: Hippocampal Activation.

Somatotopic mapping in the human somatosensory motor cortex along with corresponding functional MRI activation patterns.

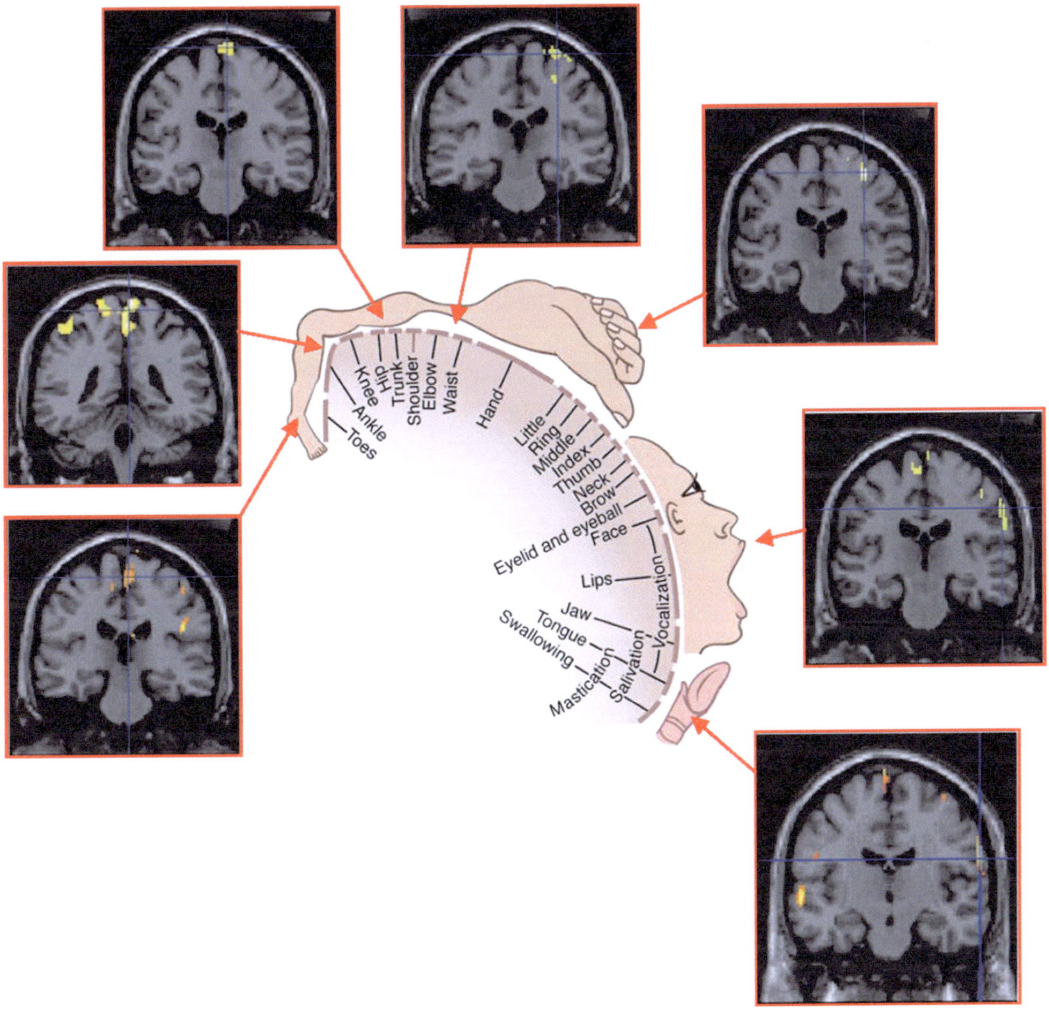

Index

A

AD. *See* Alzheimer's disease

Aging
BOLD fMRI changes and, 263
HRF and, 263
memory
activation and, 164
episodic, 161–162
remote, 165
semantic, 170–173
tasks for, 174
working, 163, 174–175
neurovascular system changes and, 262

Alzheimer's disease (AD). *See also* Dementia
episodic, 168–171
fMRI, 104
memory, 168–171
semantic, 174
task difficulty, 104

Aphasia, 104

Arterial spin labeling (ASL), 86–88

Asymmetric spin-echo (ASE), 32

B

Blood oxygenation level-dependent (BOLD), 72
brain mapping, 122
cognitive conjunction, 142
functional fMRI, 3
tactile stimulation, 124

BOLD fMRI, brain
age-related changes in, 263
auditory tone representation on
high, 280
low, 280
Broca's motor area on, 284
cerebellum, coordinating motor task, 284
data preprocessing, 63
different temporal structures of, 61–63
distortion correction, 63
face representation, 279
foot representation, 278
hand representation, 279
hippocampal activation, temporal lobe represented
on, 285
HRF and, 263
inferior frontal gyrus, frontal lobe represented on, 282
knee representation, 278
limbic lobe (anterior and posterior cingulate
regions), 281
medial frontal gyrus, frontal lobe represented on, 282
motion correction, 64
noise and, 261
normalization, spatial, 64–65
parietal lobe represented on, 284
slice acquisition correction, 63–64
spatial smoothing, 65
statistical analysis for, 65–69
superior frontal gyrus, frontal lobe represented
on, 282
temporal lobe represented on, 282
tongue representation, 280
trunk representation, 278
visual cortex activation, 281
Wernicke's area, temporal lobe represented on, 283
wrist representation, 279

Brain activity
semantic, 266, 267
task for, 265

Brain-behavior relationships, 249

Brain mapping
Astonishing Hypothesis, 119
N back task, cognitive theory, 146–148
BOLD, 122
brain structure visualize
history, 122–123
MRI, 122

Brain mapping (*cont.*)
  calcarine sulcus, functional specialization, 125
  cognitive conjunction, 141–142
  cortical imaging
    anatomy, topography, 140
    positron emission tomography (PET), 120–121
    visual field defect, 132
  ERP integration, 150
  fMRI, 7
    development, 122
    event-related, 152–153
    oddball task, 153–154
    task battery, 127
    vs. visual fields, 132
    vs. Wada and intraoperative language
        mapping, 132
  functional differentiation, 143
  functional mapping, cortical areas
    identification, 126
    preservation, 126
  functional neuroanatomy
    attention processes, 144–145
    language processes, 143–144
    separate, combined systems, 149, 150
    very high level cognitive processes,
        154–156
    working memory, 146
  Go-No Go task, 151
  integrative mapping
    language functions, 133, 135
    sensory and motor functions, 133–134
  language mapping cases
    cortical responses, 132–133
    early bilingual patient, 137
    late bilingual patient, 135
    motor mapping, 137–139
  multifunction task
    healthy volunteer, 128
    procedure, 128
  neuroscience, cognitive, 249–269
  postsurgical status, 134
  spatial information, 151–152
  statistical parametric mapping (SPM), 141
  Stroop task, 147–150
  task battery, sensitivity
    healthy volunteers, 129
    vs. intraoperative electrophysiology,
        131–132
    patients and healthy volunteers, 131
    surgical population, 129–131
  task sensitivity, evaluation, 130
  temporal integration, 151–152
Broca's motor area, 284

C
Cerebral blood flow (CBF), 3

Cerebral metabolic rate of glucose
    (CMR$_{glu}$), 3
Cerebral metabolic rate of oxygen
    (CMRO$_2$), 3, 81
Cognition
  epilepsy patient, 220
  neural basis of, 252
  neurodevelopmental abnormalities
        in, 238
Cognitive subtraction, 58–59
  assumptions for, 258
  brain mapping, 141
  brain region inactivation disruption of, 268
  brain systems associated with, 250
  inference in, 250–252
  neuroimaging study of, 261

D
Dementia. *See also* Aging
  semantic memory, 171–173
  working memory, 163, 174–175

E
Echo planar imaging (EPI), 44–52
  gradient echo-recalled, 48–49
  methods, 44–45
  pulse sequences
    echo-formation mechanisms, 48
    gradient coils, 48
    intrinsic decay, 46
    k-space transversed and, 46
  spin echo-recalled, 49–50
  spiral-echo, 50–52
Echo train length (ETL), 33
Electroconvulsive shock therapy (ECT), 216
Electroencephalography (EEG), 254
EPI. *See* Echo planar imaging

F
FAIR. *See* Flow-sensitive alternating inversion recovery
False-discovery rate (FDR), 68
Fast imaging with steady precession (FISP), 41, 85
Fast Low Angle SHot (FLASH), 38
FDR. *See* False-discovery rate
FISP. *See* Fast imaging with steady precession
Flow-sensitive alternating inversion recovery (FAIR), 7
fMRI. *See* Functional magnetic resonance imaging
Free induction decay (FID), 38
Functional magnetic resonance–adaptation (fMR-A), 257
Functional magnetic resonance imaging (fMRI)
  activation patterns, 194
  AD, 104
  advantages, 93
  analysis techniques, 104
  BOLD, 24
  brain mapping

vs. functional MRI, 94
    perfusion-based, 94
    transcranial magnetic stimulation (TMS), 94
challenges/limitations of
    brain activation, 77
    brain system dependent, 78
    functional spatial, 77–78
    MR physics-based, 72
    physiological-based, 76–77
    pulse sequences for, 83–86
    SNR and field strength in, 74
    static field inhomogeneities in, 74–76
    subject movement as, 80–81
    threshold effects and localization as, 81
clinical challenges, 93–112
clinical planning
    signal localization, 110
    signal reliability, 111
cognitive theory, 264–265
conjunction analysis, 107–109
contrast to noise ratio, 15–17
dependent measures
    activation paradigms, 106
    language lateralization (LI), 107
    Wada testing, 104
development, 122
draining vein problem in, 78–80
echo planar imaging
    gradient echo-recalled, 48–49
    methods, 44–45
    pulse sequences, 45–48
    spin echo-recalled, 49–50
    spiral-echo, 50–52
electrophysiological relationship, 112
event-related potential studies combined with, 268–269
experimental design and data analysis for, 55–69
extravascular component
    dephasing effects, 13
    R_2 and R_2 changes, 14
    spin-echo and gradient-echo image, 12
    static averaging, 13
functional integration, 265–266
gradient-echo technique
    formation mechanism, 36–38
    imaging pulse sequence, 38–41
    spin-echo and, 25
hemodynamic based mapping
    cascade of, 95
    studies, 94–96
hypotheses tested with, 263
imaging contrasts, 6
intravascular component, 9–11
    issues in, 258–260
language maps *vs.* cortical stimulation maps, 200–201
lesion studies combined with, 266–268
neuroscience, cognitive applications with, 249–269

oddball task, 153–154
oxy/deoxyhemoglobin signal mapping, 100
PET *vs.,* 252
physiological changes
    BOLD contrast, 6
    CBF *vs.* CBV, 5
    vascular hemodynamic response, 4
practice effects, 102–103
principles, 3–18
prototypical, 258
pulse sequences for, 83–86
reproducibility, 109–110
scanning methodologies, 23–52
scan sequence and susceptibility
    echo planar imaging (EPI), 97
    echo time (TE), 98
    gradient echo *vs.* asymmetric spin echo, 98–99
sensitivity of, 88
sequences of
    flow effects, 35–36
    vascular effects, 33–35
SNRs, 23
k-space coverage, 30, 31
spatial resolution, 17, 256–257
specialization, 264
spin-echo technique
    formation mechanism, 25–27
    gradient-echo *vs.,* 14–15, 36–38
    imaging pulse sequence, 27–33
statistical techniques for analyzing,
        260–262
study/task designs, 100
within subject *vs.* group analysis, 105
T_2 and T_2 based fMRI, 9
task battery, 127
task difficulty
    AD, 104
    aphasia, 104
task selection, 100–101
technical considerations, field strength
    contrast-to-noise ratio (CNR), 96
    signal-to-noise ratio (SNR), 96
temporal resolution
    hemodynamic response, altered and, 254
    heterogeneity, 18
    issues in, 256
    neural activity, exact time, 17
    statistical analysis in, 260
temporal resolution, BOLD response, 81–83
T_1 weighted fMRI
    applications of, 9
    ASL, 6
    CBF changes, 7
    hypothetical longitudinal magnetization, 7
    intravascular and extravascular signal
        contributions, 10

vs. visual fields, 132
vs. Wada and intraoperative language
    mapping, 132
Wada test, 215–241
Fusiform face area, 264

G
Gaussian random field theory, 67, 261
Gradient-echo technique
    formation mechanism, 36–38
    imaging pulse sequence, 38–41
    spin-echo and, 25

H
Hemodynamic based mapping, fMRI
    cascade of, 95
    studies, 94–96
Hemodynamic response function
        (HRF), 59

I
Independent component analysis (ICA), 69
Inference
    functional neuroimaging studies, 250–252
    to population, 141
    types, 56–58
Intracarotid amobarbital test (IAT). *See also* Wada test
    background/history and, 216–218
    data interpretation for, 219
    discrepancies, fMRI, 220
    epilepsy, 217
    fMRI language paradigms and, 220–229
    fMRI replacing
        clinical concerns for, 238–239
        memory tasks for, 231
        technical concerns for, 235–238
    language function assessment with, 223
    language lateralization, 216
    language mapping, 229
    limitations of, 218, 219
    neuroimaging techniques for, 229
    protocol
        language testing in, 218
        memory testing in, 219
        recall testing in, 219
        recognition tasks in, 219
    results, fMRI, 221, 229

L
Language lateralization
    epilepsy, 225
    fMRI, 225
    IAT, 224, 225
Language systems
    fMRI, surgical planning usage of, 202–205

language mapping
    aphasia predicted outcome with, 184
    clinical applications, 183–184
    normative studies, 195–197
    presurgical applications, 184
    reliability/validation/outcome prediction studies, 195
    treatment effects monitored with, 185
    Wernicke–Broca neuroanatomical model of, 183
Language task, passive listening
    semantic decision, 193
    sentence/word reading, 191, 193–195
    visual object naming, 192
    words, 191–192
Larmor frequency, 41
Linguistics
    effects of task states, 190
    stimuli effects, 189

M
Memory
    episodic
        AD and, 168–171
        age related changes in, 162–167
        neural basis models for, 162
    hemispheric encoding and retrieval asymmetry
            (HERA) model, 162
    pictorial, 165
    remote, 165
    semantic
        AD and, 174
        brain activation patterns, 170
        fMRI measure of, 171
        neural basis of, 162
    tasks
        face-recognition, 169
        fMRI, 170
    testing, 161
    TLE assessment, fMRI, 171
    working
        brain activity related to, 174
        delayed-response tasks for, 174
        neural activity, persistent and, 175
        sentence-comprehension task for, 174
        tasks for, 174
        visual, 173
MR angiography (MRA), 25

N
Neuroanatomical atlas, 277–285
Neuroanatomy, functional
    attention processes, 144–145
    high level cognitive processes, 154–156
    language processes, 143–144
    separate, combined systems, 149–150
    working memory, 146

P

PET. *See* Positron emission tomography
Point spread function mapping (PSF), 84
Positron emission tomography (PET), 56, 120–121
Presurgical language mapping, 204, 205
PSF. *See* Point spread function mapping

S

Scanning methodologies. *See* Echo planar imaging;
        Gradient-echo technique;
        Spin-echo technique
Signal-to-noise ratios (SNRs), 23, 73
SNRs. *See* Signal-to-noise ratios
Spin-echo technique
    formation mechanism, 25–27
    gradient-echo *vs.*, 36–38
    imaging pulse sequence, 27–33
    sequences of
        flow effects, 35–36
        vascular effects, 33–35
SPM. *See* Statistical parametric mapping

Statistical parametric mapping (SPM), 141

T

Test-retest reliability, 197–198

U

Ultra-fast low-angle RARE imaging
        (UFLARE), 85

V

Voxel volume, 73

W

Wada test
    comparisons, 199–200
    fMRI, 106
    language lateralization, 221–222
Wernicke's area, 283

Z

Z-shimming, 75